REVIEWS

Yoga and Resilience: Empowering Practices for Survivors of Sexual Trauma is ess[...] [...]rdless of their level of experience, to be able to skillfully teach yoga and facilitate a [...] [...]auma; which includes so many of our students. This book is also a blueprint for yoga teachers who spe[...] [...]ach to survivors, which hasn't been available until now. I'm grateful that yoga has evolved to produce texts like this so that survivors can heal in our classes rather than be re-traumatized because of ignorance or lack of fundamental training. As yoga teachers, it is so important that we learn the necessary skills to understand the specific needs of sexual violence survivors and work towards creating a classroom experience that is informed, mindful and responsible. This book is a resource that can do that. I highly recommend it.

Seane Corn, co-founder of Off the Mat, Into the World; author of *Revolution of the Soul*

This book is timely and important; it's a piece of yoga's contribution to the #MeToo movement. Many of our students have experienced sexual trauma whether we know it or not, so this book is a necessary read for all yoga teachers so that we can make sure our students are safe in our classes. This book is a collaboration of leaders in the field who also weave in some of their own personal insights as survivors themselves. This should be on the book shelf of every yoga teacher.

Hala Khouri MA, SEP, E-RYT, co-founder of Off the Mat, Into the World

This book is an act of love and respect. Created collaboratively to quicken consciousness for people seeking yoga as a practice that is free from sexual harm, this book places survivor wisdom at its center. The book teaches us that trauma-sensitive yoga makes yoga deeper and safer for all of us. The best practices in each chapter are strings of light, illuminating why cultural humility and deep listening are promises and a way of life. From prisons to schools, from temples to military outposts, the authors identify how yoga can be twisted to cause harm and provide steps to ensure healing. While *Yoga and Resilience* is written by/for an expansive yoga community, it is also for preachers, parents, activists, mapmakers and healers – all of us seeking a violence-free world. In the tradition of Tarana Burke, Angela Davis, and Leslie Salmon Jones – those who have long stood up against racist and gendered violence – *Yoga and Resilience* asks us to see the practice of yoga and struggles for freedom as a perfect eagle pose, elegantly intertwined. Read this book, pass it on, whisper, sing, pray, honor its capacious words.

Becky Thompson PhD, RYT-500

We are living in a time of things falling apart, when our emotions seem big and real while the hatred and fear seems so sweet and tempting. This is also a time when we have forgotten that the earth is an extension of our bodies and our bodies are an extension of the earth. Both the earth and our bodies are saturated with trauma. The land is saturated with centuries of violence and neglect. Our bodies are saturated with various expressions of trauma including transhistorical, intergenerational, and vicarious traumas on top of the traumas from surviving emotional and physical abuse. These experiences of trauma have knocked us out of our bodies as an expression of disassociation and disembodiment. If there is disembodiment then there is some disconnection from our emotions as well as a deep disconnection from the earth. For me, this situation translates into a profound social, environmental, political, and spiritual crisis. We have to call in what we need to liberate us. *Yoga and Resilience* is one of the vital texts we need to cultivate deepening relationship with our bodies, identities, trauma, and the earth. *Yoga and Resilience* reminds us of the liberatory power of yoga and calls the tradition in to foster our relationship with our bodies, and offers a clear path towards freedom and connection during these intense times.

Lama Rod Owens, author of *Love and Rage,* co-author of *Radical Dharma*

This best practices book is mandatory reading for anyone offering yoga in any setting. While often unseen, there are survivors of sexual trauma in all places where yoga is practiced and taught. The authors have comprehensively and bravely laid out a detailed framing for understanding sexual violence, and importantly, how to overcome the effects of trauma and grow stronger using yoga. Founded in the science behind the traumatic response, with both personal and professional experience on the topic spanning multiple decades, the writers and editors capture the nuance of working with survivors in detail and with practicality. This work celebrates survival and challenges practitioners to deliver yoga that is as safe as possible and inclusive for every survivor. It offers hope, movement towards healing, and genuine celebration. The best practices here are thoughtful, well-researched, and practical: techniques that can be used every day to help people facing the damaging effects of sexual violence as they journey towards their own fullest well-being.

Thordis Elva, author, TED speaker, survivor and yoga enthusiast

Yoga and Resilience: Empowering Practices for Survivors of Sexual Trauma offers a groundbreaking integration of embodied practices for understanding and healing from sexual trauma with a deep foundation in the practices and commitments of social justice activism. Grounded in the science of trauma and resilience, and the expertise of millennia of healing practices, it is an innovative contribution with the potential to heal the many wounds quietly rippling through so many of our communities. May it be read and shared widely.

Rhonda V. Magee, Professor of Law, University of San Francisco School of Law

This book is a must-read for those interested in best practices for trauma-sensitive yoga. With case studies and quotes from survivors, it provides a compassionate framework dedicated to understanding the scope and context of sexual trauma and sexual violence, its impacts, and working with survivors. In a highly accessible manner, *Yoga and Resilience* includes practical and accessible guidance (i.e., suggestions for language use, check lists, visual aids, and safety plans) that is both strengths-based and resilience focused. Written by contributors specializing in areas across the fields of trauma, substance abuse, pediatrics, psychiatry, religion, and criminal justice, this book is a wellspring of resourceful information. It tackles difficult issues, including abuse within religious and yoga communities, as well as the unique experiences of pregnant women, children and teens, queer people, the elderly, people with physical, developmental and intellectual disabilities, military members, and incarcerated survivors. The authors carefully engage with the deep history of activism in combating sexual trauma and violence by providing a resource to confront the foundations of contemporary yoga practices and facilitate empowering yoga experiences.

Meredith G. F. Worthen, Professor of Sociology, the University of Oklahoma

Reading this book by experienced teachers and therapists in the field of yoga and therapy, puts my own journey in context and offers much valuable information for teachers who are bravely out in the world of education, prisons, cultural communities, hospitals, children, care-givers and more; a way to become aware of trauma and the importance that yoga is not what we do but who we are and how we meet each person and their needs. Each chapter offers practical help, for many different situations that as teachers we may find ourselves meeting. Yoga and Resilience constantly emphasizes the importance of the way we meet our own trauma as a guide to recognize and be there for our students. I salute Danielle and her co-writers for this important book on yoga and trauma.

Angela Farmer

With the emergence of trauma-informed yoga, this volume provides an accessible and research-informed guide to critical issues in sexual violence and trauma. Its continuous turn to contexts and attention to vulnerable communities moves beyond thinking of yoga in terms of 'tools and techniques' for healing and reframes yoga spaces as critical spaces for justice work. Each essay opens up new angles of analysis, inviting readers to consider the communal, intersectional, and historical dimensions of trauma. This is a necessary guide for *all* care providers – social workers, chaplains, clinicians, and first responders – who are working with persons and communities impacted by sexual violence.

Dr. Shelly Rambo, Boston University

This is an important book as it focuses on assisting those who are often forgotten or overlooked. I am glad that there is a resource that exists so that people can learn about trauma, healing and resilience. It is a book that I will personally utilize and suggest to survivors.

Dr. Shelly Clevenger, Illinois State University

YOGA
AND
RESILIENCE

Contributors

Keyona Aviles
Jacoby Ballard
Lisa Boldin
Maya Breuer
Regine Clermont
Colleen DeVirgiliis
Alexis Donahue
Pamela Stokes Eggleston
Jennifer Cohen Harper
Dani Harris
Nan Herron
Daniel Hickman
Diana Hoscheit
Sue Jones
James Jurgensen
Mark A. Lilly
Jana Long
Anneke Lucas
Amanda J.G. Napior
Amina Naru
Danielle Rousseau
Emanuel "Manny" Salazar
Austin K. Sanderson
Lidia Snyder
Nicole Steward
Rosa Vissers
Kimberleigh Weiss-Lewit
Ann Wilkinson

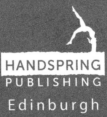

HANDSPRING
PUBLISHING
Edinburgh

YOGA
AND
RESILIENCE

Empowering Practices for Survivors of Sexual Trauma

Editor **Danielle Rousseau**

Forewords
David Emerson
Amy Wheeler

HANDSPRING PUBLISHING LIMITED
The Old Manse, Fountainhall,
Pencaitland, East Lothian
EH34 5EY, Scotland
Tel: +44 1875 341 859
Website: www.handspringpublishing.com

First published 2020 in the United Kingdom by Handspring Publishing
Copyright © Handspring Publishing 2020

ISBN 978-1-912085-93-4
ISBN (Kindle eBook) 978-1-912085-94-1

British Library Cataloguing in Publication Data
A catalogue record for this book is available from the British Library

Library of Congress Cataloguing in Publication Data
A catalog record for this book is available from the Library of Congress

Notice

Neither the Publisher nor the Authors assume any responsibility for any loss or injury and/or damage to persons or property arising out of or relating to any use of the material contained in this book. It is the responsibility of the treating practitioner, relying on independent expertise and knowledge of the patient, to determine the best treatment and method of application for the patient.

All reasonable efforts have been made to obtain copyright clearance for illustrations in the book for which the authors or publishers do not own the rights. If you believe that one of your illustrations has been used without such clearance please contact the publishers and we will ensure that appropriate credit is given in the next reprint.

Fig 1.1 Model of yoga service reproduced with kind permission from Childress T and Cohen Harper J (2016). **Box 2.1** Adverse Childhood Experiences Study (ACES) study measures reproduced with kind permission from Felitti, et al. 1998. **Fig 2.1** HPA axis and our normal stress response reproduced with kind permission from Stoller C (2019). **Fig 2.2** Autonomic nervous system reproduced with kind permission from Stoller C (2019). **Fig 2.4** Window of tolerance. © 2019 The National Institute for the Clinical Application of Behavioral Medicine. **Box 3.1** Post Traumatic Growth (PTG) in participants in a trauma-informed yoga curriculum reproduced with kind permission from Yoga 4 Change 2019. **Fig 3.1** Historical trauma impacts on health reproduced with kind permission from Mohatt NV, et al. (2014). **Fig 3.2** Four components of consent reproduced with kind permission from Worthen MGF (2016). **Table 3.1** Reasons survivors may not report sexual violence to authorities reproduced with kind permission from Worthen MGF (2016). **Fig 8.1** Sample safety plan reproduced with kind permission from Stanley B and Brown GK (2011).

Commissioning Editor Sarena Wolfaard
Project Manager Morven Dean
Copy Editor Laura Booth
Designer Bruce Hogarth
Indexer Aptara, India
Typesetter DSM Soft, India
Printer CPI Group (UK) Ltd, Croydon CR0 4YY

The
Publisher's
policy is to use
paper manufactured
from sustainable forests

CONTENTS

FOREWORD *by David Emerson*

Yoga and Resilience is a testament to the persistence and dedication of everyone involved, as well as to the organizational skills of the editors. It takes on a very important topic that deserves all of our attention – the realities of sexual violence in our world and the need for healing from the violence – with the mission to render yoga a safer, more accessible practice for survivors.

While providing lucid context, practical assessment, and an array of best practices for care providers that offer yoga in the context of healing sexual trauma, in its very construction the book itself reflects a core value that is at its textual center. By utilizing the framework of an edited volume, *Yoga and Resilience* provides an opportunity for multiple voices to share space rather than for the voice of a singular "expert" to dominate. The structure of the book itself provides an implicit challenge to the hierarchical model that over-invests power into the singular person while syphoning power away from others, the root of trauma.

As is pointed out repeatedly throughout the book, abuse and coercion thrive in environments of unequal power. In response to this endemic pattern that is present in all the various forms of sexual violence outlined in *Yoga and Resilience*, the authors suggest collaboration: care providers joining with survivors or people engaged in healing and, together, eliminating these insidious power dynamics that make sexual violence possible in the first place.

Along with heaps of sound practical advice, and intriguing empirical evidence, what makes *Yoga and Resilience* so successful is that it returns again and again to the necessity of questioning power dynamics as they are showing up *right now*. By learning to see/feel what is happening with power and skillfully respond to it in the moments that we are offering our yoga service, the authors collectively suggest that it is possible to create healing environments that "[take] care of the most vulnerable in a traditional yoga setting." Care-taking in this way is not paternalistic or pathologizing, but rather empowering, collaborative and healthier for everyone involved.

Finally, in *Yoga and Resilience*, there is an appeal for what the authors term "universally inclusive yoga," which is an attempt to reimagine the potential of yoga as safer, more welcoming, more trauma-informed and more intentional; places where power is shared rather than hoarded and abused. The authors of this thorough, honest, highly readable book have made a very important contribution to our shared understanding of a critical problem while offering some real ways forward.

David Emerson TCTSY-F
Co-founder and Director of the Center for Trauma
and Embodiment at the Justice Resource Institute
Author of *Trauma Sensitive Yoga in Therapy*
Co-author of Overcoming Trauma through Yoga
Cambridge, Massachusetts
February 2020

FOREWORD *by Amy Wheeler*

Yoga and Resilience is the book I wished I had read decades ago, when I first began to understand the impact of trauma on the mind, the nervous system and heart.

This book will help all yoga teachers and yoga therapists properly organize the classroom and communicate in a trauma-informed style, in order to facilitate their students in healing from sexual traumas.

The book outlines all the different populations that have been strongly impacted by the varied experiences of sexual trauma. The revelation of how many students are affected by these experiences is shocking, even to me, someone who has been hearing about sexual trauma from her students for three decades. This book has helped me to understand how it is even possible so many people have been adversely impacted by sexual abuse.

Sexual trauma is often characterized as being experienced only by women, as a result of abuse by their intimate partner or childhood incest. *Yoga and Resilience* shows the prevalence of sexual abuse in the following populations: gender and sexual minorities, men of all ages, the elderly, people with disabilities, college students, those serving in the military, sex trafficking victims, and people who are incarcerated. Sadly, we all know how rampant it is in religious and spiritual organizations and institutions. It makes one wonder, is there anyone who has not been closely impacted by the trauma of sexual abuse? The victims might include the survivor, an intimate partner of the abused, a best friend, a student or even the formerly abused who has now become the abuser.

One of my favorite parts of *Yoga and Resilience*, is learning about the developmental impact that occurs when the abuse happens at different times of the lifespan of an individual. In other words, the expression of childhood abuse and adult onset abuse may be very different. As well, we need to see the person/ survivor as an individual in order to create the map for their unique healing journey.

The "Best Practices" for creating a trauma-informed yoga experience is an essential part of this book. It describes over and over how clear and direct communication is very important. An example being, telling the student why and how the class is organized in a trauma informed way is crucial to building trust with the student. The text boxes with "Best Practices" are so simple and easy to read. Any teacher/ therapist (yoga or otherwise) could glance through the book and find helpful information. Conversely, any teacher or therapist could sit down, and have a very deep and meaningful reflection about how they structure their classroom, communication and relationships.

The book also focuses on a strength-based resilience approach, instead of focusing on only the injury or trauma. These strength-based guidelines help us as teachers and therapists to understand how our communication and words impact the student and just how mindful we need to be. We can learn to watch for what triggers the student and find more effective ways to relate in ways that make him or her feel safe. This book lays out how creating a safe space, setting proper boundaries, having compassionate leadership and cultural humility are keys to healing.

In summary, it is our job as yoga teachers and yoga therapists to become trauma informed and take responsibility in our healing spaces, classrooms, in our student-teacher relationships and even within our friendships. It is our job to stand up and speak when we suspect that students are not being treated well. It is our job to walk away from teachers who are abusing students. We cannot learn to do this until we learn about trauma-informed yoga. *Yoga and Resilience* is a remarkable offering that our yoga community will welcome, and I hope that everyone will read it carefully and apply the knowledge that they gain.

Amy Wheeler PhD, C-IAYT
President of the International Association
of Yoga Therapists
Southern California
January 2020

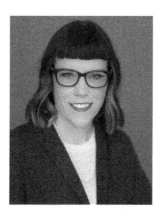

Danielle Rousseau PhD, LMHC

Danielle Rousseau, PhD LMHC, is a Boston University faculty member, licensed therapist and certified yoga teacher. Dr. Rousseau's professional focus has been in trauma service and gender advocacy. She is a scholar activist and justice educator. Dr. Rousseau worked in the field of forensic mental health as a therapist in correctional facilities and served communities through crisis response and victim advocacy. Her research, teaching and practice focus on justice, trauma, gender, mental health, mindfulness, inclusivity and resilience. She is an advocate of integrative, holistic approaches that support embodied self-care. Dr. Rousseau has received multiple grants; she is currently part of a project developing, implementing and evaluating an opioid specific yoga curriculum. Her work is published in many academic books and journals. She is a sought-after national speaker and trainer and has developed a diverse range of curricula and trainings.

Best Practices Project Manager

Amina Naru E-RYT, YACEP, Executive Director

of the Yoga Service Council, is the founder of Posh Yoga LLC in Wilmington, Delaware, and co-founder of Retreat to Spirit. Amina is a trauma-sensitive yoga instructor, workshop facilitator, and YSC Best Practices project manager. Amina served three terms as secretary for the YSC Board of Directors and is a contributor for Best Practices for Yoga with Veterans and Best Practices for Yoga in the Criminal Justice System. She served as project manager for *Yoga and Resilience* and *Yoga with People in Addictions and Recovery*. Her expertise is in the field of yoga service for communities, juvenile detention centers and adult prisons. Amina has been featured in *Yoga Journal, Yoga Therapy Today* and on the J. Brown and Yoga Alliance podcasts. She served as Executive Director of the nonprofit Empowered Community and is the first black woman to implement curriculum-based yoga and mindfulness programs for juvenile detention centers in the state of Delaware. Amina Naru's work is deeply informed by her studies with master teachers Johnny Gillespie of Empowered Yoga, James Fox of Prison Yoga Project, B.K. Bose of the Niroga Institute, Nikki Myers of Y12SR, and Jennifer Cohen Harper of Little Flower Yoga.

AUTHORS

Pamela Stokes Eggleston MBA, E-RYT500, MS, C-IAYT
is Executive Director of the Yoga Service Council and Founder of Yoga2Sleep. She is a certified yoga therapist with specialized training in plant-based nutrition, cognitive behavioral therapy for insomnia (CBT-I), and yoga for trauma. Pamela has worked with the Substance Abuse and Mental Health Services Administration, the Veterans Administration, the Department of Labor, as a yoga therapy intern for Johns Hopkins Hospital, and as an advisor on Congress supported publications centering on substance abuse, mental health, criminal justice and military and veteran caregiver matters. Pamela is a contributing editor of *Best Practices for Yoga with Veterans* (YSC/Omega, 2016) and researcher/author of *Yoga Therapy as a Complementary Modality for Female Veteran Caregivers with Traumatic Stress: A Case Study* (Maryland University of Integrative Health, March 2018). Her work and writing have been featured in *Yoga Therapy Today, Gaiam, Military Spouse Magazine, Yoga Journal, Mantra Yoga and Health, Essence, the Huffington Post,* and she has appeared on Ellen and MSNBC.

Dani Harris
has provided leadership in the field of mindfulness, resilience and yoga in the US, Canada and the UK. She has taught breath based resilience practices, as well as yoga, to youth who have experienced diverse trauma in high priority neighborhoods for over a decade with particular focus in First Nations, Metis and Inuit youth, queer youth and those recovering from sexual violence. Dani has worked extensively in the Toronto District School Board with administrators, superintendents, executive superintendents, public health nurses and mental health groups. She is also the co-creator of Rebel Breath, a social enterprise ensuring all people have access to front-line resilience practices. Dani is also an advisor to Each Amazing Breath, and has worked closely with both the Yoga Service Council and Street Yoga on various projects. She currently lives in Toronto, Canada.

Nan Herron MD
completed a residency combining pediatrics, child and adult psychiatry, followed by a fellowship in PTSD with Dr. Bessel van der Kolk – the field of PTSD has always been her passion. Nan is a trained yoga teacher, and has her "doctor's bag" filled with tools gathered from many schools of mindfulness: Dialectical Behavioral Therapy, EMDR, Mindfulness-based Stress Reduction, Mindful Self-compassion, Trauma-informed Mind-body Program, and Positive Neuro-plasticity Training. Three years ago, she left Boston and moved to her own piece of paradise in Sonoma County, Northern California. Nan continues to work full-time on locked in-patient wards in a psychiatric hospital, working with folks of all ages who are in acute crises of every kind (75% have documented trauma histories). She offers her patients a myriad of options: not just meds, traditional "talking therapy" or ECT, but also EMDR, many varieties of meditation, TIMBo mind-body flashcards, yoga, etc. In addition, she does out-patient consultations for veterans and firefighters and police who are struggling with PTSD. In the past, few years Nan has traveled with Sue Jones (who created TIMBo) to Kenya to address PTSD in Maasai women and teach skills to the Kenyan yoga teachers of Africa Yoga Project.

Daniel Hickman

teaches meditation/adaptive yoga in the Military Advanced Training Center and Adaptive Recreation Center at the Walter Reed National Military Medical Center via the Exalted Warrior Foundation. He dircts his Multidisciplinary Yoga Teacher Training at The Center for Mindful Living in Washington, DC. He mentors with the Insight Meditation Community of Washington, and is a Yoga Service Council board member. He partnered with Howard University Cancer Center/Hospital – restorative yoga interventions for African-American breast cancer survivors (pilot study), Friendship Place/La Casa – meditation/yoga for the recovering homeless (in Spanish), and the Defense and Veterans Center for Integrative Pain Management – yoga for patients with chronic back pain (US Military). He authored instructional videos – Yoga Beginnings & Vets Yoga, and worked at the now defunct Nosara Yoga Institute (Guanacaste, Costa Rica). In his past life, he was an artist-educator with The Smithsonian Institution's Discovery Theater, The Kennedy Center for the Performing Arts, and studied at El Estudio Busqueda de Pantomima Teatro (Guanajuato, Mexico). Daniel is a traditional rock climber and native Washingtonian.

Beth Jones

is a 300-hour certified Trauma Center Trauma Sensitive Yoga Facilitator, offering trauma informed yoga practices to Family Violence Project's emergency shelter, Day One Recovery classroom, sexual assault support groups, and in private classes. She also leads modules and workshops on trauma-informed approaches for yoga teacher trainings, the UNE School of Social Work, and mental health conferences throughout Maine. Since 2010, Beth's work in trauma has given her a more hopeful, grounded approach to facilitating embodiment and self- empowerment through yoga. FMI about classes, please visit www.bethjonesyoga.com.

James Jurgensen

is a consultant and researcher. He specializes in experience design, data analytics, program monitoring and evaluation, and change management. James has worked collaboratively with several public, private, and nonprofit institutions to understand their respective digital maturity; explore the untapped potential of data collection and analysis; and develop and implement a clear roadmap toward more informed and impactful operational and strategic decisions in the realms of data management and stakeholder engagement. James utilizes his expertise in statistics and human-centric design to perform robust data analysis and translate outcomes into a dynamic, scalable, and sustainable stakeholder engagement strategy.

Amanda J.G. Napior MDiv

is an ordained minister and doctoral candidate in religious studies at Boston University, where she is writing her dissertation on rehabilitation and religion in modern Corrections. With a background as a yoga instructor, teacher and tutor in prisons, and hairstylist, Amanda has consistently turned scholarly attention to phenomena she has noticed in practice. In addition to her collaborations with contributors to this present volume, Amanda has co-authored chapters in *Sensory-enhanced Yoga for Self-regulation and Trauma Healing* and has articles forthcoming in *The Journal of Ritual Studies* and *Journal of Correctional Education*. Amanda holds an MDiv from Harvard Divinity School with a focus in Christianity and a BA in religion, with an emphasis in American religious history, from the University of California at Santa Barbara.

Danielle Rousseau PhD LMHC

is a Boston University faculty member, licensed therapist and certified yoga teacher. Dr. Rousseau's professional focus has been in trauma service and gender advocacy. She is a scholar activist and justice educator. Dr. Rousseau worked in the field of forensic mental health as a therapist in correctional facilities and served communities through crisis response and victim advocacy. Her research, teaching and practice focus on justice, trauma, gender, mental health, mindfulness, inclusivity and resilience. She is an advocate of integrative, holistic approaches that support embodied self-care. Dr. Rousseau has received multiple grants; she is currently part of a project developing, implementing and evaluating an opioid specific yoga curriculum. Her work is published in many academic books and journals. Dr. Rousseau was a contributing editor for the Yoga Service Council's *Best Practices for Yoga in the Criminal Justice System*. She is a sought-after national speaker and trainer and has developed a diverse range of curricula and trainings.

Lidia Snyder

is a Licensed Master Social Worker (LMSW), Registered Yoga Teacher (RYT) and Certified Trauma Center Trauma Sensitive Yoga Facilitator (TCTSY-F) and a firm believer in the capacity of yoga to enhance and change lives. After conducting numerous interviews, she co-authored a book in in the 1990's examining the experiences of homeless families, including shared histories of trauma. Working in the child welfare and juvenile justice systems Lidia repeatedly witnessed the trajectory of unaddressed trauma. A personal yoga practice had brought many benefits to Lidia and she began to understand the mind/body connection on a deeper level. She combined her passion for social justice and yoga eventually completing her teacher training at the Himalayan Institute followed by a 300-hour Certification from the Trauma Center. She teaches in both traditional practice spaces as well as less traditional settings such as residential treatment centers and hospitals, homeless shelters for women and children, housing for formerly incarcerated males and as part of clinical treatment teams for trauma survivors. Lidia provides continuing education seminars to better understand how yoga can be part of a healing process for trauma survivors. She continues to practice, study and give thanks.

Kimberleigh Weiss-Lewit MA, IBCLC, E-RYT 500, CD/CDT

has served as Liberation Prison Yoga's Program Director, as a teacher trainer and on their board. She continues to develop curriculum for LPY and for other organizations and teachers looking to incorporate trauma-informed prenatal yoga into their work. Most recently, she partnered with Yoga Behind Bars to offer prenatal yoga teacher training to their certified yoga teachers living at Washington Corrections Center for Women. She provides support for the prenatal and postpartum yoga programs, as well as breastfeeding and new parent support, at Rikers Island Jail in New York City. She is a registered yoga teacher, certified prenatal yoga teacher, International Board Certified Lactation Consultant, birth doula, and birth doula trainer. Kim is part of the teacher training team at the Hudson Yoga Project in Hoboken, NJ. After obtaining an MA in Drama Therapy from New York University, she began prison-based work over a decade ago with Rehabilitation through the Arts serving people in both men's and women's prisons in New York. She also served families affected by domestic violence and sexual abuse at Clifford Beers Clinic in New Haven, Connecticut. Kim was honored to work on the YSC's last book: *Best Practices for Yoga in the Criminal Justice System* (2016–2017).

CONTRIBUTORS

Keyona Aviles LMHC

practices privately from her home-based wellness boutique in Boston, Massachusetts, Inspired Release. She specializes in Restorative Practices, Circlekeeping, and is also a TIMBo lead trainer and facilitator. Her belief in the body as instrumental in mental and emotional healing led her to become an ACE certified personal trainer in 2003, AFAA certified Group Exercise Instructor in 2006, Vinyasa Yoga instructor in 2009, and to train with Project Adventure in Adventure Based Counseling. When she is not counseling, circle keeping, or consulting, Keyona enjoys spending time with her family, dancing, and creating expressive art pieces. Find out more about Inspired Release at inspiredrelease.com

Jacoby Ballard

has been working at the intersection of contemplative embodied practice and social justice for 20 years, and currently teaches in Salt Lake City, Utah. He is a co-founder of Third Root Community Health Center in Brooklyn, a worker-owned cooperative expanding access to holistic healing modalities for marginalized communities that now continues on without him. His writing can be found in four anthologies: *Yoga Rising: 30 Empowering Stories from Yoga Renegades for Every Body; Mindfulness for Beginners; Yoga, the Body*, and *Embodied Social Change: an Intersectional Feminist Analysis*, and most recently, *Transcending: a Trans Buddhist Anthology*. Jacoby has worked within queer community for 12 years, deepening compassion, connection, courage, and resilience through weekly classes and retreats. He offers mindfulness and yoga tools in schools and college campuses, prisons, hospitals, recovery centers, and now Huntsman Cancer Institute in Salt Lake City. Jacoby serves on the Advisory Council of the Yoga Service Council, and is on Faculty at Off the Mat, Into the World and can be found at jacobyballard.net

Lisa Boldin MSW, MBA, TCTSY-F

is the Coordinator of the Trauma Center Trauma Sensitive Yoga (TCTSY) Certification Program based at the Center for Trauma and Embodiment at JRI in Boston. Additionally, she provides supervision to students who are seeking certification in this evidence based practice. Lisa has offered TCTSY as an integral part of psychotherapy in outpatient and residential behavioral health facilities, working extensively with survivors of sexual trauma and violent crime. Lisa is an Ayurvedic Practitioner and a past board member and conference manager for the National Ayurvedic Medical Association. Lisa practices trauma informed therapy and works in a variety of settings on New Hampshire's Seacoast.

Maya Breuer E-RYT 500

is Vice President of Cross-Cultural Advancement for the Yoga Alliance, co-founder of the Black Yoga Teachers Alliance, and founder of the Santosha School of Yoga. In 1999, Maya created the Yoga Retreat for Women of Color™. An activist, an author and a consultant to many community-based/non-profit organizations, Maya co-authored an NIH funded study: "Back to Health: Yoga vs. Physical Therapy for Minorities with

Chronic Low Back Pain"; conducted at the Boston Medical Center and published in the *Annals of Internal Medicine*, July 2017. She contributed to Stephen Cope's, *Will Yoga and Meditation Really Change My Life?* and is currently writing a book on yoga and meditation.

Regine Clermont MSW, RYT

is a certified Usui Reiki II Practitioner and an Integrative Health Coach. For over 27 years, she has worked with families, adults, and the elderly. Regine has worked in the fields of mental health, trauma, abuse, homelessness, affordable housing, and gerontology. Currently, she works for Seabury Resources for Aging's Care Management Program as a Life Enrichment Specialist. Regine's yoga journey started 17 years ago. In 2013, she became certified in Reiki; in 2014 she received a certificate as an integrative health coach. In 2018, she received her 200-hour yoga teacher certification from Sky House Yoga in Silver Spring, Maryland. Regine's passion is to be of service and teach others through yoga, how to listen and trust their body for optimal healing. As David Frawley says in *Yoga and Ayurveda: Self-healing and Self-realization*, "Restoring wholeness in the body, mind, and spirit, is what we are all seeking, both individually and collectively."

Colleen DeVirgiliis

has been teaching yoga in Chester County, PA since 2004. She is the Director of Training for the Transformation Yoga Project, a Greater Philadelphia based nonprofit offering trauma sensitive yoga and mindfulness programs in recovery centers, correctional institutions and behavioral health settings. Colleen has participated in numerous trainings focused on trauma sensitivity, accessibility and inclusion and has been active in yoga service since 2010.She is a trained facilitator with the Alternatives to Violence Project and is a member of the Think Tank at State Correctional Institute Chester in PA. In addition to leading classes in the community, she is a mindfulness provider in schools and has co-facilitated several 200-hour Yoga Instructor Trainings within the Pennsylvania prison system. Her work in yoga service continues to be a source of inspiration, joy and growth.

Alexis Donahue

completed her 200-hour Yoga Teacher Training at The Light Within Yoga Studio and continues her yogic education by attending classes, workshops, and specialized training sessions. As the Creative Director for Transformation Yoga Project, Alexis offers a unique perspective on the cultural, emotional, and philosophical aspects of mindfulness. Due to her own personal experiences within the children and youth services system, sharing yoga and mindfulness with adolescents who've been impacted by trauma has become her life's purpose. Her work for Transformation Yoga Project gives her the opportunity to teach within the juvenile justice system while also utilizing her social media expertise to bring awareness to the issues impacting today's incarcerated youth.

Jennifer Cohen Harper MA, E-RYT, RCYT

is the Immediate Past President of the Yoga Service Council, and is dedicated to making yoga and mindfulness practices accessible to all people, and especially to all children. Jennifer is the founder of Little Flower Yoga and The School Yoga Project, author of *Little Flower Yoga for Kids*, and coeditor of *Best Practices for Yoga in Schools*.

Diana Hoschiet

is the founder of Harmony Yoga Therapy in Wilmington, DE. A Certified Yoga Therapist and Experienced Registered Yoga Teacher, she has been teaching and developing Yoga Therapy based wellness programs for individuals and special populations since 2006. Diana has made it her life's mission to empower people to improve their physical, mental, emotional, and spiritual health through the practices of Yoga.

Sue Jones

is well-known in the field of yoga and trauma and has presented numerous workshops and talks on the subject of trauma, yoga, hands-on healing, and TIMBo at Omega Institute, Kripalu, Mental and Behavioral health facilities in the greater Boston Area, multiple Massachusetts Department of Mental Health Symposiums, National Conferences and New England area yoga studios. She has been profiled on CNN, on FOX news, and in numerous publications, including *Yoga Journal*, the *New York Times, Shape, Whole Living*. Sue was interviewed most recently by author Rick Hanson as a trauma expert for his Foundations of Well-being online course. Since beginning her journey in somatic-based healing, she has trained and delivered TIMBo to over 4,000 women globally. She writes a blog for both the The TIMBo Collective and *Elephant Journal*. She oversees a world-wide community of women connected via online platforms to support one another and build continued capacity to help others with TIMBo. Her first book, *There is Nothing to Fix* was published in 2019.

Mark A. Lilly

is a writer, and mindfulness and communication trainer who has taught workshops all over North America to widely diverse audiences including physicians, nurses, social workers, police officers, therapists, mental health workers and countless others. Mark is the founder of Street Yoga, an internationally recognized non-profit which provided yoga and mindfulness classes to at-risk populations in Portland and Seattle. Mark has extensive expertise in community- as well as hospital-based mindfulness practices, and has initiated Mindful Communication workshops for physicians, along with similar trainings for nurses and social workers. He is also the co-founder of Rebel Breath, and has developed the practice of Body-Mind Rehab Therapy for use in in-patient settings. Mark also is co-founder of Each Amazing Breath: a UK social enterprise which has brought breath-based resilience practices to over 10,000 students, teachers, and school staff. He is also co-creator of the Mindful Parents & Caregiver program which serves social workers and their client families with practical, everyday mindfulness.

Jana Long E-RYT-500, C-IAYT

is the co-founder and Executive Director of the Black Yoga Teachers Alliance, Inc., and director of Power of One Yoga Center in Baltimore, MD. She is a yoga teacher and therapist specializing in the application of yoga to support the health and wellness of older people and the management of acute and chronic disease. As an

Ayurvedic life style consultant, she focuses on self-care practices and ancestral wisdoms for preventive health. She is a certified Master Gardener in Baltimore City and a community educator who raises awareness around ecological sustainability and urban farming. Jana travels nationally and internationally with the Global Peace Initiative of Women as part of a global contemplative movement to help young adults awaken the spiritual resources to restore earth's balance and to create a more compassionate and life sustaining world community. Jana embodies all the roles of feminine energy – daughter, sister, mother, aunt and grandmother. She is former media professional who had a long career at *The Washington Post*. She is a writer, gourmet cook and astrologer.

Anneke Lucas E-RYT-500

founded Liberation Prison Yoga (LPY) in 2014 and serves as its executive director. LPY works with an average of 35 trained volunteer teachers to offer more than 20 weekly trauma informed yoga programs at Rikers Island, the Manhattan Detention Complex, Bedford Hills Maximum-Security Prison, Taconic State Medium-Security Prison, and Wallkill Medium-Security Prison, in New York State. LPY additionally runs jail-based programs for transgender women, those in drug rehab, and severely mentally ill women; studio-based weekly community classes for formerly incarcerated students; and programs at reentry facilities. A survivor of child sex trafficking and extreme violence, Anneke has used elements of her own 30-year healing journey to develop programs based on how she would have wished to be treated in her young adult life. Currently, she is designing a 200-hour Yoga Alliance-registered teacher training for Liberation Prison Yoga, focusing on bringing yoga to traumatized populations. She's writing a book about her healing journey, *Seeds Beneath the Snow: Post-traumatic Growth and Purpose in Dark Times*.

Emanuel "Manny" Salazar

is a 24-year military veteran and a clinical social worker specializing in working with youth who have experienced trauma. During this time, he received his 200 hour RYT from Vetoga, completed a 100-hour training with Mindful Yoga Therapy, and attended a 52-hour yoga nidra training with Amrit Desai all with the purpose of supporting those who have experienced trauma. Inspired by both his military experience and work with youth as a licensed Social Worker, Emanuel founded Mindful Warrior Retreats, LLC in May 2017 with the mission to empower underserved communities, including veterans and vulnerable youth, to overcome trauma and hardship through mindfulness education and cultivating emotional resilience. Manny's practice is rooted in the philosophy of empowering clients to find meaning in their traumatic experiences through a strength-based perspective, asking not "what's wrong with you?" but "what's right with you?" He views healing as a collective effort, reframing culture as a central feature in well-being.

Austin K. Sanderson

moved to NYC in 1998 to attend New York University's Tisch School of the Arts, Design and Production Department. After graduating with his Masters degree in set and costume design, he has spent the next eighteen years working as a designer in the American theater. In 2008 he was introduced to Jivamukti Yoga in a yoga class at Club H Fitness with yoga teacher Susan Steiner. As he continued to take class with Susan and other Jivamukti teachers, he wanted to learn more and share with others his life changing experience brought about while practicing the Jivamukti Yoga Method. In 2011, Austin attended the Jivamukti 300+ hour teacher training program at the Omega Institute. In 2012, he completed his 800-hour Jivamukti Teacher Certification at The Jivamukti Yoga School NYC. Austin is extremely grateful to all his teachers, but most of all to Sharon Gannon and David Life for the amazing gift of Jivamukti Yoga. Austin is the co-owner of Jivamukti Yoga Center Jersey City and if the co-producer of Yoga Fest Jersey City, a free public yoga, music and vegan food festival held in the heart of downtown Jersey City NJ during the summer equinox.

Nicole Steward, MSW
is a social worker and yoga instructor with a focus on community engagement, public education, foster youth advocacy, and trauma-informed yoga. With more than two decades of social work practice in non-profits and accountability work in K-12 education, Nicole has noticed the need for radical self-care to discharge toxic stress we absorb through our work. This awareness drives her to study the ways yoga and mindfulness affect our brains and bodies, keeping us engaged and renewed. Nicole teaches yoga and offers self-care workshops to social service agencies and non-profit organizations. Nicole believes self-care is a radical tendency we must adopt if we are to sustain ourselves as service providers and human beings. She has been a CASA for more than 15 years, is a proud former foster parent to three amazing kids and a "grandma" of two.

Rosa Vissers MFA, E-RYT-500
sees movement as a powerful pathway to connect to our resilience, experience our aliveness, and build community. She has been part of Seattle-based Yoga Behind Bars for over a decade, and served as its Executive Director for over 6 years. During her time as ED, she spearheaded yoga teacher trainings for people who are incarcerated, and partnered with Birth Beyond Bars and Kimberleigh Weiss-Lewit to offer prenatal yoga teacher training at Washington Corrections Center for Women. She was honored to contribute to YSC's Best Practices for Yoga in the *Criminal Justice System* book. Originally from the Netherlands, Rosa has an extensive background as an international dance artist and continues to create and perform.

Ann Wilkinson BA
is the Director of Mentoring Services at My Life My Choice, a program of Justice Resource Institute. Since 2002, My Life My Choice has offered a unique continuum of survivor-led services aimed at preventing the commercial sexual exploitation of children. Since coming to My Life My Choice in 2006, Ms. Wilkinson directs the Survivor Mentoring program in which commercially sexually exploited and high risk youth are paired with trained adult survivors for a one-on-one, long-term relationship. Further, Ms. Wilkinson works with service providers to augment and fine tune their services for this vulnerable population. Ms. Wilkinson brings a wealth of personal and professional expertise, including over twenty years in the fields of trafficking, domestic violence, addiction, and HIV services.

PREFACE *by Robert "Skip" Backus*

Since our beginning, Omega's mission has been to awaken the best in the human spirit and to provide hope and healing for individuals and society. Yoga and service have always been core components of our offering, and they continue to serve as transformative tools toward our personal and collective growth and well-being.

Over the years, an ever-widening network of people and organizations that share our deep commitment to service has enriched our community. Through this experience, we have learned that the power of working together is much stronger than walking the path alone. When we combine our energy and intentions, we extend our reach and have a greater positive impact in the world. That's why it's only natural that the Yoga Service Council and Omega have partnered together on a path to offer and support yoga service.

This partnership began in 2009, when Omega offered space for a group of yoga teachers to come together and talk about ways to support those who work with vulnerable and underserved populations. The YSC emerged from this initial gathering and offered the first annual Yoga Service Conference at Omega in 2011.

During each Yoga Service Conference at Omega, we have discovered and rediscovered that the YSC Board of Directors and others who choose to be involved in this work are some of the most compassionate people we have met. Yoga service truly is a practice of the heart – and a specific path of yoga that fully aligns with Omega's mission and ideals.

As a result of our shared commitment to yoga and service, the YSC and Omega decided to formally partner in 2014 to bring yoga into the lives of more individuals and communities that have limited access to these vital teachings. We are excited to continue this partnership with the YSC and all its member organizations.

Helping people heal from trauma through trainings and retreats focused on complementary and alternative healing modalities has been an area of focus at Omega for more than 20 years. We know sexual trauma can affect the mind, body, and spirit, bringing unique challenges to the healing process.

Yoga and Resilience: Empowering Practices for Survivors of Sexual Trauma is the fourth title in our Yoga Service Best Practices series. In 2017 and 2018 we hosted two symposiums where leaders in the field gathered at Omega to share experience, wisdom, and aspirations for the project. We offer a special thanks to Yoga and Resilience project leaders Amina Naru (project manager and co-executive director of the Yoga Service Council), Danielle Rousseau (editor), Pamela Stokes Eggleston (co-executive director of the Yoga Service Council), and all the writers and contributors.

We are honored to have helped in the development of this essential new guide.

Robert "Skip" Backus
Chief Executive Officer
Omega Institute, Rhinebeck, NY
February 2020

PREFACE *by Yoga Service Council Board*

Welcome to the fourth Yoga Service Council's Best Practices Book.

We would like to acknowledge, where we held our symposium in Rhinebeck, NY, is situated on traditional territories. The territories include: The Lenape and the Mohican. We would also like to recognize the enduring presences of all Indigenous Americans on this land.

What happens when over two dozen service professionals of specialized vocations, come together to collaborate, research, investigate, debate and ultimately create? A hugely resourceful rough draft is forged. This draft, full of potent information, intricate formulations, crucial studies and findings, becomes thoroughly refined over a year-long process, into a much needed book that is in your hands right now.

Some might say a distinct reference on this particular subject is well overdue. Some might say it is actually right on time, considering the #MeToo movement. Some might say they are just relieved that this subject continues to be brought forth into a larger topic of conversation.

We would like to acknowledge the symposium participants who travelled from all around North America to make this happen. Every contributor volunteered their expertise, experience and time away from their home to meet, dig deep, and give clarity to such dark subjects. As with past symposiums, yogis, psychologists, psychiatrists, listened social workers, academics, certified yoga instructors, activists, writers, yoga studio owners, school teachers, mothers, fathers, sons & daughters, and survivors of sexual assault, met for five days during the month of October, in Rhinebeck upstate New York.

This would not have been possible without the generosity of the Omega Institute, the Yoga Alliance and Lululemon. The tremendous support of these three organizations, for this particular symposium, was held in great appreciation. A seamless experience was made for participants to meet as strangers and leave as friends.

As well, we would like to acknowledge the spirit of seva found in the many generous souls, both past and present, who have made up the greater body of the Yoga Service Council. It is often said that seva, also known as selfless service, is the heart of karma yoga (selfless action). We are blessed to know that this spiritual pathway is very much alive and continuing to thrive.

Deep Regards,
The Yoga Service Council Board
February 2020

PREFACE *by Amina Naru*

In 2017 I was presented with the opportunity to manage the *Best Practices for Yoga with Survivors of Sexual Trauma* book project for the Yoga Service Council. The timing was ripe with the developments of the #MeToo movement, and the need for standards within the mainstream yoga community.

Each contributor of this book was carefully selected based on professional and personal experiences, and expertise within the field of sexual trauma. The amazing people that came to contribute their knowledge and years of experiences volunteered a week of their time, away from their families and careers at the Omega Institute carving the outline and content of this book. It was no small feat. The nature of the subject matter is quite sensitive and required all hearts and minds to be open to the magnitude of the task before us.

In 2018, we held another gathering of volunteers at Omega to bring more voices into the work. The project had evolved into a living breathing entity which rendered deliverables such as the Universally Inclusive Yoga Agreement, #thepledge, Universally Inclusive Yoga Community Resource Paper, YSC Sexual Trauma webinar, and meetings with the Yoga Alliance. The project gained national as well as global attention and support.

I, a survivor of sexual trauma, have a heartfelt deep connection to this work and have my own personal attachments to the need for all people to be treated with respect and dignity in spaces where yoga is being taught and practiced. Through this work my hope is that standards around consent, touch, and creating safe communities will be uplifted and held with great reverence and responsibility. Through this work may we all be more informed, educated, and compassionate for the suffering and safety of others.

I would like to thank the Yoga Service Council Board of Directors and the Omega Institute for recognizing the need and taking on the task of providing the foundation for a groundbreaking, community changing manuscript to be written. I have unwavering love and gratitude for all of the writers and contributors for their commitment and undying passion to see this project to completion. I want to thank Here to Be, and the Yoga Alliance Foundation for their financial support and for believing in us to carry out this mission. I want to thank my co-executive director Pamela Stokes-Eggleston for emotional and spiritual support, and co-facilitating the magical symposium experiences at Omega. Lastly, I have great honor and respect on top of the mounds of gratitude to the Editor of this book, Dr. Danielle Rousseau, who helped provide the glue and vision not to mention hard work to see this project completed and in the hands of renowned publisher, Handspring.

I stand within the company of utmost brilliance and greatness.

Warmly,

Amina Naru
Project Manager
Yoga Service Council
February 2020

PART
1

Understanding Sexual Trauma

Introduction: Setting the Context

Authors *Danielle Rousseau and Dani Harris*

To begin, we wish to set the context of this project. The journey that has led us to this final project is unique – in some way innovative, in others, not new at all. This text is unique in its collaborative voice. It was born of the Yoga Service Council's (YSC's) Best Practices for Yoga with Survivors of Sexual Trauma project, at the time, a next step in a series of guides offering best practices for bringing yoga service into being for various populations and contexts. We will discuss this model in greater detail in a moment, but first wanted to clarify our "we" and share some fundamental beliefs that set the context for this work.

The writing shared in each of the chapters that follow goes far beyond the work of the individual Chapter authors. As we will detail, the foundation of this work lay in a co-creation process involving leading voices in the yoga service field. Together, a collaborative journey has resulted in the work presented in this text. While we acknowledge that our joint perspective is still not comprehensive, we strive to pursue this inquiry in as inclusive a way as possible, knowing that we still have much to learn. We recognize that, despite our efforts, there are people and voices not represented here, deepening some silences to which we were hoping to give sound. Nevertheless, we authors hope the extant silences of this text might spark curiosity and encourage our readers to pursue more learning and collaboration, beyond these pages. And learning beyond these pages is precisely what this book encourages.

We share some foundational beliefs:

It is our belief that everyone can access yoga no matter what they have been through and that those who have survived, as well as those surviving and trying to break the cycles of their own trauma, can, as safely as possible, move towards healing in a variety of ways using many different modalities.

We believe that the safest experiences of yoga can bring people back to themselves, and give them a chance to experience their bodies not only with less fear, but eventually with immense connection and joy.

We also believe that feelings of strength, joy, empowerment, safety, and deep connection to self and others can exist in *any* offering of yoga – not just when one feels "healed" but throughout one's entire journey. It is no longer optional that we approach our teaching with anything except the greatest care and the deepest love for ourselves and those we share yoga's offerings with.

We acknowledge that, as a whole, we are working from the broad understanding and conceptualization of modern Western yoga. We as a group have roots in a diverse scope of lineages and practices. We approach our discussion of yoga and related practices with a deep cultural humility and acknowledge the fundamental importance of engaging conversations concerned with issues of cultural appropriation. We will discuss this in more detail in future chapters, but want to acknowledge the scope of perspectives, backgrounds, and practices that shape this discourse, and acknowledge the importance of engaging discussions of complicated histories and abuses within the yoga community. Forefronting issues of power, privilege, and justice is fundamental to this work.

We are motivated by the highest sense of safety and care around the sharing of yoga, as well as by the desire to make yoga accessible to every person. Yoga is a practice of discovery and self-discovery, as it often fosters vulnerability in one's own body and self. When we share yoga with others, we cannot know their full history or vulnerabilities. We have a sacred responsibility to be as safe as possible at all times, so that each person can participate in the practice of yoga, no matter their circumstance. In order to be accessible, we believe that the offering of yoga should strive to be trauma-informed, universally inclusive, and be rooted in a discussion of strength-based resilience. This work is an attempt to begin a discussion of best practices to support accessibility, inclusion, and awareness of the specific impacts of sexual trauma.

Setting the Context

The current text arose from the Yoga Service Council's Best Practice series. The Yoga Service Council is a 501 (c) (3) nonprofit organization formed in 2009 in collaboration with the Omega Institute. Committed to strengthening the field of yoga service, the YSC works to: (1) facilitate collaboration and community building, (2) promote excellence in education and training, (3) support leadership and organizational development, and (4) advocate for social responsibility and ethical action.

The mission of the YSC is to maximize the effectiveness, sustainability, and impact of individuals and organizations working to make yoga and mindfulness practices equally accessible to all. Through this mission, they envision a world where everyone has equal access to yoga and mindfulness practices that support healing, resilience, self-development, community building, and positive social change.

The YSC defines yoga service as "the intentional sharing of yoga practices that support healing and build resilience for all regardless of circumstances, taught within a context of conscious relationship rooted in self reflection and self-inquiry" (Childress & Cohen Harper 2016). The theoretical conceptualization of this is depicted in Figure 1.1.

In this model, intention and a commitment to conscious relationship are the center of offering yoga in service. Conscious relationship "asks people to educate themselves about social justice issues (e.g., privilege, race, violence, gender, poverty) as well as to listen openly and with curiosity

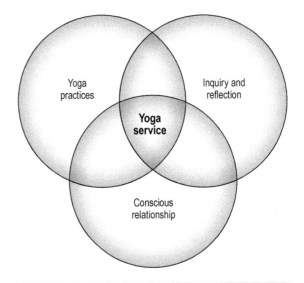

Figure 1.1

Model of yoga service

Source: Childress T and Cohen Harper J (2016) What is yoga service? A working definition [Online] Available: https://yogaservicecouncil.org/community-resource-papers

to each other's perspectives" (Childress & Cohen Harper 2016: 1). Conscious relationship fosters the development of authentic relationship.

Embodied mindfulness practices represent an effective strengths-based approach for fostering resilience, and ameliorating the many impacts of traumatic stress, with benefit for diverse populations. The Yoga Service Council has developed a model for accessibility to mindfulness practices that highlights yoga practices, inquiry and reflection, and conscious relationship. Through reflection and self-inquiry we acknowledge the impacts of our own history, privilege, bias, and wisdom. YSC defines yoga practice as including "physical postures, breath work, meditation, and deep relaxation," while acknowledging that other ethical, spiritual, and philosophical perspectives and practices play a role. Overall, yoga service works to support empowerment and well-being through sharing the practice of yoga.

The YSC has also established a unique and accessible methodology for developing guides that share knowledge and resources supporting those who wish to share yoga service. The YSC developed a book series that represents a co-creative and innovative model for fostering best practices in embodied mindfulness. The first three books in this series were the *Best Practices for Yoga in Schools* (2015), *Best Practices for Yoga with Veterans* (2016), and *Best Practices for Yoga in the Criminal Justice System* (2017). The current work represents the fourth book in this project series.

The best practices project is dedicated to uplifting the field of yoga and has two major components: an annual symposium and best practices text. At the symposium, teachers, researchers, therapists, medical professionals, policy makers, and others in the yoga service field share insights, experiences, and knowledge through a collaborative process. Through qualitative data gathering and supported by the research literature, best practice are distilled. Resultant best practices support teaching yoga and mindfulness in ways that are as safe as possible, effective, inclusive, and supported by experiential and research-based expertise. An edited volume is published that integrates the knowledge generated at the symposium.

The best practices texts are co-creative projects. Each text draws on the embodied wisdom of diverse experts in the field, who together attend a five-day symposium. At the symposium, subgroups are established and data are gathered on specific topics. Through a qualitative and exploratory process, group members engage in an iterative process of establishing best practices that are rooted in both experiential and empirical knowledge. A writer is designated for each group; it is the role of the writer to record the group's process and synthesize findings into a best practices chapter for the group's specific topic. After the writer authors their chapter, the co-creative process allows for feedback and input from group members and project contributors as a whole. The final text represents the culmination of an iterative collaboration among project contributors, chapter authors, and the editor.

Best Practice for Yoga with Survivors of Sexual Trauma

The most recent symposia addressed yoga for survivors of sexual trauma. The importance of addressing the many impacts of sexual trauma is undeniable. This project works to give voice to survivors and create an environment that fosters resilience in the wake of trauma through support of an inclusive yoga community. We recognized a need for work in this area and that the practice of yoga service needed to be informed by a comprehensive understanding of the impacts of sexual trauma and violence specifically. Because many seek or are referred to yoga in the aftermath of sexual trauma and acknowledging the fact that not all yoga is healing and that yoga contexts themselves have the potential to be traumatizing, we recognized the need for exploration of best practices for offering yoga to survivors. Recognizing the deep history of activism, service, policy, and education in combating sexual trauma and violence, we knew that more needed to be done specifically in the field of yoga service.

As we prepared for and gathered as a group for the first symposium, an explosion of media and public disclosures tied to the #MeToo movement was occurring. While we recognize that sexual trauma has long been pervasive, existing across both time and place, we also began to acknowledge an undeniable call to action and accountability.

As we convened for the symposium in the fall of 2017, it became clear that the scope of the work we were doing was greater than prior projects. There existed an opportunity to rise to the current moment and actively seek justice and acknowledge the systemic impacts of abuses of power and privilege. If we were to live up to the definition of yoga service, we needed to actively pursue change, including change within the yoga community itself.

At the same time, we recognized that there were important voices who were underrepresented. As a result, the decision was made to gather for a second symposium. Some participants returned and we invited additional voices to the table. The scope of the project grew, and we are grateful that the significance of this expanded vision was recognized and supported by our stakeholders. The expansion of the project resulted not only in a broadened discussion of the topic, but also in additional deliverables, including a pledge for studios and other yoga spaces, multiple articles, and the decision to more formally pursue a published book. From the efforts of these two best practices symposia, we offer you the current best practices text.

Sexual trauma devastates the whole person, families, relationships, communities, tribes, and nations, often for many generations forth. The mechanisms of power and control shape legislation and policy within systems. Violence spurts from that ill.

The good news is that we can right this shift; the tumult is here, and we are still standing, together, at the moving edge of a deep shift in how we think, feel, believe, and talk about sexual violence. We claim its impacts and celebrate how yoga, if shared with deepest grace, can move in highly profound ways to create spaces where acceptance, healing, and action take place.

Structure of this Text

We have the profound opportunity to make yoga as safe and accessible as possible and, with this, people can heal, and generations can be uplifted; cycles of violence can lessen to the point of extinction. The work of yoga service necessitates a strong foundation in self-inquiry and an embrace of both experiential and empirical wisdom. In tandem with such a foundation, a strong personal practice is mandatory before sharing any modalities in the yoga service field. Throughout this book, you will be invited to consider new perspectives as to how the practice of yoga can be offered in a way that is deeply informed by both self-inquiry and conscious relationship.

Following this chapter, Chapter 2 and Chapter 3 establish a foundational context for the text. Chapter 2 provides an overview of trauma and Chapter 3 a contextualization of sexual trauma specifically. After these two chapters, each subsequent Chapter offers best practices for putting this work into the world. The chapters of Part 2 provide more general best practices including best practices for trauma-informed yoga (Chapter 4), best practices for working with survivors of sexual trauma (Chapter 5), and relational wisdom for self-care, boundaries, and cultural humility (Chapter 6). Following these more general best practices, we move into best practices that address more specific populations and contexts. Part 3 speaks to development discussing specific work within the context of pregnancy and postpartum (Chapter 7) and best practices for working with children and adolescents (Chapter 8). Part 4 addresses identity and intersectional perspectives, including working with the gender and sexual minority community (Chapter 9), men who are survivors (Chapter 10), and working with elders and those with disabilities (Chapter 11). Part 5 speaks to contexts of sexual trauma, including best practices for working with sexual trauma on college and university campuses (Chapter 12), military sexual trauma (Chapter 13), intimate partner violence (Chapter 14), sex trafficking (Chapter 15), working with incarcerated survivors (Chapter 16), and abuse in religious, spiritual, and intentional communities (Chapter 17). We conclude looking forward with a discussion of what we can do within the yoga community to address sexual trauma and promote universally inclusive practices (Chapter 18).

Each of the chapters offering best practices begins with a brief introduction about context, potentially offering definitions, statistics, and other information to provide readers some footing.

Often a narrative or case study is shared to help establish this context. Each introduction is followed by an offering of best practices as they have been co-created and collaboratively developed by project contributors. As noted above, some chapters address best practices for specific populations and contexts. These are developed and offered by experts in each area. You may recognize some repetition in recommended best practices among sections and chapters. These commonalities reflect our desire to offer content chapters that can stand alone for those looking for understanding around a specific topic. We do recommend that if you seek specific best practices for individual populations or contexts, you first root yourself in Chapter 2 through Chapter 5 as a foundation. We also offer the book as a text that can be read in whole for a more comprehensive exploration.

Although the authors of each Chapter have been afforded space for their individual voices and artistic expression, we also acknowledge the collaborative voice that runs throughout. All contributors to each of the two symposia have had the opportunity to review the work as a whole to have input and ensure that each of their individual voices has been accurately represented as part of the collective. Further, we have worked collaboratively to shape editorial decisions that impact the text as a whole. For an example, we have chosen to use "they" as a representative and inclusive pronoun throughout the text. This was a collaborative decision and will be reflected throughout to maintain a common voice and natural flow between chapters. Additionally, we use writing that reflects the language best practices we recommend throughout the text; for example, we use the term "form" (instead of pose or posture) to describe the physical forms that make up yoga asana. That said, and despite the co-creative process, you as a reader will also recognize the unique voice that each of our writers brings.

We acknowledge and honor all of the wisdom that has made this work what it is. We respect all of the unique ways contributors have "labored" as part of this project. We value both empirical and experiential, written and lived knowledge. We honor the wisdom and expertise of all of our contributors, while also acknowledging that, at the most basic level, none of this knowledge belongs to us, for knowledge is shared. For each chapter, you will notice that the byline reflects all contributions, both those of participants who engaged in writing and those who shaped the best practices in a multitude of ways including group facilitation, holding of space, and sharing of lived knowledge and wisdom. As part of our offering, we suggest the fundamental importance of universal inclusivity. We want to clearly embody this: that we, through our work and offering, are a model of universal inclusivity and resilience building through true co-creation.

This text is but a beginning, a tool to encourage self-inquiry and inspire action. As you, the reader, encounter this information and the best practices that follow, you may find yourself stepping into waters you know very well and others that are entirely new. Practitioners (yoga instructors, agency administrators, clinicians, social workers, and other trauma-informed service providers) must then seek more and ongoing education and training in order to do justice in their work with people who have experienced sexual violence and trauma. These best practices in this text are informed by the authors' own diverse experiences as service providers or researchers in these contexts, and, in many cases, as survivors themselves. We cannot give voice to all experiences or best practices, but we have tried to speak loudly from the depths of our own. Learning and inquiry are a journey. The call to activism, empowered connection, and conscious relationship is not discrete, but continuous. We challenge you to continue to ask questions, seek learning, and engage in critical inquiry. We urge you to seek the connection that will empower change.

We want to remind our reader that you are not alone in this work, and that the people whom you serve have a capacity for healing and resilience that is wide and deep. We invite practitioners to work from the conviction that you are supported even when colleagues are absent or unknown, and to teach to your student's resilience, while trusting in their capacity to heal. May your communities, as well as the brilliance and love that draws you to this work, be your fuel. Know that over time, you will gain more tools and greater proficiency in what you do, if you do not already feel up to the tasks that demand your attention. At our best, we are always in inquiry, always learning. New and experienced practitioners must remember to lean on what they may not be able to see but rather can feel, or intuit. New practitioners must be willing to step back and learn from the wisdom of people in their organization. Experienced practitioners must continually seek support and ongoing inquiry. All must forefront conscious relationship building. Your connection to your community of support is vital to the sustainability of your work. Your commitment to radical self-care will fuel your capacity for service.

Our world is one of incredible suffering, but our capacity for healing, creativity, relationship, and resilience is something beautiful. We hope this text will support you in your cultivation and practice of that beauty.

Understanding Trauma

Authors *Lidia Snyder and Danielle Rousseau*

While the focus of this text is primarily rooted in addressing the impacts of sexual trauma, first having a contextual understanding of trauma more generally becomes fundamental. It is our belief that embodied practices, such as yoga, play an important role in addressing the impacts of trauma, and sexual trauma more specifically. In this chapter, we aim to provide an understanding of trauma that will set the foundation for our work in relation to delineating best practices utilizing yoga and mindfulness practices with and as survivors of sexual trauma.

Increasingly trauma is being noted as a contributing factor in mental, physical, and behavioral health care. During the late 1990s the landmark Adverse Childhood Experiences Study (ACES) revealed clear linkages between childhood traumatic experiences and subsequent health problems ranging from diabetes to substance abuse (Felitti, et al. 1998).

ACES Study Items
- Verbal abuse
- Physical abuse
- Sexual abuse
- Physical neglect
- Emotional neglect
- Family member diagnosed with a mental illness
- Family member addicted to alcohol or other substance
- Family member who has been incarcerated
- Witnessing a mother being abused
- Losing a parent to separation, divorce, or other reasons

The data available to date suggest that childhood trauma is associated with adverse brain development in multiple regions that impact emotional and behavioral regulation, motivation, and cognitive function (De Bellis & Zisk 2014). Additionally, functional Magnetic Resonance Imaging (fMRI) has shown how the brain responds to trauma, as well as what impact various interventions have on the brain's structure and function. Functional Magnetic Resonance Imaging measures and reveals post-traumatic enlargement of the amygdala along with diminishment of the hippocampus leaving many with a chronic state of hypervigilance and a sense of reliving their trauma (van der Kolk 2006). Interestingly, preliminary research reveals how particular types of yoga and mindfulness can alter and support the repair of various brain regions (Streeter, et al. 2010). As a result, the topic of trauma is an expanding theme for researchers as well as a consideration for service providers, educators, and others, including yoga instructors and practitioners.

Due to the plethora of lineages, styles, and schools of yoga, it can be challenging to identify precisely how the practice of yoga impacts various components of physical and mental health.

Yoga is gaining increasing acceptance in health-care settings and exists alongside traditional Western medicine as some health care providers now support yoga as an adjunctive treatment approach. The benefits of yoga have been long touted by practitioners, but more recently advances in technology have allowed for research to reveal a host of benefits linked with the practice of yoga. With a growing body of literature to support its validity, yoga now represents a valid strategy for the treatment of trauma. Because yoga practices vary greatly, practicing yoga in the wake of sexual trauma can have both beneficial and deleterious impacts. The selection of or referral to a yoga class, particularly in the wake of trauma, must be done in an informed and intentional way. This includes seeking yoga practices that are inclusive, trauma-informed, and strengths based, with teachers who are rooted in an understanding of the impacts of trauma. There are many considerations for referral to yoga in the wake of trauma. Clinicians seeking to recommend yoga for survivors should seek appropriate and informed referrals, prepare their clients for what to expect from yoga practice, and work to expand their personal awareness, education, and practice as related to yoga (Rousseau, Weiss-Lewit, & Lilly, 2019).

Yoga that is adapted to the unique needs of individuals working to overcome trauma-related symptoms may help ameliorate symptoms by creating a safe space for students to learn how to respond to, rather than to be overwhelmed by, their symptoms and circumstances. Yoga not thus adapted, on the other hand, may inadvertently increase reactivity and activate PTSD symptoms.

(Justice 2018: 39)

It is of fundamental importance that we root our work in the field of yoga in a foundation of education in relation to both trauma and sexual trauma specifically. It is through education and bearing witness to and wholeheartedly believing survivors that we can best support and be held accountable. In Chapter 3, we will discuss important specifics regarding sexual trauma, including the importance of defining and understanding sexual trauma and consent. In this chapter, we set the foundation of understanding trauma more generally, exploring the trauma and stress response and discussing how trauma impacts our mind and body. We will also address the impact that trauma can have for those working with survivors. This chapter, combined with the next, aims to set a contextual foundation for the best practices offered in the remainder of the text.

Understanding Stress and Trauma

Stress occurs "when an organism perceives a threat to its existence or well-being" (Mate 2003: 29).

According to the work of Gabor Mate, stress has three primary components. It is composed of:

1. The event, physical or emotional, that the organism interprets as threatening. This is the stress stimulus, also called the stressor.

2. The processing system that experiences and interprets the meaning of the stressor. (For humans, the nervous system and the brain.)

3. The stress response, which consists of the various physiological and behavioral adjustments made as a reaction to a perceived threat (Mate 2003: 31).

The stress response has a very real and often negative influence on our physical self and overall well-being. Chronic stress is connected with disease (dis-ease). It is also important to note that it is not only an actual threat but also perception of a threat that can lead to a stress response.

There are three factors that universally trigger stress: (1) uncertainty, (2) loss of control, and (3) lack of information (Mate 2003: 34). We respond to these triggers biologically and our perception of stress influences how we experience it. The stress response can be positive. Some level of stress is necessary in order to help us achieve and accomplish goals. Picture the experience of stress as falling on a bell curve, with optimal performance occurring with a moderate and acute (passing) experience of the stress response. You benefit from the stress response and release of stress hormones when you need to perform – say just before a big presentation. However, too much stress can be detrimental. Our systems were not made to exist in a chronic state of stress response. When we are unable to return to homeostasis or our state of "normal," our system is unable to balance itself and this leads to chronic stress and disease.

Acute stress is the immediate short-term body response to threat.

Chronic stress is activation of the stress mechanisms over long periods of time when a person is exposed to stressors that cannot be escaped either because she does not recognize them or because she has no control over them.

(Mate 2003: 35; emboldening added)

Trauma occurs in response to an inescapably stressful event that overwhelms people's existing coping mechanisms; trauma represents exposure to a threat or perceived threat of some kind.

According to the *Diagnostic and Statistical Manual of Mental Disorders, Fifth Edition* (DSM–5) such threats would include death, threatened death, actual or threatened serious injury, or actual or threatened sexual violence. This threat could come through direct exposure, witnessing the trauma, learning that a relative or close friend was exposed to trauma, or indirect exposure to adverse details of trauma, usually in the course of professional duties (American Psychiatric Association 2013). A trauma response is a normal response to an abnormal situation; responses are rooted in primitive neurobiology for the express purpose of keeping us safe. The problem comes when a continual feedback loop of stress and trauma response takes hold. This perpetuates a state of chronic stress and trauma in the body, and contributes to the incapacity of the mind and body to accurately assess a true threat of danger.

We must remember that stress and trauma responses are biological responses that serve important, and potentially lifesaving, functions. We have many physiological adaptations to stress and trauma. These adaptations can allow us to escape danger, or to foster a sense of connection that can promote resilience. It is only when our stress responses become chronic and out of balance that they become detrimental and potentially toxic (Levine 2008).

Trauma responses can lead to extremes of avoidance or reenactment, fear, anxiety, hyperarousal, hypoarousal, or numbness, which can all contribute to a diminishing of one's opportunities for experiencing life's fullness (Levine 2008). For example, avoiding public spaces (including public transportation) is a common coping mechanism that can have social, educational, and economic consequences. Isolation can result as social invitations are declined. All of these responses are protective mechanisms. However, they can remain in place over time and become maladaptive.

Depending upon the lens one uses to explore trauma, differing consequences may receive a stronger focus. For instance, if taking a psychological approach, the quote below from the American Psychological Association may resonate as it highlights the emotional aspect of trauma.

> Trauma is an emotional response to a terrible event like an accident, rape or natural disaster. Immediately after the event, shock and denial are typical. Longer term reactions include unpredictable emotions, flashbacks, strained relationships and even physical symptoms like headaches or nausea. While these feelings are normal, some people have difficulty moving on with their lives. Psychologists can help these individuals find constructive ways of managing their emotions.
> (American Psychological Association 2019)

Alternatively, Peter Levine, originator of Somatic Experiencing (SE), points to the impacts beyond emotions. SE is a trauma therapy that aims to take into account the thwarted, biologically based, self-protective, and defensive responses that emerge in the wake of trauma, as well as the discharge and regulation of excess autonomic arousal that results (Levine 2008).

A more expansive conception of trauma is offered by the Substance Abuse and Mental Health Services Administration (SAMHSA) in that it identifies the myriad impacts of trauma: "Trauma results from an event, series of events, or set of circumstances experienced by an individual as physically or emotionally harmful or life-threatening with lasting adverse effects on the individual's functioning and mental, physical, social, emotional, or spiritual well-being" (SAMHSA 2019).

> My path to reconciliation with my past involved several lengthy in-patient, locked ward hospital treatment stays. The methods of treatment devised by very well-meaning doctors and therapists, were clinically focused, based on the DSM. In this, there was no room for any Indigenous spirituality practices. In order to receive treatment, I had to conform to practices that were linear, where black and white, right and wrong, treatment maintenance or treatment resistant were the only options. My traditional teachings however were based on the medicine wheel, circular and forgiving; they allowed to movement between the directions, East (awareness), South (understanding) West (knowledge) and North (wisdom). In order to receive treatment, I had to accept the medical world's ways as greater than the teachings I was given from elders and ancestors. I was unable to burn sage or sweetgrass, lay tobacco or use cedar as a medicine. As a result, I lost my practices. This type of treatment, away from community, drums, singing, the wisdom of my people, led me down paths of frequent relapse. It wasn't until I reconnected with the resilience and voices within my community that I truly began to heal from my sexual trauma.
> – Trauma-informed yoga student

While having an understanding of how trauma is defined is important, we would suggest that a more holistic perspective is warranted. Labeling the trauma response as a disorder lacks a strength-based focus. Survivors are not broken; our job is not to fix them. How we talk about trauma shapes our response to it. Individualistic and disorder-based definitions of trauma fall short in recognizing the collective impact of trauma and a narrow focus fails to recognize the tremendous impacts that historic and intergenerational trauma can have. We must recognize that there are intersectional and systemic factors that shape how people experience trauma and impact their capacity for response. We need to be inclusive of diverse perspectives and experiences in our attempts to understand and respond to trauma. A holistic, embodied, and strength-based conceptualization of and response to trauma is needed; we must work to foster and support resilience in survivors. At its core, trauma represents a loss of connection – disconnection from self and one's sense of community. Healing can only come in reconnection and reintegration.

The potential impacts of trauma are complex. While these impacts do vary from person to person, there also exists a common and deeply rooted response to the experience of stress and trauma that we as humans share at both a physiological and emotional level. Our bodies and minds have a tremendous capacity for resilience, and it is important to understand the impacts that trauma can have on the mind and body. We will briefly address these in the upcoming sections.

HPA and Our Hormonal Response to Stress

Humans are able to survive based on our ability to respond in the face of threat or danger. Central to this reaction is the hypothalamic–pituitary–adrenal (HPA) axis (see Table 2.1). The HPA axis is comprised of the hypothalamus and the pituitary gland located in the brain, and the adrenal glands, which sit just above the kidneys, and serves as the primary central stress response as the human body strives for homeostasis. The HPA axis is responsible for the transmission of stress hormones and activates in response to real or perceived threats. The primary job of the HPA axis is to regulate the stress response (Figure 2.1). The HPA axis is also involved in regulating diverse systems such as digestion, immunity, and body temperature. With real or perceived stress, the hypothalamus releases the hormone corticotropin-releasing factor (CRF), which signals the pituitary gland to release the adrenocorticotropic hormone (ACTH). ACTH travels to the adrenal gland where it signals the release of the hormone cortisol, causing changes that help the body to manage stress.

In a well-regulated system, this activation comes on and off line appropriately in response to times of threat. However, for some traumatized individuals, the stress response becomes habituated even when there is no actual threat, resulting in flooding the body with stress hormones. Researchers have explored the role of the HPA axis in autoimmune disorders, irritable bowel syndrome, chronic fatigue syndrome and anxiety linking chronic inflammation due to excessive HPA response to central nervous system (CNS) sensitivity (Borsini, et al. 2014).

It is worth noting that traumatic impact on brain architecture and functioning, such as stress hormone secretion, is related to the age at which trauma is experienced with children being more susceptible as the brain is arguably developing up until age twenty (De Bellis & Zisk 2014).

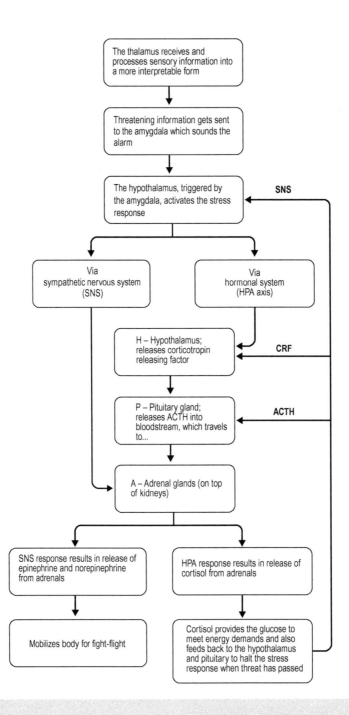

Figure 2.1

HPA axis and our normal stress response

Stoller C (2019) Sensory-enhanced yoga for self-regulation and trauma healing, Edinburgh: Handspring Publishing LIM.

This last point is important to understand in addressing sexual trauma with yoga because a student's presentation/affect/behavior may represent the lasting impact of trauma suffered decades ago. Surviving trauma may also leave an individual in a stunted state of psychological development whereby their chronological age and psychosocial developmental stage are not in synch (Fergusson, et al. 2013).

The Autonomic Nervous System

It is well documented that trauma impacts a person on multiple levels, including changes in neurobiology and altering the form and functionality of the nervous system, both central and peripheral. The brain and spinal column make up the central nervous system (CNS). Signals from the CNS are transmitted to the body via the peripheral nervous system and including the autonomic nervous system. The autonomic nervous system is made up of the sympathetic and parasympathetic nervous systems. The sympathetic nervous system and parasympathetic nervous system work together, balancing activation to meet our ongoing needs. This ongoing balance is jeopardized in the face of a significant threat or stressor, at which point there is an imbalance in favor of the sympathetic nervous system. See Figure 2.2 for illustration of the autonomic nervous system and its functions. A dysregulated nervous system can impact daily functioning as well as long-term health. A healthy, properly functioning nervous system allows for times of activation "fight or flight" (sympathetic nervous system) to be countered by times of stabilization "rest and digest" (parasympathetic nervous system). The stress response becomes habituated and begins to experience perceived threat, even before the body is consciously aware. The following offers a very abridged description of the autonomic nervous system and the role it plays in regulating our body including mobility, respiration, and vital functions.

The *sympathetic nervous system* (SNS) is essentially the body's emergency response system, activating the body's response when it meets threats. When you become frightened, a rush of hormones is released increasing alertness and heart rate and sending blood to muscles in preparation to run or put up a fight. Breathing accelerates, your heart beats faster, your digestion processes stop, and the bronchial tubes in your lungs expand. These functions provide more oxygen to your body. Your pupils dilate, which increases your field of vision, and your mouth becomes dry due to the lack of production of saliva. Your body prepares for immediate response – to fight or flee.

The *parasympathetic nervous system* (PNS) has one general function, to control homeostasis and the body's rest and digest response. In short, it is responsible for conserving and maintaining physical resources. The PNS works much more slowly than the SNS, slowing heart rate, returning pupils to their normal size, regulating skin temperature, and reactivating all of the responses that have been paused by the SNS in response to stress. The PNS allows us to find calmness, connection, and compassion. Although it operates on its own, there are ways that you can help the PNS return you to homeostasis after an "emergency," real or imagined. For example, deep mindful breathing stimulates the vagus nerve, which is the main nerve in the PNS, and can help you self-regulate and return to homeostasis more quickly.

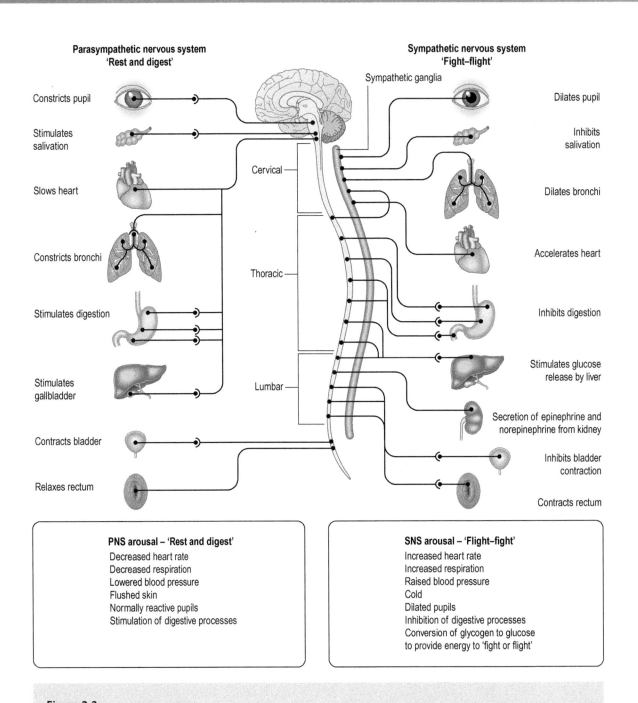

**Parasympathetic nervous system
'Rest and digest'**

**Sympathetic nervous system
'Fight–flight'**

Constricts pupil

Stimulates
salivation

Slows heart

Constricts bronchi

Stimulates digestion

Stimulates
gallbladder

Contracts bladder

Relaxes rectum

Sympathetic ganglia

Cervical

Thoracic

Lumbar

Dilates pupil

Inhibits
salivation

Dilates bronchi

Accelerates heart

Inhibits digestion

Stimulates glucose
release by liver

Secretion of epinephrine and
norepinephrine from kidney

Inhibits bladder
contraction

Contracts rectum

PNS arousal – 'Rest and digest'
Decreased heart rate
Decreased respiration
Lowered blood pressure
Flushed skin
Normally reactive pupils
Stimulation of digestive processes

SNS arousal – 'Flight–fight'
Increased heart rate
Increased respiration
Raised blood pressure
Cold
Dilated pupils
Inhibition of digestive processes
Conversion of glycogen to glucose
to provide energy to 'fight or flight'

Figure 2.2

Autonomic nervous system

Stoller C (2019) Sensory-enhanced yoga for self-regulation and trauma healing, Edinburgh: Handspring Publishing LIM.

The Vagus Nerve

- Cranial nerve, connects brain and body

- The principal nerve of the parasympathetic nervous system

- A total of 80 percent of fibers of the vagus nerve run from the body to the brain; only 20 percent of fibers run from the brain to the body

- The vagus nerve is responsible for various tasks in the body, such as heart rate, breathing, and digestion

- Other vagus nerve functions include communication between the brain and the gut, relaxation, anti-inflammation, lowering heart rate and blood pressure, fear management

- Vagul stimulation has been used to aid patients with major depressive disorder who are medication resistant, and is additionally seen to impact anxiety and bipolar disorders

- Mindful breathing stimulates the vagus nerve

The aftermath of trauma can involve symptoms of impairment, including hyper and hypo arousal of the nervous system. This can range from mild bouts of fear or withdrawal to chronic experiences of terror or emotional numbness. Experiences of being on "high alert" or "immobile" can place someone beyond a space in which they can cope effectively. When this happens physical and functional impairments lead to misinterpretation and exaggerated reactions to otherwise tolerable or non-threatening experiences. Our nervous system becomes trapped in a chronic state of stress response. The good news is that we have the capacity to modulate our stress response and positively support self-regulation.

Trauma and the Brain

In the wake of trauma, our bodies may continue reliving and reenacting traumatic stress, a response that is rooted in our brain and experienced in our bodies. The experience of trauma directly impacts our brain and can change neural architecture and functioning. With trauma, the capacity for the brain to integrate sensory input diminishes. We see decreased capacity for executive functioning and over-activation of the more primitive parts of the brain.

> The most important job of the brain is to ensure our survival, even under the most miserable conditions. Everything else is secondary.
>
> (van der Kolk 2014: 55)

Dating back to the late 1960s, the American neuroscientist Paul MacLean presented the triune or three-part brain reflecting the evolutionary growth and function of the human brain. This triune structure identifies the historic reptilian brain (instinctual), the limbic or mammalian brain, and the neocortex, which is responsible for the executive functions of rational thinking, planning, and managing behaviors. See Figure 2.3 for detail. Our brains develop from the bottom up. The reptilian brain is comprised of our spinal cord and hypothalamus and sits at the lowest part of our brain. This part of the brain controls all of our basic functions, those things that happen automatically without our thinking about them (breathing, digestion, sleep, temperature regulation, and so forth). Our limbic or mammalian brain is located in the middle of our brain structure; we share the limbic part of our brain in common with other mammals. This structure deals with

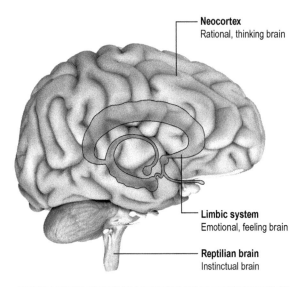

Neocortex
Rational, thinking brain

Limbic system
Emotional, feeling brain

Reptilian brain
Instinctual brain

Figure 2.3
Triune brain

emotion and the ongoing assessment of danger and risk. Together, the reptilian brain and limbic system make up the emotional brain, in charge of modulating our survival. The neocortex includes the higher functioning of our rational brain and includes the prefrontal cortex. The functions of the neocortex include sensory perception, spatial reasoning, conscious thought, language, creativity, and sense of self. The neocortex, and the prefrontal cortex specifically, is the site of executive functioning in humans, including working memory, cognitive flexibility, and inhibitory control. Executive functioning includes our ability for self-control, planning, decision making, and problem solving.

Trauma is especially impactful on the emotional brain (the limbic and reptilian brains) and this has a tremendous influence on how we respond to trauma and on our capacity for self-regulation. As Bessel van der Kolk (2014: 57)

describes, "The emotional brain is at the heart of the central nervous system, and its key task is to look out for your welfare." Traumatic stress impacts functions such as arousal, sleep, breathing, chemical balance, and basic "housekeeping."

The experience of trauma, and specifically chronic trauma, impacts the alarm system of our brain. Part of the limbic system, the amygdala, is responsible for our perception of emotion, including anger, fear, and sadness. The amygdala assesses and alerts us to the emotional valence of stimuli; it is what triggers the fight-or-flight response. With trauma, the balance between the amygdala and neocortex shifts dramatically. A high degree of activation in the amygdala and related structures generates emotional response and sensory impressions based on fragments of information – the executive functioning of the prefrontal cortex is bypassed. People become emotionally activated and initiate a stress response before cognitive evaluation of a situation can occur. The activation of the limbic system also impacts how memory is stored. Trauma is experienced and encoded through the senses – sensory input that is interpreted by the limbic system. Traumatic memories are not stored in a logical or language-centered way. This is why people often remember trauma as sensation, or why survivors may not accurately relate key details in an interview with law enforcement.

With chronic stress and trauma, individuals can become stuck in a continual state of alert (fight or flight). Survivors react in instinctual response originating in the emotional mind and not the thoughtful, rational mind. With compromises to our neocortex, we lack the integration, planning, and assessment needed to accurately assess whether or not we are in danger. When emotions run high (as is often the case after trauma) the executive function capacity of the brain is diminished. When sights, sounds, smells, or touch trigger a survivor's senses, there is a response including a flush of hormones and physical changes that leave many experiencing the same stressed reaction as when actually facing a threat, even when there may be no current threat present. Many trauma survivors experience chronically overwhelming physical and emotional states, long after the actual trauma has passed, without the capacity to manage the complex experiences of the trauma response.

> No matter how much insight and understanding we develop, the rational brain is basically impotent to talk the emotional brain out of its own [trauma] reality.
>
> (van der Kolk 2014: 47)

Technological advancements and access to functional Magnetic Resonance Imaging (fMRI) have offered visual depictions of how the brain can be physically altered after traumatic experience. Areas of the brain impacted by trauma include the amygdala (increased function), hippocampus (becomes diminished), and prefrontal cortex (diminished structure and functional, decreased emotional regulation). There are also impacts on stress hormone levels for norepinephrine and cortisol. A very simplified explanation is that in the aftermath of trauma, the fear alert center (amygdala) becomes overactive and perceives threat where there is none. Simultaneously, the hippocampus is diminished in its ability to store and recall memories in a time-sequenced manner. Diminished access to the prefrontal cortex decreases executive function and capacity for reasoning. These physical changes coupled with dysregulated stress hormones mimic a chronic, threatening encounter and leave many survivors in a suspended or prolonged state of threat, sometimes known as hyperarousal.

The hopeful and empowering part is that our brains have the capacity for healing through neurogenesis. This relies on a literal rewiring of our neural pathways. In order to rewrite our response to stress, we have to review, renew, and rewire the habituated responses that our system has to stimuli, both from inside and outside of the body. This "new learning" is limited for several reasons, the first of which is that neurogenesis, the process by which neurons are created in the brain, is negatively correlated with stress, and positively correlated with learning or enriched experience, which can be challenging when our system is responding to stimuli before we can assess its actual context or meaning (Gazzangia, et al. 2018). Without decreasing stress, the stress hormones and chemicals will continue to damage neurons in the hippocampus and prefrontal cortex, limiting our capacity to create new memories. Decreasing the stress response is a crucial first step and relies on balancing the autonomic nervous system, which, as we have discussed, can get stuck in sympathetic activation. There is no way to repair the molecular building blocks to learning without this first step.

We know that recovery and new ways of responding are possible because our brains have plasticity – the ability to change. But without adequate neuronal bodies with which to realize new affinities and connections we continue to stay "stuck." With resilience, we can rewire the fear center of our brain and change our response to stress and trauma. Yoga and mindfulness practices can offer an effective tool for self-regulation.

Trauma and Yoga

Through the practice of trauma-informed yoga, participants are offered opportunities to experience a sense of safety, or what Dr Dan Siegel

(2010) refers to as the "window of tolerance." The concept of the "window of tolerance" sets the stage to understand the range of responses that are possible when facing stressful situations and establishes the foundational concept that there is a "sweet spot" in which we are best able to handle stress. Each individual has their own window of tolerance, which is impacted by the state of our central nervous system. As shown in Figure 2.4, the window of tolerance, which lies in the center of the diagram, allows for maximized, positive response to stress.

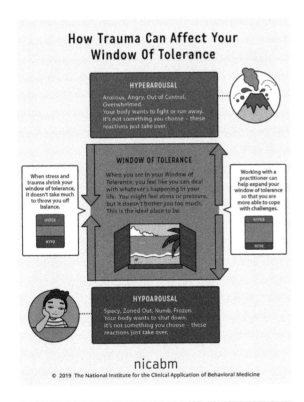

Figure 2.4

Window of tolerance. © 2019 The National Institute for the Clinical Application of Behavioral Medicine

Window of Tolerance, The National Institute for the Clinical Application of Behavioral Medicine [Online] Available: http://www.nicabm.com [1 November 2019].

Beyond the window of tolerance is a zone or border where struggles may arise that bring about feelings of unease, lack of connection, and challenges responding to stress. This is not a full-on danger zone, but certainly is not a place for optimal response due to dysregulation. Beyond that zone of dysregulation lies hyper and hypoarousal. Readers are reminded that one of the impacts of surviving trauma is an altered nervous system. When feeling hyper-aroused, it is far more challenging to successfully manage stressful events in a calm demeanor due to increased activation of the HPA axis. Likewise, being in a state of hypoarousal will make it extremely difficult to respond as emotional and physical capacity is diminished. Trauma survivors benefit from re-establishing or widening their window of tolerance.

Engaging with trauma-informed yoga provides individuals an opportunity to move closer toward their window of tolerance, to widen the window. Trauma-informed yoga encompasses awareness of felt internal sensations and for many this results in an increased tolerance for awareness. Someone who was triggered by a change in body temperature or increased heart rate can progress to notice these changes without a reactive response. Research suggests that over time students can expand their awareness and regulation of the central nervous system, which helps to widen their window of tolerance (Siegel 2010).

Trauma survivors often describe social and emotional challenges that we know are linked to trauma-impacted neural circuits and brain structures. From research, we know that the brain's function is impacted by prior experiences and that these past experiences serve to frame current beliefs and behaviors (Clark, et al. 2013). An individual who has experienced sexual trauma in the context of a relationship may anticipate a recurrence in future relationships and as a result will avoid intimate contact. Similarly, a survivor of rape by a stranger might limit instances where they are out in public unaccompanied out of fear of repeated assault. Based on a meta-analysis of eleven research publications on yoga and healing trauma, Telles, et al. (2012) concluded that certain changes in neurotransmitters following yoga practice may be responsible for the improved psychological state, including decrease in fear, anxiety, sleep disturbances, and feelings of sadness in survivors.

A trauma-informed yoga practice impacts both higher and lower level functions of the brain. Yoga has been shown to impact nervous system functioning and emotional regulation, two key factors in moving survivors from stress reactive to mindfully responsive (Taylor et al., 2010). Simply stated, trauma-informed yoga is a mechanism for recalibrating a survivor's capacity for self-regulation. This occurs through two potential mechanisms, top-down and bottom-up regulation. A bottom-up approach alters the threat detection system and autonomic nervous system functioning and a top-down approach modulates messages from the prefrontal cortex improving access to executive function. As van der Kolk (2014) points out, bottom-up regulation can be accessed through breath, movement, and touch, and top-down regulation through mindfulness meditation and yoga. In order to be optimally self-regulated, we need to be able to clearly observe, know, predict, organize, and modulate our responses to what we experience (stimuli and sensory input). Through a trauma-informed approach to yoga, survivors may improve the efficiency and integration of the brain networks responsible for sensing and managing threats and regulation of cognitive, emotional, and behavioral responses.

Seeking Trauma-informed Practices

Recognizing the multi-faceted impacts of trauma for the populations with which we work becomes fundamental. No matter where yoga is offered or who it is offered to, classes will include survivors of sexual trauma. Accordingly, it is important for all people offering yoga to seek an understanding of trauma and its impacts and to offer practices that are informed by and respond to this understanding.

While there has been a movement toward "trauma-informed" training and practices, there lacks a consensus of what this precisely means for yoga. Many trauma-informed yoga trainings are being offered, but with little oversight or consistency. Is such training informed by experiential and empirical knowledge? Are offerings and information presented accurately? Is the training enough?

In addition, many working in the yoga field lack awareness of the impact that trauma can have. Those of us at the forefront of this work have all shared accounts of interactions with professionals in the field of yoga who have yet to hear of trauma-informed practices or trauma-focused work. This certainly suggests we have a long way to go. We must acknowledge and respond to this dearth of a common understanding of concepts including trauma and trauma-informed practices.

In 2014, the Substance Abuse and Mental Health Services Administration advanced the position that because people who have experienced trauma (single episode, repeated, or chronic) are more likely to show consequences that are physical, mental, and behavioral the need to address trauma should be elevated to a public health priority. As the popularity of yoga continues to expand in the West, it becomes increasingly important to acknowledge the intersection of body-based interventions (including yoga) and the need for awareness of and response to the impacts of trauma.

The term "trauma-informed" refers to practices that integrate an awareness of and responsiveness to the many potential impacts of the trauma response. According to Hopper, Bassuk and Olivet (2010: 82), "Trauma-informed Care is a strengths-based framework that is grounded in an understanding of and responsiveness to the impact of trauma, that emphasizes physical, psychological, and emotional safety for both providers and survivors, and that creates opportunities for survivors to rebuild a sense of control and empowerment."

Trauma-informed care emerged from the expanding role of domestic violence and rape survivors in the early 1970s (Burgess & Holmstrom 1974). As the voice of female survivors of interpersonal violence became elevated in the late 1970s, in line with the expanding momentum of the Women's Rights movement, awareness of trauma and the beginnings of a trauma-informed approach were taking hold. As the struggles of Vietnam War veterans gained increased clinical attention, through treatment and research, a shift took place that reframed understanding the aftermath of traumatic events from asking, "What's wrong with you?" to asking, "What happened to you?"

Dating back to the late 1990s, trauma-informed care evolved to move from the domain of therapeutic care to being woven into settings as diverse as schools, medical, and carceral settings. In 1998, the Substance Abuse and Mental Health Services Administration conducted a multi-year study examining women with trauma histories who experienced substance and mental health problems. The result of this study produced trauma-informed care guidelines and raised awareness for the need for trauma-informed care for all adults. In 2001, the National Child Traumatic Stress Initiative and the National Child Traumatic Stress Network were created, expanding the need for trauma-informed care for all. Advances in trauma-specific scientific research, including trauma assessment tools, have both broadened the understanding of trauma's impact and the availability of effective post-traumatic treatments and strategies.

The model of the Five Principles of Trauma-Informed Care can be a valuable resource in thinking about developing trauma-informed yoga and mindfulness programming. According to Fallot and Harris (2009), the Five Principles of Trauma-Informed Care suggest ways we can inform our work with an awareness of trauma. See Figure 2.5 for detail.

Five Principles of a Trauma-informed Care

- **Safety** – ensuring the greatest level of physical and emotional safety

- **Trustworthiness/Transparency** – maintaining appropriate boundaries and making tasks clear

- **Choice** – prioritizing individual control and choice; having small choices makes a big difference

- **Collaboration** – maximizing collaboration with service providers and therapists to create opportunities for full participation

- **Empowerment** – prioritizing survivor empowerment, skill-building, and self-efficacy

---

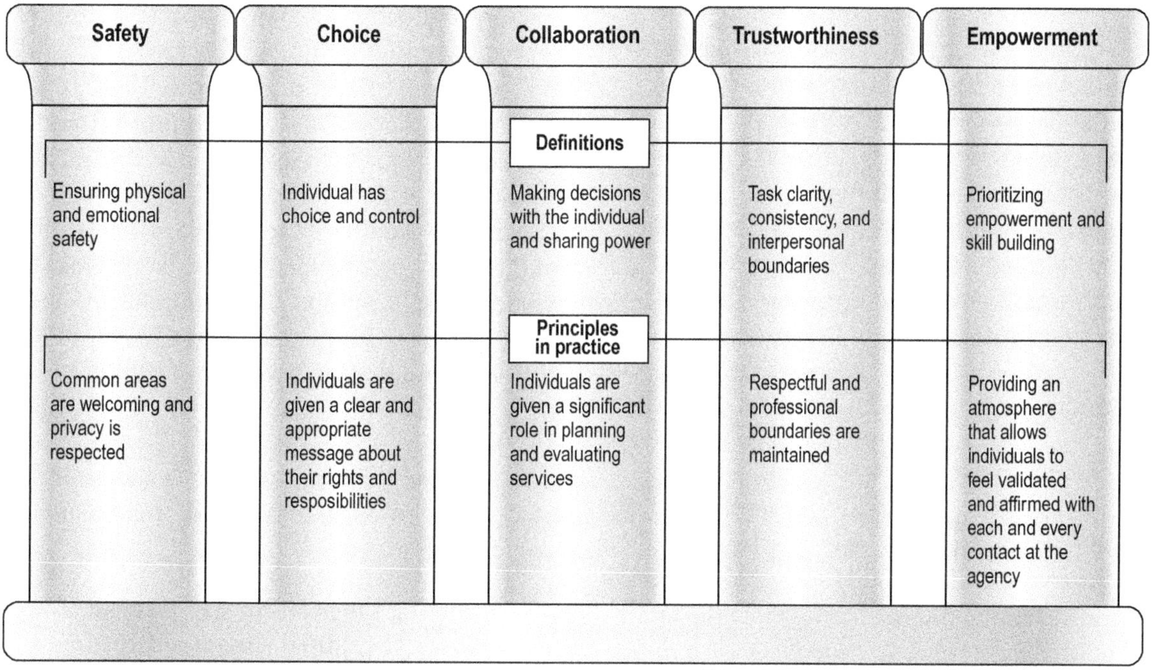

Safety	Choice	Collaboration	Trustworthiness	Empowerment
		Definitions		
Ensuring physical and emotional safety	Individual has choice and control	Making decisions with the individual and sharing power	Task clarity, consistency, and interpersonal boundaries	Prioritizing empowerment and skill building
		Principles in practice		
Common areas are welcoming and privacy is respected	Individuals are given a clear and appropriate message about their rights and resposibilities	Individuals are given a significant role in planning and evaluating services	Respectful and professional boundaries are maintained	Providing an atmosphere that allows individuals to feel validated and affirmed with each and every contact at the agency

Figure 2.5

The five principles of trauma-informed care

The Five Principles of a Trauma-informed Care can serve as a guide in designing an experience for yoga students that begins the moment they enter a physical space or visit your website. Whether in a school, community center, or studio, written materials as well as the physical space can serve as a reflection of your understanding and application of the principles of trauma-informed approaches.

Trauma-informed yoga specifically and intentionally takes the impact of trauma into account and recognizes the ways that yoga itself has the potential to traumatize and even retraumatize. Yoga that is trauma-informed forefronts the needs of participants, creating an environment that is as safe as possible.

Trauma-informed yoga offers yoga practice in a way that is consistent and predictable, while offering instruction in an invitational and non-directive manner. The primary focus is not on the physicality and exactness of bodily movement but instead on the internal experience of the student. Trauma-informed yoga takes into account the most vulnerable person in every setting and is structured around practices of orienting, containment, and body and brain positivity. It also builds on the great strengths that each person – including survivors of every sort – brings to their practice. Trauma-informed yoga recognizes that trauma is both individual and collective, and that trauma carries impacts both in the present moment and across histories and generations.

Chapter 2

> Trauma-informed yoga is a discipline of nuanced seeing and heightened understanding of how each yoga participant is experiencing the practice at any given moment, in any circumstance. It considers the safest possible experience of yoga to be the surest path for each person to become a stronger, more alert, and discerning individual.
>
> (Rousseau, et al. 2018)

Trauma-informed yoga works to engage both the sympathetic and parasympathetic nervous system as participants gain (or re-gain) their ability to notice their bodily sensations and emotional states and increasingly tolerate the totality of their present moment experiences. An important piece of this awareness is interoception. Interoception refers to the mechanisms by which the brain senses and integrates signals from inside the body to provide an ongoing, changeable perception of one's internal state. Interoception is an individual's total experience of their being. By using the physical body, trauma-informed yoga can offer the opportunity to monitor and tolerate discomfort inherent in the bodies of survivors of sexual trauma. Interoception is:

> The perception and integration of autonomic, hormonal, visceral and immunological homeostatic signals that collectively describe the physiological state of the body.
>
> (Barrett & Simmons 2015: 422)

A trauma-informed yoga practice respects and integrates interoception as a means to establish a sense of personal safety, allow for choice, initiate empowerment, encourage collaboration, and work toward building an internal sense of trust.

In recognizing the many impacts of trauma, it becomes important to integrate a trauma-informed approach in the work that we do. Careful considerations surrounding a trauma-informed approach should be made, recognizing that trauma-informed practices exist on a continuum. A trauma-informed yoga curriculum and instruction intended for sexual trauma survivors must meet specific requirements along with having programmatic and teacher-flexibility to address unpredicted behaviors, different abilities, and changing moods.

A trauma-informed approach is multifaceted and can include some of the following components:

- **Realizing** the prevalence of trauma; awareness is the initial step in digesting the impact that trauma has, and education is of fundamental importance.

- **Recognizing** how trauma exists along a continuum and that its impacts can present differently for each individual; we must work to ensure that survivors are seen and heard.

- **Resisting** re-traumatization by reducing triggers and teacher authority, while using invitational language and universally inclusive practices.

- **Responding** appropriately by putting knowledge into practice, staying up to date on research to continually improve content, and taking informed and intentional action.

Trauma-informed yoga works with the needs of the student in the moment. In some cases, this includes a physically rigorous class and in others a more restorative approach. Additionally, a trauma-informed approach to yoga takes into consideration far more than merely session content. Consideration should be taken in relation to staffing, physical design, hours of operation, and types of classes offered. This text will provide many examples of best practices supporting trauma-informed approaches to yoga and mindfulness practices. In the final chapter, we will engage a deeper discussion of how the yoga community can respond in trauma-informed and universally inclusive ways.

Vicarious Trauma

In committing to this work, it is important to recognize that holding space for survivors can have an impact on service providers. The term *vicarious trauma* was first used by McCann and Pearlman (1990) to describe pervasive changes that occur within clinicians over time as a result of working with clients who have experienced trauma. These include changes in sense of self, spirituality, worldview, interpersonal relationships, and behavior. While we are not conflating the experiences of clinicians with those of yoga instructors, all who work with sexual trauma would benefit from an understanding of the potential impact of vicarious exposure to trauma.

> Vicarious trauma is the experience of bearing witness to the atrocities committed against another. It is the result of absorbing the sight, smell, sound, touch and feel of the stories told in detail by victims searching for a way to release their own pain. It is the instant physical reaction that occurs when a particularly horrific story is told or an event is uncovered. It is the insidious way that the experiences slip under the door, finding ways to permeate the counsellor's life, accumulating in different ways, creating changes that are both subtle and pronounced. Vicarious trauma is the energy that comes from being in the presence of trauma and it is how our bodies and psyche react to the profound despair, rage and pain. Personal balance can be lost for a moment or for a long time. The invasive and intrusive horrors infiltrate and make their mark. The waves of agony and pain bombard the spirit and seep in, draining strength, confidence, desire, friendship, calmness, laughter and good health. Confusion, apathy, isolation, anxiety, sadness and illness are often the result.
>
> (Richardson 2001: 7)

The book *Trauma Stewardship* (Van Dernoot Lipsky 2009) delineates sixteen warning signs of trauma exposure response. It is important to recognize that the emotional experience of trauma response can lead to intense and potentially chronic stress reactions. The signs and symptoms of vicarious trauma are similar to PTSD and can include the potential for experiences of hypervigilance, guilt, sleeplessness, illness, avoidance, and social withdrawal. Traumatic experiences, even those experienced vicariously, are embodied, meaning we hold the impacts of trauma in our physical bodies, a fact that can have a direct impact on health and well-being. In reviewing the characteristics of trauma exposure, you may recognize some signs in your colleagues or even yourself. There is nothing wrong in recognizing the impacts of trauma exposure; the problem comes when we ignore these signs. When we do not respond to these warning signs, well-being can be significantly impacted and our capacity to effectively work with others can diminish.

Sixteen Warning Signs of Trauma Exposure Response:

- Feeling helpless or hopeless
- A sense that one can never do enough
- Hypervigilance
- Diminished creativity
- Inability to embrace complexity
- Minimizing
- Chronic exhausting/physical ailments
- Inability to listen/deliberate avoidance
- Dissociative moments
- Sense of persecution
- Guilt
- Fear
- Anger and cynicism
- Inability to empathize/numbing
- Addictions
- Grandiosity – an inflated sense of importance related to one's work
                    (Van Dernoot Lipsky 2009)

Self-compassion, sustaining appropriate boundaries, and self-care are important in effectively doing this work. Connection, peer support, and supervision are also key. It is essential for a yoga teacher working with trauma populations to have a regular, personal practice to reset a neutral mindset and awaken a sense of self. Teachers should seek ongoing self-inquiry and an awareness of the potential that they may be experiencing vicarious trauma or residual impacts of their own trauma history. We will discuss this in greater detail in Chapter 6 when we explore relational wisdom and address self-care, boundaries, and cultural humility.

Conclusion

Understanding trauma and becoming trauma-informed are not about knowing individual, personal trauma histories. Rather, this process involves recognizing the reality that many people have had traumatic experiences and for some the aftermath involves wide-ranging and long-lasting impacts. While trauma is widespread, it is important not to conflate stress with trauma and to differentiate these two based on severity. Trauma is much more than the event itself, whether it was physical or emotional in nature. Traumatic experiences can carry a legacy of emotional, behavioral, psychological, and neuropsysiological imprints that can emerge across time.

Our role as those in the field of yoga service is to hold space for all that trauma entails. In understanding and responding to trauma we must seek active practice, self-inquiry, and conscious relationship to others. Offering yoga in any context requires education on trauma and its many impacts and appropriate approaches for trauma-informed care because whether we are aware of it or not, trauma survivors are present in all yoga settings. We cannot ignore the importance of trauma-informed practice – doing so is ignorant and invites the potential for harm. Instead, we are called to ongoing inquiry and action. True yoga service is a call to action; it is both personal and political. We must know better in order to do better, and this should be each of our goals. In the upcoming chapters, we offer an ongoing discussion and exploration of best practices for engaging in yoga service holding as centered intentional trauma response and promoting resilience. As noted previously, our discussion is not exhaustive but meant to be a starting point to encourage your ongoing inquiry, questioning, discussion, and action. The next chapter will provide some context of sexual trauma specifically before we launch into these best practices.

Understanding Sexual Trauma

3

Authors *Dani Harris and Danielle Rousseau*

In sharing this work and the guidelines in the chapters to follow, we believe that it is first necessary to set a context of understanding regarding the topics we will be addressing. Sexual trauma is a complex topic. Both historically and in the current time it can represent a taboo topic, one rich with silence, misperceptions, and misunderstanding. A discussion of sexual trauma ultimately involves legal definitions, social constructs, and systemic impacts as well as individual experiences, perceptions, and responses.

In engaging this work, we must understand and hold the multitude of complexities and perspectives that exist related to the subject. We must also consider those voices that are not at the table. In this vein, we do not offer answers, but instead hope to encourage inquiry and conversation. There remains so much to consider and much yet to be discovered.

With this invitation to conversation and openness to perspective, we also recognize that this is an area in which survivors have frequently been silenced. We recognize the importance of discussion and breaking down stigma, shame, and silence. Recognizing limitations in language, we know that we need to talk about sexual trauma in all of its iterations.

In this text, we use the term "sexual trauma" as a comprehensive term to discuss any violation of a sexual nature. This can include sexual harassment, sexual abuse, and sexual violence. In the next section, we share a definition of sexual trauma that one member of the project spent

significant time co-creating. While this definition is neither comprehensive nor perfect, we offer it as part of this important discussion and encourage its use in engaging, thinking about, and discussing sexual trauma.

In this chapter, we provide an overview of sexual trauma and its many impacts. While this discussion, like our definition, is not comprehensive, we believe it is important as a step in setting the context for what is to come in the book ahead. We begin with an understanding of historical and integrational trauma and its repercussions and continue to define and address the many impacts of sexual trauma.

Historical and Intergenerational Trauma

Historical trauma, including sexual trauma, is carried by ancestors, elders, nuclear and adoptive, foster, and chosen families, and it can last lifetimes. Power imbalanced governments, religions, lineages, and organizations have perpetuated abuses that have devastated cultures, communities, and individuals.

Historical trauma represents "a complex and collective trauma experience over time and across generations by a group of people who share an identity, affiliation, or circumstance" (Mohatt, et al. 2014: 128). While initially used to describe the intergenerational impact of the mass murder of European Jewry in the Holocaust, this term is also used in discussion of oppression including other genocides, colonization, slavery, internment, forced relocation, destruction of forbiddance of cultural practices, languages, and traditions as well as other forms of mass trauma and structural violence.

Historical trauma can include the intergenerational impacts of trauma as well as the collective impacts of ongoing oppression. According to Mohatt, et al. (2014), intergenerational trauma contains three key elements: the presence of a trauma, shared or experienced collectively, and spanning multiple generations. In this conceptualization, contemporary members of a group can experience the impact of trauma, as a secondary survivor.

The experience of historical trauma for all stakeholders is far-reaching and has a significant influence on the world(s) in which we live. Both historically and contemporaneously our laws and policies, educational and academic discourses, the use of natural resources, health care, as well as the structure and practices of justice systems, have been shaped by the experiences of historical trauma (Wolfe 2006).

Research shows that historical trauma contributes to the development of post-traumatic stress disorder (PTSD), anxiety, depression, shame, fear, disrupted interpersonal relationships, and other health issues (Mohatt, et al. 2014). The impact of intergenerational trauma is distinct in comparison to acute trauma. Impacts include but are not limited to:

- historical trauma continuing intergenerationally

- patterns of parental abandonment

- generational distrust in organizations that have perpetuated the abuse (schools, governments, churches, yoga lineages, and so forth)

- cultural abandonment/disinterest

- internalized racism

- epigenetic transmission of behavioral patterns

- group suicide/suicide pacts

- communal silence.

Mohatt et al. (2014) suggest an approach that focuses on addressing contemporary impacts of historical trauma (Figure 3.1). Individual and collective effects of trauma are complex and diverse and are experienced within an ongoing context of systemic disadvantage. In focusing on the contemporary manifestations of historical

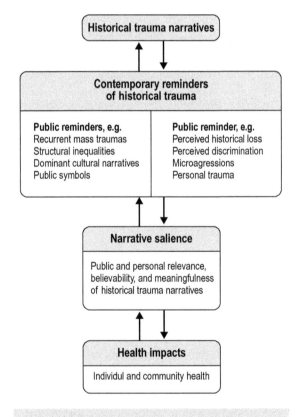

Figure 3.1

Historical trauma impacts on health

Source: Mohatt NV, et al. (2014) Figure 1 Narrative model of how historical trauma impacts health, in Historical trauma as public narrative: A conceptual view of how history impacts present-day health, New Haven, CT: Yale University School of Medicine, p. 132.

trauma, yoga can be well suited to help ameliorate negative impacts, including those related to sexual traumas specifically.

We note that narratives show up in different ways for different people and are regularly experienced in the body. Practices such as yoga, meditation, and mindfulness if guided and practiced with attention to safety, can reconstruct the trauma story. This integration happens on both personal and historical levels, leading to increased capacity for equanimity, offering a path towards healing and resilience. Mohatt, et al. (2014) suggest that when people's histories contain historical trauma, how we understand and respond as communities and individuals can both impact and promote resilience.

As discussed in the first chapter, the Yoga Service Council defines yoga service as the intersection of the practices of yoga, self-inquiry and reflection, and conscious relationship. It is through educating and holding oneself accountable in creating transparent and conscious relationships with all stakeholders that change begins. In holding oneself responsible for both, including students and their histories, we can help create safer spaces for those enduring the long-lasting effects of trauma.

While discussion of historical trauma is, in general, unlikely to arise in a yoga class, it is essential to understand that the lasting impact of historical trauma can be present in subtle and authentic ways. You can expect that participants injured by perpetrators of historical violence will be in your yoga classes. With this knowledge, you can also be a witness in celebration of the profound bravery, wisdom, and resilience that survivors of historical and intergenerational trauma carry with them. In Chapter 6, we will share some best practices for addressing historical trauma. Also, we would recommend seeking to educate yourself on the topic further. As with other forms of trauma, it is essential to remember that the experience of historical trauma, while impactful in many harmful ways, also offers a profound potential for resilience in both individuals and communities.

Defining Sexual Trauma

The following definition represents the Yoga Service Council's understanding of sexual trauma. It was born from the efforts of project contributors rooted in collaborative exploration of both empirical and experiential data.

> *Sexual trauma* is an experience in which an individual is overpowered, manipulated, violated, betrayed, or controlled by another in a position of power. The experience often includes feelings of powerlessness, fear, and a lack of agency or choice. The impacts of sexual trauma can result in the person's relationship to their sexual self, sexuality in general, and sex in society being influenced by the power differential of the original event or events.

The collaborators have come to understand, through a variety of experiences, communities, and lenses, that a sexual violation is the act perpetrated against the survivor, and the trauma experienced is the consequence of that violation. Sexual violence is a tool of oppression. In its most distilled form, the tool of sex is manipulatively used to overpower another; the predominant driving motivator of sexual trauma is power and manipulation. What defines a sexual trauma is not the sexual act per se, or the degree of arousal of a perpetrator, but instead the redefinition of sex through the lens of power and control or lack thereof. When sex is used by someone in a position of power over another who is made powerless, we can call this sexual trauma.

We live in a world where we are surrounded by mass sexual messaging. These messages not only affect how we process sexual violations, but also how we talk about them, define them, and treat them. Sexual trauma affects an individual's body, mind, and spirit. Trauma is embedded in the body, impacted by how the individual who has experienced the violation perceives the event(s). Living after sexual trauma not only requires the person to learn and create skills in basic survival but also to deal with multiple internal belief systems. These beliefs can alter the survivor's perception of beliefs to do with one's self-worth, beauty, sexuality, cleanliness, capabilities, and strength.

What differentiates sexual trauma from other traumas is that a sexual trauma can impede a survivor's ability to develop healthy sexuality. When filtered through the traumatic experience, a survivor's experience of sex, desire, sexual likes and dislikes, sensuality, intimacy – nearly everything relating to bodily and emotional intimacy is affected.

It is important to have a foundational understanding of sexual trauma and its impact. Every ninety-two seconds, someone in the United States is sexually assaulted. One in six women and one in thirty-three men have been the victim of an attempted or completed rape. Transgender college students are at a higher risk for sexual violence as compared to their peers. Indigenous Americans are at the greatest risk of sexual violence, with rates of sexual assault twice that of other races. It is estimated that 80,600 people who are incarcerated are sexually assaulted each year. Thousands of military members experience sexual violence, but the incidences often go unreported (RAINN 2019).

Table 3.1 Reasons survivors may not report sexual violence to authorities

Reasons survivors may not report sexual violence to authorities

Lack of recognition of rape
- Do not believe that what happened is actually "rape" (either in a legal or cultural sense).
- Do not think they will be believed.
- Feel it is not important enough to report.
- Do not feel the perpetrator meant to harm them.

Emotional responses
- Embarrassment or shame about the assault.
- Guilt or self-blame about the assault.
- Do not want anyone to know this happened.
- Friendly, loving, or otherwise positive emotions directed toward the perpetrator.
- Placing the needs of others (for example, children) above the desire to report.

Perceived negative social repercussions of reporting
- Fear the negative stigma attached to being labeled and viewed as a rape victim.
- Fear retaliation/reprisal from the perpetrator(s) or from their friends/family.
- Fear being ostracized from their family, social, or religious group.
- Do not want to get the perpetrator in trouble.

Perceived negative legal repercussions of reporting
- Believe that going through the reporting experience with law enforcement officials might be too traumatic or damaging.
- Believe that they cannot provide enough evidence to prove that an unwanted sex act occurred (that is, the burden of proof is on the victim).
- Fear that past sexual experiences will be revealed as a result of legal procedures. Although, in many places such as Australia, Canada, and the United States, "rape shield laws" protect victims by limiting the admission of evidence of past sexual experiences in criminal proceedings.
- Fear being punished for other infractions that took place during the rape such as underage drinking or illicit drug use.
- Do not think that anything will be done about it even if they do report.

Utilization of non-law enforcement-based responses
- Decided to deal with it on their own (that is, it was a personal matter).
- Decided to report to another source (friend, counselor, teacher, social worker, and so forth).

Source: Worthen MGF (2016) Sexual deviance and society: A sociological examination, London: Routledge.

In understanding the scope and context of sexual trauma and sexual violence, we must recognize that the data we do have are significantly underreported; many survivors of sexual trauma do not report to authorities. There are a variety of reasons survivors do not report, including fear, stigma, fear of not being believed, and the impacts of traumatic stress. Table 3.1 presents Meredith Worthen's (2016) discussion of reasons survivors would be hesitant to report rape to law enforcement authorities.

Definitions of rape and sexual violence more generally are complicated by the impacts of place, time, and systemic power differentials. Legal definitions and public perception of sexual violence are shaped by culture, context, and social construction. Sexual violence is a nonlegal term that refers to a variety of sexual-based crimes. It is important to note that legal definitions of sexual offenses differ from state to state and among different countries. The Rape, Abuse & Incest National Network (RAINN) has a database at www. rainn.org that allows for comparison of sex crime statutes by state.

Through the Uniform Crime Reporting (UCR) Program, the Federal Bureau of Investigation (FBI) collects national level data on crime, including rape. From 1927 to 2012, the FBI defined rape as "the carnal knowledge of a female forcibly and against her will." This definition is clearly problematic; it silences the voices of, and denies the experience of, many survivors. In response to advocacy including lobbying and grassroots efforts, the definition of rape was modified in 2013. The current FBI (2019) definition is "penetration, no matter how slight, of the vagina or anus with any body part or object, or oral penetration by a sex organ of another person, without the consent of the

victim." A clear distinction here is that the new definition does not specify gender for victim or perpetrator, thus not limiting discussion of rape to a man penetrating a woman. The definition also includes rape by an object and invokes the concept of consent. According to the FBI and UCR reporting procedures, attempts to commit rape are included in reporting but statutory rape and incest are not. While this definition is an improvement and takes steps to recognize the diversity of survivors, it remains limited in its scope and impact.

According to the FBI, rape is: The penetration, no matter how slight, of the vagina or anus with any body part or object, or oral penetration by a sex organ of another person, without the consent of the victim.

Sexual assault refers to sexual contact or behavior that occurs without explicit consent of the victim (RAINN 2019). In addition to rape as defined above, sexual assault can include: attempted rape, fondling or unwanted sexual touch, or the forcing of a victim to preform sexual acts. Sexual harassment includes "unwelcome sexual advances, requests for sexual favors, and other verbal or physical conduct of a sexual nature … when this conduct explicitly or implicitly affects an individual's employment, unreasonably interferes with an individual's work performance, or creates an intimidating, hostile, or offensive work environment" (RAINN 2019; EEOC 2019).

Conceptualizing Consent

Understanding sexual trauma necessitates a discussion of consent. There is no single definition of consent, with each state defining its own regulations around capacity to consent. In general, consent represents agreement between participants to engage in sexual activity. An individual's

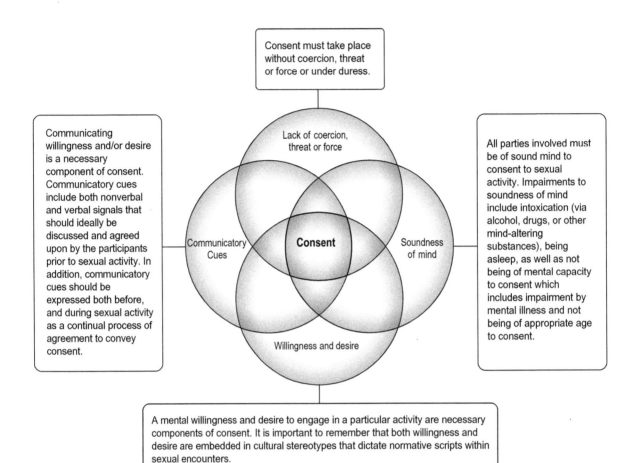

Consent must take place without coercion, threat or force or under duress.

Communicating willingness and/or desire is a necessary component of consent. Communicatory cues include both nonverbal and verbal signals that should ideally be discussed and agreed upon by the participants prior to sexual activity. In addition, communicatory cues should be expressed both before, and during sexual activity as a continual process of agreement to convey consent.

Lack of coercion, threat or force

Communicatory Cues

Consent

Soundness of mind

Willingness and desire

All parties involved must be of sound mind to consent to sexual activity. Impairments to soundness of mind include intoxication (via alcohol, drugs, or other mind-altering substances), being asleep, as well as not being of mental capacity to consent which includes impairment by mental illness and not being of appropriate age to consent.

A mental willingness and desire to engage in a particular activity are necessary components of consent. It is important to remember that both willingness and desire are embedded in cultural stereotypes that dictate normative scripts within sexual encounters.

Figure 3.2

Four components of consent

Source: Worthen MGF (2016) Figure 12.5: Four necessary components of consent, in Sexual deviance and society: A sociological examination, London: Routledge, p. 340.

capacity to consent can be impacted by a variety of factors, including age, developmental ability, intoxication, physical ability, relationship of victim and perpetration, consciousness, vulnerability status, and incarceration. Consent is about communication and should happen any time sexual activity occurs. Consent is also dynamic; the decision to consent can change at any moment. For more information, visit www.rainn.org.

Meredith Worthen presents a model of consent that involves four fundamental components. (See Figure 3.2 below.) These include mental willingness and desire; communicatory cues; occurrence without coercion, threat, force, or under duress; and soundness of mind. Mental willingness and desire to engage in activity is a fundamental component of consent, but we must also recognize that culture and social scripts influence our conceptions of consent. For example, physically or verbally abusive relationships often have victims choosing to engage sexually with partners as a way to "buy time" between the abuse. While it may be a mental choice of the survivor, the accumulated physical and psychological impacts have a damaging effect. This trauma is often unrecognized by "outsiders," but when abuse is measured in decades, rates of PTSD can soar.

As a second component, participants must communicate willingness and desire. Communicatory cues can be both verbal and nonverbal, and should be discussed prior to sexual activity. Further, communicatory cues should be present both before and during sexual activity with ongoing consent. Consent must take place without coercion, threat, force, or under duress, which must take into account context. For example, some people, such as those who are incarcerated, may not have the capacity to give consent. Finally, all participants must be of sound mind. Impairments to this could include intoxication, being asleep, lacking mental capacity, or not being of appropriate age. It is important to note that each of these factors can be impacted by situational and cultural factors (Worthen 2016).

Understanding the Impacts of Sexual Trauma

The impact of trauma is vast, and our understanding of effective responses to trauma continues to grow. The current discussion is not exhaustive or comprehensive but can provide a context, and, therefore, an understanding of where to start. We cannot know the experience of any survivor in our class, but we can know a range of possibilities. The best practices help minimize risk for further damage and maximize bodily agency, empowerment, and insight. We additionally recognize that trauma responses exist in support of

survival. We use the practice of yoga to ease the somatic and emotional toll that many survivors pay as a result of their trauma.

The current *Diagnostic and Statistical Manual* (DSM-5) (APA 2013) of the American Psychiatric Association (APA) recognizes an entire category of trauma and stressor related disorders. These disorders develop a picture of psychological distress following exposure to a traumatic or stressful event. A common conceptualization of the long-term impacts of traumatic stress is the diagnosis of post-traumatic stress disorder (PTSD). In the wake of trauma, PTSD characterizes the potential for intrusive symptoms (distressing memories, dreams, flashbacks, psychological distress in reaction to reminders of the event, and psychological reactions to internal and external cues), avoidance (efforts to avoid memories, thoughts, feelings, and external reminders), negative alterations in cognitions and mood (inability to remember, negative cognitions, persistent negative emotional states, diminished interest in significant events, feelings of detachment, inability to experience positive emotion), and alterations in arousal or reactivity (irritable behavior, angry outbursts, self-destructive behavior, hypervigilance, exaggerated startle response, difficulty concentrating, and disturbed sleep).

The DSM-5 informs much of medical and mental health practice in the United States and beyond. However, as a clinical definition, the DSM-5 delineation is limited. There are many and diverse ways in which people experience trauma; reactions to trauma are complex. The DSM-5 model can be seen to oversimplify complex human reactions. Diagnoses of the DSM can be stigmatizing and can pathologize normal coping behavior in the wake of trauma.

In general, the model of the DSM does not support a strength-based perspective. While a person can experience the symptoms discussed above, they may also experience positive transformation and growth. Further, it is important to acknowledge that trauma responses are normal life-saving responses to abnormal or distressing life events.

In developing yoga programming that is responsive to trauma, it is important to recognize the negative impacts of trauma, but at the same time to seek examples of the potential for resilience and strength. It is important to remember that distress and growth are not mutually exclusive.

In the following sections, we will illuminate some of the potential impacts of the experience of trauma. This discussion is not meant to be exhaustive, but instead to allow teachers and practitioners a perspective of how trauma can be experienced. Understanding both the emotional and embodied ways we experience trauma can help to inform how we shape yoga and mindfulness offerings for students and guide students in the type of practice they seek.

Dissociation

After an experience of sexual trauma, and sometimes for many years forward, survivors can experience periods of dissociation. Survivors can find themselves in a perpetual state of being triggered, re-experiencing aspects, and symptoms of trauma. They can also experience periods of dissociation. With dissociation, a survivor psychologically and physiologically becomes disconnected from their senses, self, and history. Within the dissociated state, there is a remarkable ability for the body and mind to tune the outside world out and to dampen emotional and physical systems such as hunger cues and executive functioning so that energy is spent resourcing for survival.

Dissociation sometimes looks like temporary emotional paralysis, but can also look like going through the motions with either a detached sense of reality, as though one experiences the world from outside oneself, or having a highly attuned focus on a few aspects of reality only. In a yoga class, this might look like an inability to retain a memory of repeated patterns of yoga forms, being receptive to adjustment cues one day and completely unresponsive to the same the next. Students who have difficulty translating language-based yoga cues into physical forms could be in a dissociative state, although this is not necessarily the case.

Control

Trauma survivors often experience a diminished sense of control and agency. As a result, survivors may feel the need for excessive control over their environment. This need for control impacts relationships and capacity for connection to their communities. The need for control can result in a high level of rigidity and the absence of spontaneity. In a yoga class, this can present as anxiety and panic at last-minute teacher substitutions, changes in class routine, including mat set up, or class starting a few minutes late.

Lack of Control

Alternately, one may find themselves on the other side of the control spectrum. If the body and mind interpreted and normalized ownership and control taken away throughout the sexual trauma, a survivor may have difficulty being able to make any decisions without the aid of others. A lack of control can result in the survivor abandoning their own needs and presenting with a decreasing capacity for bodily and emotional self-knowledge. Sometimes a decreased awareness of the way that the body takes the shape of yoga's forms and movements presents as a lack of proprioception or awareness of body position and movement. In yoga classes, the experience might look like attempting forms that are beyond the participant's ability simply because they are "following instructions."

Reenactment and the Experience of Intrusive Symptoms

The stress response is a biologically derived reaction to a life-threatening event. With trauma, survivors can become stuck in the stress response, reacting even when they are not currently in threat of danger. Survivors may have stress reactions to everyday events and experiences. Further, reenactment and re-experiencing trauma can occur at any point, even during what may seem to be an otherwise ordinary and non-threatening circumstance.

Intrusive symptoms can include distressing memories, dreams, flashbacks, and re-experiencing aspects of the traumatic event. Distress symptoms can be brought on by specific cues or sensory reminders of past trauma. In the context of a yoga class, we can hold the awareness that students may be having an experience that we are entirely unaware of. We can note that seemingly simple cues or prompts can be triggering. We can never create a space that is entirely safe or that avoids triggering. We can create spaces that are intentional, informed with awareness, and designed to minimize risk. A teacher can offer flexibility and a range of options to meet students where they are, and allow students to co-create a practice that supports mindful well-being.

Numbness

Many people who have experienced sexual violence report feeling numb at some point. Survivors may avoid stimuli and reminders connected to the traumatic event. This avoidance of thoughts, feelings, and experiences numbs out negative stimuli, but one is also left numb to positive thoughts, feelings, and experiences. Additionally, when one is no longer numb, a wide range of emotions and somatic experiences become overwhelming and intolerable. This experience can be jarring, un-grounding, and frightening, causing students to flinch or jump. We can avoid judgment when a student's response differs from what we might expect.

Developing a Belief System that the Event(s) are Your Only Worth

People in trauma-heavy situations will often find thoughts of failure crowd their usual sense of self and worth. Survivors often come to believe the lies maliciously told by perpetrators. Trauma can significantly impact cognitive thought processes. Impacts can include exaggerated negative beliefs or expectations about oneself, others, or the world (for, "I am bad," "No one can be trusted," "The world is perilous," "My whole nervous system is permanently ruined") (American Psychiatric Association 2013). Survivors of sexual trauma commonly blame themselves, and negative self-talk is common. These feelings can lead to detachment and disengagement. In yoga, aim to offer an invitational approach that seeks inclusivity while promoting individual agency.

Abandoning Self

Reconnecting with the body can initially be a very uncomfortable and frightening experience. As a safety mechanism during times of highest threat, the body and mind will often "check out" from the current experience, to create a buffer between the self and the horrors being endured. This practice of abandoning self is so common among trauma survivors that frequent, expressive, re-association methods can be beneficial to return people to greater habitation in their self, for example, a cue such as "you might notice the corners of your feet as they press into the floor."

Memory

Common to trauma survivors are memory disturbances. After a traumatic experience, the events encode themselves in the brain, changing the way one interprets memories. In different stages of recovering from trauma, memory can be incomplete or seemingly distorted. Flashbacks to the event(s) and poor executive functioning in survival can look like impaired decision making and problems with concentration. In yoga, a student may not remember specific repeated sequences, phrases, or classroom norms, even if they have returned frequently to your class. Be patient and go gently.

Emotion

People who have experienced sexual violence, when not numbed or dissociated, often have heightened feeling states emotionally and physically. Trauma responses can include irritable emotions, reactions, or outbursts of anger. Feelings of resentment can arise from several sources. Examples include: seeing other people's lives as perfect, comparing recovery successes, and/or feeling that more could have been done to protect an individual from being violated. Know that a full range of emotion may be present in the wake of traumatic stress. Within the context of yoga, we can hold space for a sophisticated experience of emotion, while at the same time sharing tools that foster emotional regulation.

Objectification

Being treated as a thing, that another person can do with what they desire, leads to feelings of objectification. A survivor can interpret any attention as objectification. Some lean into this,

having associated their worth with being an object, while others hide, ultimately hoping not to be noticed at all. Teachers and those working with survivors should work to avoid judgment of a student who they perceive to present as over-sexualized. In yoga, each person will have unique experience of being seen or not seen, being the center of attention or always on the margins. This is largely due to how people were treated in their trauma. Be present, without judgment, to a wide range of potential experiences and presentations.

Shame

Shame is a reliable hallmark for those who have experienced sexual trauma. Shame can come from the many messages we receive about sex and sexuality. The perpetrator can reinforce shame. A sense of shame may also have roots in cultural, religious, and community ideas and practices whereby the shame has moral implications for the survivor. In a yoga class, this can present as feelings of embarrassment or anxiety. Shame can look like anxiety about not meeting the teacher's expectations or fearing being called out for doing yoga "wrong." A survivor may experience feelings of shame in a yoga class as they regain a sense of embodiment, perhaps for the first time in a long time. Again, it is vital to offer a practice that is invitational and provides a variety of options. Teachers should be aware that a student may not feel empowered to opt for a modification or an assist and have this awareness inform their language and modeling of the practice.

Betrayal

Often, perpetrators of sexual violence are known to the victim as someone who the survivor thought was safe. One can feel betrayed by the very people who were supposed to protect them. Reenactment of this can be seen in the yoga classroom when there is teacher inconsistency, student favoritism, and an unwillingness to examine the physical safety of the forms we teach in relation to the readiness of the student.

> I was a woman abused by men, but had much more anger and resentment for the women in my life who didn't protect me. This made me distrust all women in my life who didn't protect me.
> — YSC symposium participant

Broken and Undeserving

When someone feels broken, coming to a yoga class that invokes ideas of self-care, health, and healing can be challenging. When one has a history of sexual violence, entering a yoga class can come with considerable risk, anxiety, pressure, and a sense of unworthiness. We have to keep in mind that not one of us is broken, ever. Further, healing is not a linear process. As students come to us to seek connection and potential healing, it has to be our intention to see each person, ourselves included, as deserving and whole.

Contamination

The words spoken and the physical nature of sexual trauma can leave survivors feeling sullied and contaminated. Devastatingly, many also view the world around them in the same way. Feelings of being contaminated or worries about contaminating someone else can quickly become a survival mechanism to protect themselves and others from the contamination they have experienced. This contamination extends to the physical spaces where we practice. We must both recognize this potential and create inclusive environments that promote acceptance. We can create spaces that offer the potential for healthy embodiment.

> When I first started practicing yoga, I would get to class early and sanitize the floor where my mat would be, as well as the mat itself. I would not, for a second, step off my mat, no matter what the form required. I was terrified of contaminating the space and other people with what I considered my spreadable disease. It took years for me to figure out that this was a traumatic response to rape.
> — YSC symposium participant

Resilience

According to the American Psychological Association, resilience is "the process of adapting well in the face of adversity, trauma, tragedy, threats or significant sources of stress" (APA 2019). Many view resilience as the capacity to "bounce back," yet we suggest that resilience represents a far more complex construct. We acknowledge the resilience of those with whom we work and see yoga as a tool that has the potential to be supportive in fostering resilience. While work remains to be done in the pursuit of defining and studying resilience, we recognize that there is value in taking a strengths-based approach to understanding trauma response and addressing the many impacts of sexual trauma.

Psychologists Hamby, Grych, and Banyard (2018: 172) describe resilience as being comprised of three primary elements. The first is adversity or "some sort of stressful or traumatic experience." The second is evidence of healthy function after such an event. The third element is the protective factor or strength(s) that foster the overcoming of adversity. As Hamby et al. (2018) pointed out, much research to date measures resilience through the absence of clinical symptoms and psychological distress. They suggest that a strengths-based approach is fundamental, and that assessment must include measures of well-being, not solely lack of distress. These researchers developed a model of resilience and related assessment portfolio that explores strengths in three primary areas: self-regulation, interpersonal strengths, and meaning making. Each factor is what they call malleable or dynamic in that it has the capacity to change (Hamby, et al. 2018; Grych, et al. 2015). Coutu (2017: 10) suggests a common understanding of three primary characteristics of resilience, including "a staunch acceptance of reality; a deep belief, often buttressed by strongly held values, that life is meaningful; and an uncanny ability to improvise."

Regulatory strengths: The capacity to control impulses, manage emotions, and persevere

Interpersonal relationships: Relationships (family, friends, community) and personal qualities that sustain relationships

Meaning making: The ability to explain and understand experiences

(Hamby, et al. 2018: 173; emboldening added)

We would suggest that resilience is dynamic and not static. Resilience is not a trait that we either have or do not have; the pathway of resilience is not linear. It is possible to experience more or less resilience at different points, and one's level of resilience does not define value. We would also suggest that both individuals and communities can be resilient. It is our hope that the field continues to explore resilience as an important aspect of trauma response. We invite yoga teachers and practitioners to explore how they might invite resilience into their practice in support of well-being.

Posttraumatic Growth

Within the wake of trauma is the profound potential for resilience. One representation of this is the concept of posttraumatic growth. Tedeschi and Calhoun (1996, 2004) developed the concept of Posttraumatic Growth, suggesting the potential for positive change after a life crisis. They define posttraumatic growth as "positive psychological change experienced as a result of the struggle with highly challenging life circumstances" (Tedeschi & Calhoun 2004: 1). Other researchers have gone on to explore and measure posttraumatic growth and discuss its role as a strength-based approach to resilience building and psychological health and well-being. Posttraumatic growth recognizes that trauma can be a shared experience, and resilience can be collaborative. As a result, posttraumatic growth can improve interpersonal relationships and contribute to social transformation.

There is evidence that yoga can promote posttraumatic growth in the wake of trauma. Universally inclusive yoga creates the space and potential for resilience and growth in survivors of trauma. When we seek practices that are trauma-informed, we can recognize the capacity for resilience and growth. For example, in one study participants in a trauma-informed yoga curriculum in three correctional facilities demonstrated significant increases in posttraumatic growth after completion of the curriculum (see text box below).

Post Traumatic Growth (PTG) refers to positive outcomes as described by individuals who have experienced adverse or stressful events. This measure assesses increased strengths, spiritual change, new life possibilities and appreciation of life. Although both voluntary and control participants showed change, the impact for voluntary participants was much greater (Yoga 4 Change 2019: 2).

A Call to Action

There remains much work to be done in combating sexual violence and addressing the many impacts of sexual trauma. Responses to and attempts to combat sexual violence have necessarily been both personal and political. Many responses have been grassroots, with support growing with increased awareness. One example is the Take Back the Night movement, an international movement to combat sexual violence and violence against women. This movement began in the 1960s in Belgium and England and has gained awareness and support since with the formation of an international foundation in 2001. To date, Take Back the Night events have been documented in more than thirty-six countries and 800 communities (Take Back the Night 2019).

> Our mission as a charitable 501(c)3 Foundation is to create safe communities and respectful relationships through awareness events and initiatives. We seek to end sexual assault, domestic violence, dating violence, sexual abuse, and all forms of sexual violence.
>
> (Take Back the Night 2019)

Much of the work in this area has come out of local rape crisis centers, including efforts to establish legal and mental health supports for survivors, activism to change legal, public policy, and definitional issues concerning rape, and attempts for community education and training concerning sexual violence and its impacts. Local, national, and international organizations offer survivor services, education, public policy reform initiatives, and consulting and training. We must acknowledge the foundational work that has been done and recognize all that remains to be done.

We view yoga as one potential tool for activism, which we will discuss further in our final chapter. Through our practice and offering of yoga, we can be of service to survivors. But this requires self-inquiry, understanding, and compassionate action. True service needs to come from a place of connection – working with, not working for. In order to change systems, including our societal reaction to sexual violence and trauma, we must change the minds and behaviors of the people within such systems. Our own awareness and intentionality can inform and influence that of others. We are called to live into this service.

Informing Our Work

We have just scratched the surface of exploring an understanding of sexual trauma. We continue an ongoing inquiry in this area. We believe that as teachers and practitioners we have an obligation to educate ourselves and to act from a place that is informed and intentional.

This book is not intended to be a comprehensive exploration of trauma or sexual trauma specifically, yet we believe it is important to introduce the discussion. This and the preceding chapter provide foundational context for the best practices that follow. In the best practice chapters ahead, we explore how an understanding of the many impacts of sexual trauma should inform our practice and service. We will explore both general best practices and best practices that target specific populations and contexts. Again, we recognize that the scope of our discussion is not comprehensive; it is our hope that the information provided will foster ongoing inquiry and discussion and inspire change.

PART
2

Introduction to Best Practices

Best Practices for Creating a Trauma-informed Yoga Experience

Authors *Lidia Snyder, Beth Jones, and Nan Herron*
Contributors *Jacoby Ballard, Sue Jones, Anneke Lucas*

Introduction

Case study

Sandra is a 27-year-old woman who works as an administrative assistant in a corporate office. She was sexually traumatized by her step-father throughout her chaotic childhood starting at age five. She tried to tell her mother, but her mother dismissed her attempts to raise the conversation. The sexual abuse stopped when Sandra entered puberty at age twelve. Since graduating from high school she has had minimal contact with her family. She has few friends and has never had a satisfying romantic relationship. She reports social anxiety, frequent bouts of depression, and waking up most nights from nightmares. She recently started therapy to address these symptoms, as well as to address her fear of intimacy and difficulty trusting people. Her therapist suggested that yoga might be helpful, so she put on sweatpants and an old T-shirt and went to a local studio to try a yoga class. She intentionally chose a class that would be taught by a woman.

When she entered the classroom she immediately felt anxious and had the sense that everyone else knew one another and that she didn't belong. The other women had beautiful yoga clothes and thin, sculpted bodies. As the class began the teacher introduced himself and stated that he was "subbing" for the usual teacher. He put on unfamiliar, "foreign-sounding" music, which distracted her from following the cues offered. The yoga forms were harder than she had expected and the teacher often insisted that students stay in physical positions that felt challenging to maintain. She began to judge herself for being weak and uncoordinated. She noticed that the large man next to her was sweating profusely and she felt upset and disgusted. In the middle of the class while walking among the students, the teacher came over to her mat when she was attempting a tree form, and put his hands on her hips, which startled her. She became angry at him and angrier at herself for her response, and was unable to think about anything else for the remainder of the class. She felt like she had "failed at yoga" and decided she would never try it again.

She was, however, able to discuss this experience at her next therapy session. Her therapist immediately apologized for not carefully providing more specific guidance regarding what yoga classes to pursue. Her therapist arranged for her to have an intake at a local Women's Center for a Trauma-Informed Yoga Class, which, after much hesitation, she decided she would try.

During the intake a woman met her at the reception desk and introduced herself as "Joan." Joan explained that she was a licensed yoga teacher who had extensive training in "Trauma-Sensitive Yoga." She stated

continued

Case study *continued*

that the classes would consist of eight women, aged twenty-five to fifty, who all had childhood histories of intra-familial sexual abuse. She described the rules and format of the classes, which would consist of twelve ninety-minute sessions with another qualified co-teacher, and she emphasized the importance of confidentiality and respect. She described that early classes would have time set aside for brief general introductions, and that there would be fifteen minutes at the beginning and end of every class for optional check-ins. During this "check-in" time, participants would have the opportunity to tell the others how they were doing and what they were feeling, but not to discuss specifics about their lives or histories, which they could continue to address with their therapists. She stated that the teachers would never touch the students, that modified forms would be offered, and that if anyone wanted to sit or lie down throughout the class they were encouraged to do so. She shared that since there would be two teachers present, one of the teachers would be available to address any unexpected challenges. Joan emphasized that the students would be expected to inform the teachers if they were unable to attend the session. She said that all the students were encouraged to be in individual therapy, since yoga often led to new insights and areas of awareness, which was not always easy or pleasant. Sandra asked Joan for information she could read to learn more about the risks and benefits of yoga, and Joan smiled and handed her a pamphlet. Joan encouraged Sandra to take a few days to think about whether she wanted to participate, and to discuss it with her therapist if she desired. Sandra left the meeting feeling welcomed, hopeful, and empowered.

The call to this work is often deeply personal. Many times, a yoga teacher feels drawn to teaching specific populations, for personal reasons or non-specific ones. People who are incarcerated, people with special needs, veterans, sexual trauma survivors, perpetrators, recovery groups – all will demand of a teacher a heightened self-awareness, balanced mental health, good self-care practices, and the ability to observe the impact of their own sensitivities and perhaps even their own trauma history. An approach of humility and receptivity is key. It is important to honestly examine personal motivation in doing this work. Serving people impacted by trauma through yoga may be part of the curriculum of your yoga studio or teacher training, yet it may not assume a readiness to teach. A desire to make a difference is a great way to begin, but be aware that if one is not personally ready, you risk causing harm and creating more suffering instead. This work cannot be done without extensive self-inquiry.

It is crucial to be especially mindful and explicit about safety for those who have survived trauma. In our experience, we have noticed that clear, direct communication outlining the reasons for our choices in constructing and leading a trauma-informed yoga class leads to a more favorable atmosphere for any class or gathering. Elements that are assumed or taken for granted in other settings (for example, "mainstream" yoga classes), should be described in a more deliberate, detailed, and transparent manner. Access to information decreases the likelihood of further traumatization and falls under the trauma-informed pillar of "transparency." Additionally, whenever possible, there should be an invitation and opportunity for input and discussion to best represent the needs of a particular group. Being aware of the unique requirements of a particular subset of students enhances the therapeutic elements of a sense of control and agency. It also presents an opportunity to be "heard," which can be a new, positive experience for some survivors.

Embarking upon the path of trauma-informed yoga brings with it a responsibility to acknowledge that, for many, the aftermath of sexual trauma brings with it challenges to multiple aspects of life: physical, social, emotional, and spiritual. Approaching yoga in a trauma-informed manner requires a strengths-based approach that is rooted in an understanding of and responsiveness to the impact of trauma that emphasizes physical, psychological, and emotional safety for both providers and clients (Hopper, Bassuk, & Olivet 2010). The best practices outlined in this chapter are not complicated, but they require a level of openness to examine how each one of us can play a role in creating and extending a trauma-informed yoga experience.

The following sections will address some common best practices in support of trauma-informed practices and trauma-informed yoga more specifically. This chapter also explores general best practices in trauma-informed programming. The recommendations are both experiential and evidence-based and rise from the collaborative process of co-creation that represents the foundation of this text. Subsequent chapters will dive deeper into specifics, including individual contexts and target populations. This chapter provides an overall foundation.

Best Practices

Seeking a Trauma-informed Approach

Best Practice

Seek an informed understanding of trauma-informed practice and reflect trauma-informed principles in curriculum content.

Preparing to teach in a trauma-informed way requires intentional review of programs and trainings that exist. Both evidence-based programming and accreditation status can be important in assessing the value of a program or training. Aligning yourself with a strong and proven program will help support you as you do outreach and networking to establish yourself in the community. Because trauma-informed practice is less about a physical expression of yoga and more about internal embodiment and awareness, it is essential to consider ways to reduce the likelihood of triggers, dysregulated behaviors, and retraumatization. In presenting recommendations for best practices, we share some practical considerations that may help to create a trauma-informed experience for students.

It is useful to briefly address the core differences between a traditional or classical yoga approach and one that is trauma-informed. Yoga teachers are trained to share their knowledge and expertise concerning anatomy, physiology, yoga philosophy, and ethics with students. Recalling that power dynamics are at the very core of a traumatic experience, readers may begin to see a conflict. Table 4.1 offers four aspects in which a traditional yoga approach conflicts with one that is trauma-informed. This is not to diminish the utility of traditional yoga training or instruction but rather to underscore how such an approach runs counter to core concepts of being trauma-informed.

Each aspect of curriculum should be rooted in trauma-informed theory. The five pillars of trauma-informed care, as discussed in Chapter 2, can provide a strong starting point. These pillars include safety, choice, collaboration, trustworthiness/transparency, and empowerment (SAMHSA 2014). All sessions should be built on a foundation that survivors are capable

Table 4.1 Contrasting traditional and trauma-informed yoga

Principle	Traditional	Trauma-informed
Locus of control	External, from the teacher	Internal, from the participant
Authority/Responsibility	External, rests in teacher	Internal, rests in student(s)
Goal orientation	Enlightenment, nonattachment	Safety, choice
Language/Communication	Command	Invitation

of recovery and that this work is not about treating trauma but rather about acknowledging the impact trauma has had. This work is done *with* participants, not *for* participants. It is an invitational and collaborative process.

Instructors and program administrators should seek out expert consultation before offering specific sessions for sexual trauma survivors. While most yoga practitioners have experienced individual benefits from their practice, there is risk in attempting to generalize such practices without regard for theory and empirical data.

Best Practice
Seek a foundational understanding of the history of yoga.

One of the main pillars of a trauma-informed approach is "transparency," and a frank discussion about the roots of yoga and its evolution to date is encouraged. In order for this to happen, instructors should themselves be educated in the vast history of yoga, its numerous schools and lineages, and changes from the classical to modern postural yoga eras. Suggested texts for exploration include: Andrea Jain's *Selling Yoga: From Counterculture to Pop Culture* (2015), Mark Singleton's *Yoga Body: The Origins of Modern Posture Practice* (2010), and Elizabeth De Mechilis's *A History of Modern Yoga: Patanjali and Western Esotericism* (2004).

Yoga scholar Georg Feuerstein (2011: 416) points out that yoga is widely understood as "a spiritual discipline" aimed at enlightenment that has been spread by missionaries, swamis, and gurus and more recently in the West by tens of thousands of trained yoga instructors. "Yoga" as we have come to know it, in studios in the West, does not hail directly from an ancient Indian past. Rather, it emerged in the late nineteenth-century interactions between Hindu reformers and Western gymnasts and bodybuilders, during a period of ongoing British colonial rule of India. "Modern postural yoga," as historians call it, was born in a context of colonialism as well as collaboration (Singleton 2010; Jain 2015).

Nearly a decade ago, the Hindu American Foundation (HAF) embarked on a campaign "Take Back Yoga" as a response to what was perceived as cultural appropriation and theft within the yoga community in the United States. Many HAF members believed that presenting yoga separate from what they define as its Hindu spiritual roots – uniting body, mind, and spirit with God – while acceptable, was a contradiction to its true aim. In the twentieth century and since, as different lineages of postural yoga have proliferated, many teachers have grounded their claims to spiritual authority in an ancient past, which historians of yoga caution is a misleading claim that essentializes Hinduism and yoga. At the same time, many contemporary Hindus, such as members of HAF, have criticized European and

American yoga teachers for appropriating their tradition. From our perspective, this history is complex and deserves our engagement. We recommend an approach to trauma-informed yoga that recognizes this history and yoga's deeper dimensions for those who practice it.

Best Practice
Mindfully address boundaries.

For the traumatized person, boundaries can be complicated and confusing. Young children learn about boundaries implicitly and explicitly. That is, children learn the rules of emotional and physical intimacy from their social interactions without explicitly being told and from limits that are explicitly explained, for example, "It is not safe to talk to strangers." Young people benefit from attuned parents who can notice and respect their child's particular comfort with interpersonal contacts. Many trauma survivors did not have the opportunity to develop self-protective boundaries. The adults that were supposed to care for, protect, and educate them may instead have focused only on their own needs and desires.

Depending on their particular experiences and temperament, some individuals may have boundaries that are experienced by others as "too close" or intrusive; others may appear to be distant, cold, or unwelcoming. Many survivors spend years figuring out how to feel comfortable and safe around others. It may require protracted, intensive therapy for them to recognize this and to learn how to express themselves in a way that feels comfortable. For some it may be an area of lifelong exploration or confusion.

Boundary violations are more common when there is an imbalance of power, which is intrinsic to the role of teacher and student. If the yoga teacher violates their student's boundaries, the student may not feel comfortable telling them; in fact, they may not even be aware of it. The trauma-informed yoga facilitator may have some students who require significant psychological and physical space to feel safe in the class. Others may seek closeness or intimacy with the teacher in a way that encroaches upon the teacher's level of comfort as well as their ability to maintain an appropriate level of professionalism. For example, a student may want to be "friends" with a teacher and may suggest socializing outside of the classroom. Whether this is ethical, wise, or good judgment depends upon many variables, deserves careful consideration, and may merit supervision with a professional or peer, or discussion with multiple parties.

A teacher's skills to maintain awareness and cultivate communication are critical to maximize the likelihood that boundary issues can be appropriately addressed. Ideally, multiple conversations will occur in the trauma-informed yoga classroom, and a culture will evolve where students feel safe to express their needs without worrying about being judged. It is important for the trauma-informed yoga teacher to create a culture that encourages candid and explicit discussions about what a boundary is and how to express this. The teacher has the responsibility of making sure they obtain an adequate education on how to do this, and to have ongoing supervision. Having more than one teacher is wise in order to increase support in the room for both teachers and students.

It is also imperative that every trauma-informed yoga teacher takes responsibility to cultivate an awareness of themselves, and their own areas of vulnerability and sensitivity. We encourage every teacher to have a personal mindfulness practice, and to responsibly pursue individual therapy if needed. The teaching of trauma-informed yoga – indeed, working with trauma survivors in any context – can only be sustained by individuals who develop an active practice of self-care and who are courageous and aware enough to notice when they need support. Even though the trauma-informed yoga teacher may not feel that they are "in the trenches" or engaging in explicit therapy, the energy required to manage the inevitable dynamics of a trauma-informed class, however implicit, requires extensive time for rest and regeneration. Be careful if you are an individual who is much more comfortable taking care of others than yourself. The potential for burnout, vicarious traumatization, and compassion fatigue should not be underestimated.

Best Practice
Know your scope of practice.

Regardless of your training outside of yoga, instructors are cautioned to perform solely within their capacity as yoga instructors, and not as counselors, clinicians, or healers of any other variety. Knowing and adhering to a legitimate scope of a trauma-informed yoga practice is vital at all times. Be sure to have completed your own self-inquiry and training prior to offering sessions, specifically those for healing sexual trauma. Because a teacher is actively building a relationship of trust with a student, boundaries can quickly get crossed, cues can be misinterpreted, and re-enactment of a trauma relationship(s) can occur. It is important to maintain a low-authority relationship while, at the same time, keeping the relationship professional. Some blurring of boundaries includes close friendship, over-sharing your personal information or narrative, and engaging with students, sexually or romantically.

Developing a professional persona that is empathetic and approachable is a constantly evolving task that takes self-awareness as well as an understanding of some typical survival behaviors. Re-enactment of trauma can present as high reactivity to sensation, music selection, and/or voice, and/or intolerance of others. By intentionally selecting clothing, creating a predictable setting and sequencing, using consistent choice of music or silence, and developing a predictable presentation of class content, a teacher can begin to establish boundaries that are clear, physical, and observable. A relationship of trust can have a healthy chance to begin. Be consistent to the measure.

There should be an explicit discussion of trauma-informed yoga as being distinct from therapy per se (unless it *is* therapy), and how this plays into the limits of the role of the teacher. Teachers should acknowledge, identify, and encourage the role of support for students outside of class. Teachers should clarify whether students are expected to be in therapy while involved in trauma-informed yoga. These issues should be reviewed and discussed in the screening process.

If a student is triggered, they should be supported in the moment and an appropriate referral should be made. If you knowingly work with individuals in an acute state, such as someone who was just released from the hospital or who is living in an emergency domestic violence shelter, you can insist that a clinician stay present during yoga and suggest that the clinician be available to process what comes up with a student after yoga, if possible. We will discuss this further in later chapters.

It may be helpful to review the concepts of transference and counter-transference. These terms are used to explain the dynamics that can evolve between a therapist and a client, or in any relationship, especially when there is a perceived imbalance of power, for example, student– teacher or patient–doctor. In brief, "transference" refers to the unconscious assumptions that a client has toward a therapist based on previous experience in relationships. For example, a student may believe, "They're always right and I'm always wrong" or, "They are only pretending to want to help me, but really they just want to have power over me." These kinds of assumptions about self with others may exist because of previous dynamics in a formative childhood relationship. Similarly, "counter-transference" refers to unconscious beliefs on the part of the therapist, based on previous experience, for example, "That client isn't listening to anything I'm saying." These dynamics can be quite complex and require maturity, as well as keen awareness in the yoga teacher. Often subtle, they deserve further understanding.

Best Practice
Make intentional and informed decisions regarding the use of touch.

Of all the challenges in delivering a trauma-informed approach to yoga, touch is certainly one of the more controversial. Human developmental and attachment theories highlight the primacy of physical human contact in the formation of secure attachments, healthy self-concepts, and capacity to navigate the world around us. However, because sexual trauma typically involves a violation through touch, the subsequent experience of touch is marred. Because this book intends to offer best practices that facilitate the greatest level of safety for most participants, the best practice is to avoid touch.

This best practice can be difficult for most yoga teachers who go through training for "hands-on assists" and who are encouraged to be the

authority in such touch experiences. In traditional yoga training, these assists are intended to induce comfort, stability, and body awareness, or to achieve alignment. However, touch assists can be intrusive. It is not uncommon for students to report that they can sense the physical presence of a teacher and that students sense, in their bodies, when the teacher is near. With survivors, this ability to sense and locate the perceived authority in the room may be heightened. This is called hypervigilance. Conversely, a survivor may experience hypovigilance, numbness, or alexithymia – the inability to feel and judge internal sensation. In other words, they may be entirely unaware and seemingly indifferent to the proximity of a teacher, let alone be aware of how they feel about being touched – with or without permission.

For survivors of sexual trauma, their right to choose between being touched and not being touched was violated. It is safe to assume that touch, particularly without permission to touch, can be re-traumatizing, most especially when given by an authoritative figure such as a teacher. Sexual abuse can leave survivors feeling a lack of boundaries and readily accepting of another's authority over their own bodies. They may also have a highly sexualized sense of themselves with others. Touch can provoke this. Even still, there are survivors who have strong aversions to touch while others may crave it.

> Safe and supportive touch is simple, intentional, noninvasive, and nondirective. As such, it is generally quite different from the postural "assists" provided in traditional yoga classes. That said, it's impossible to guarantee that touch won't be perceived as invasive, despite our best intentions.
>
> (Jones 2017: 5)

Some yoga teachers simply avoid offering touch assists of any kind, as it can disrupt the hard work of yoga's internal focusing and, perhaps, trigger a fear response or retraumatization. Having a "no-touch" rule simplifies this issue, and creates a clear boundary (Emerson 2015). Conversely, other trauma-informed programs use touch that is non-directive and grounding. This type of touch is notably different from more traditional assists or adjustments. And it requires the permission of each student. Offering choice is paramount and can be done in a discreet way. For instance, a teacher may give each student a token or object to put on the mat as a means of communicating whether or not touch is welcome. Once introduced, that technique should be consistently used, which invites independent experience, while also providing a direct experiment with choice and touch. A teacher should only deliver touch options and techniques after an intensive, supervised training. Careful steps are taken to introduce touch only after the student has familiarity with the teacher and the class format (Jones 2017). The decision to use touch should be an informed and intentional decision. If there is any question, touch should be avoided.

Teacher Qualification Considerations

Best Practice
Program administrators and studio owners should establish a proper plan for hiring and supporting teachers.

Program administrators or studio owners should develop a contract with yoga instructors outlining expectations and requirements. This may include responsibilities, professional conduct, compensation, grounds for termination, and confidentiality issues. There should be clear identification of what constitutes appropriate training and verification of training. Continuing education and professional development programs are important components of any specialty; a plan for ongoing training and education could be clearly delineated in the hiring process.

With regard to hiring staff, background checks and references will enhance safety, be helpful in identifying professional demeanor, and lead to successful experiences. Ongoing evaluation and support of teachers should occur. It is important for teachers to be explicit regarding their own support and self-care practices. Teachers must maintain a high level of professionalism and self-awareness, and be able to receive feedback effectively. It should also be clear as to whether and what kind of insurance teachers are expected to carry.

Presenting as a professional, a teacher should build a trauma-informed wardrobe, one that is conservative and modest. For example, choose a crew neck T-shirt versus a V-neck top. Darker or neutral colors work well. In all cases, a loose, comfortable pair of pants and a top work best as they do not reveal body-shape or leave a teacher overly exposed. Studios and special programs may wish to consider a specific dress code or uniform for teachers, particularly if teachers are employed in institutional settings.

Program guidelines should be clear about whether teachers practice along with students. Students often benefit from observing the modeling of the instructor. However, practicing along with students may compromise a teacher's attention. Teaching trauma-informed yoga often includes unanticipated moments when students become triggered and overwhelmed. A teacher who is absorbed in a self-directed yoga practice may miss signs. If there is more than one teacher this can be minimized. A second teacher or facilitator increases safety and can step in to give support to someone who is struggling or who needs to leave the room. The decision of how a teacher should present yoga must be explicitly considered when a program is in the planning stages.

Additionally, vicarious traumatization in teachers is common, even when the details of a student's trauma are not made explicit. Even experienced instructors and therapists face situations when they are at a loss for how to proceed. Studios and programs hiring teachers should be aware of the signs and symptoms of vicarious trauma and have a plan in place to support teachers who are experiencing it. Having a peer support group, either online or in person, as well as building a strong sub-list of other teachers are good ways of acknowledging the challenges inherent in this work – and may extend a teacher's health and creative vitality.

Best Practice
Trauma-informed yoga practitioners should consider not teaching alone.

As stated above, it is ideal, although not always possible, for a studio, special program, or institution to have at least two practitioners in a trauma-informed classroom. This not only supports the teachers but enhances the safety of the students. This will also allow for one teacher to help a participant who needs one-to-one attention for any reason. In addition, if complicated dynamics arise, the different perspectives and skills of the teachers will enhance a fuller understanding and increase the likelihood of a favorable outcome. If the teachers have different roles, this should be made clear to students before class.

If there is only one teacher in the room, a support person in the facility should be identified, at the very least, in the event of a safety issue or challenging behaviors – such as a violent outburst or an emotional flooding – and should remain nearby, within view. If a facility cannot provide a support person for the yoga class, a teacher should consider not teaching the class if safety is a concern.

A protocol for students who need special attention during or outside of class should be identified. This should occur in a confidential, non-judgmental manner. If the kind of help that is needed outside yoga class is beyond the skill set of the teacher, a referral should be provided. This may be a referral to therapists, lawyers, advocates, and/or doctors.

Best Practice
Educate yourself about vicarious trauma and burnout.

The work of intentionally engaging in trauma-informed practices and working with people who have experienced trauma can be triggering for teachers. Bringing the yogic principle of *ahimsa,* non-harming, to people who are vulnerable and open to retraumatization and reenactment behaviors can require teachers to put aside their own needs. By becoming aware of the signs of vicarious trauma and burnout, a trauma-informed teacher can learn much about boundaries and self-compassion. Tending to your own mental health outside work is an ongoing challenge and a professional requirement. Anyone teaching from their own trauma histories may be a very effective trauma-informed yoga teacher but should be encouraged to sustain therapy and to have a support circle of other professionals from which they can draw helpful, reflective, constructive observations, supervision, and support. Everyone working in this field should become familiar with their own triggers as well as their own symptoms of over-commitment and over-exposure to injustice and violence.

> We can try so hard to keep from hitting rock bottom that we feel exhausted from the effort. We may be so invested in minimizing and ignoring the many consequences of trauma exposure and proving that we are still up for any challenge that we push ourselves hard and harder. Instead of taking the break we need, we may take on another project or commit to another campaign – listening to our bodies is a direct way to gain insight.
>
> (van Dernoot Lipsky 2009: 83)

It is important to be familiar with the signs of vicarious trauma and burnout and to engage in ongoing self-inquiry regarding this topic. Isolation, diminished creativity, and despair are just some signs that a teacher has need of time away from trauma work. Finding substitute trauma-informed teachers for your students may be tricky but seeking them out in advance, as a precaution, is wise. Having a regular yoga practice has many benefits and, in this context, it provides a trauma-informed teacher with a good mirror. When that time for self-care is shortened, or avoided, everything becomes harder.

Developing Trauma-informed Classes

Best Practice
Care should be taken to identify appropriate student populations.

Teachers should explicitly identify what population they intend to teach, for example, teenage girls, survivors of childhood trauma, incest survivors, or trafficking survivors. Different populations have different needs. Mixing genders, ages, or any other types of cultural groups can lead to unanticipated, complicated, and potentially adverse dynamics. It may be wise to review ideas with a professional or experienced teacher to anticipate or avoid problematic outcomes. Each teacher will be drawn to a particular group for personal and professional reasons, but they will still require training for that group. All teachers should seek this specialty training, information, research, and direct experiences before teaching.

Once established in a teaching capacity, teachers must identify any exclusion criteria, for example, psychosis, substance abuse, frequent absences, suicide attempts, active suicidality, and/or dissociation. Using a referral process and forms can aide a teacher in preparing for a student on the mental health spectrum or in deciding not to teach a person. For example, psychosis and suicidality may be reasons for postponing someone's participation in a class. Dissociation, which can look like "spacing out" or inappropriate, withdrawing behavior, is a defensive strategy that many trauma survivors develop to deal with intolerable experiences. However, there are degrees of dissociation that may complicate or preclude participation. Questions of this nature must be discussed with a clinician and managed appropriately within that professional skill set. A teacher should not teach alone or extend boundaries into someone else's wheelhouse of expertise. Good, strong clinical referrals and transparency are critical. Safety of the teacher and other students relies upon collaborations such as the one between a yoga teacher and a clinician.

Once a group is established, teachers should be clear about whether or not participants are required to be in individual therapy with a professional while attending trauma-informed yoga classes. If students are required, it should be made explicit when and why the therapist would be contacted and, if indicated, a Release of Information should be obtained. The size of the group should be carefully chosen, keeping in mind that trauma-informed yoga classes often work best in groups that are smaller than typical yoga classes.

Ideally, the teachers should make every effort to arrange for accommodations to facilitate inclusion of any special needs, such as students with vision, hearing, or physical impairments. In private, teachers should inquire about students' preferred pronoun/s and then again with others in the group setting. A teacher can model gender awareness during introductions, identifying their own preference by stating name and preferred pronoun. Then, if they choose, students can introduce themselves, likewise. This process can help to create a culture of inclusion. Additionally, teachers should accommodate a student's cultural norms, such as clothing, head covering, definition of trauma and its management in another culture, relationship to authority or language barrier. If available, interpreters help increase fuller participation. To the extent that it is possible, teachers should stay current on culturally relevant pedagogy with regard to a specific population. For example, if classes are happening in an area where Somalian refugees have settled, or the student make-up is refugees, a teacher is wise to learn about refugee life and different cultures and co-cultures and to perhaps seek out a bilingual or multilingual advocate who can help educate and elucidate. This great need for improved cultural humility and available support to refugees varies widely, region to region; there is far less awareness of different cultures in rural areas. A rural teacher must dig deep.

> **Best Practice**
> Use invitational language that allows for choice.

Invitational language that facilitates choice making is a benchmark of a trauma-informed approach in all settings. Phrases such as "if you like" or "maybe you choose" are examples that allow for choice. While it may seem as though invitational language cannot offer clear, safe guidance, it does, in fact, place authority within the student to become aware of and independent in the choices they make for their own bodies. This can encourage a sense of competency, free-will, and, potentially, an internal sense of safety resulting from heightened self-awareness. A spoken invitation to students to make choices within a form, as in micro-movements, or to make a decision to do a whole different form can open a new path of healing through internal sensation, choice, and personal agency.

Language is likely the biggest adjustment for instructors to make in trauma-informed teaching. Using Sanskrit names of forms may cause confusion and move focus away from the internal. A best practice here is to use simple language, directed to body movements, with a calm tone and at a reasonable pace for each form. Below are some ways that language and the use of silence can influence tone, authority, and experiences in a classroom:

- Use of adjectives such as "slow" and "gentle" may be too directive for a student who needs a quicker pace or more high-pressure experience in a form. Adjectives also suggest that an experience is supposed to be a certain way.

- Choose the possessive pronoun "your" instead of the definite article "the" when referring to a part of the body. "Your arm" versus "the arm" versus "our arm." "Maybe you move your arm over your head" puts focus and authority within the student.

- Lengthy silences can potentially cause activation or hyperarousal of the central nervous system. Let students know how long silence will be. You can introduce it as an experiment with quiet and by keeping it brief, you can reduce the likelihood of disturbing imagery or body memory activation. As noted by Bessel van der Kolk (2006: 13), "if you are traumatized, being in silence is often terrifying. Memory of trauma is stored, so when you are stilled, demons come out."

- Invitational language examples include: "I invite you to …"; "If you would like to …"; or "If you feel ready …"; "In your own time …"; "As you are ready …"; "Maybe you'd prefer to try a different form …"; "If it works for you …"

- "Pose" or "position" can be loaded words for sexual trauma survivors, in general, as posing can be part of an abusive experience. It is recommended that the word "form" or "shape" be used instead.

- Avoid assumptions and phrases such as "You are safe here," "This room is safe," "You are grounded," or "This is healing."

- Avoid abstract descriptions, intangible imagery, or flowery language (for example, "Imagine yourself floating down a sea of compassion.") Such language distracts from each individual participant's internal, felt experience and may support disembodiment or confusion or may be experienced as triggering.

Consider the importance of body language. As a form of communication, a teacher's qualities are reflected in how they hold their bodies. Arms folded, leaning, slouching, or otherwise, an instructor's posture, stance, and general appearance are far more deeply studied by a group of survivors than what is said. Over time, a teacher who has gained practice and exposure to different groups of students will develop a personal and interpersonal way of communicating with diverse people through both spoken communication style and body language awareness.

Best Practice
Offer choices at every possible juncture.

Creating opportunities for students to make choices within their yoga practice reinforces their independence, agency, and relationship with their bodies. Trauma-informed teachers not only use invitational language and phrases such as, "You may want to try …" but they set an example by practicing with students while exercising their own choices within any given form. A teacher's visible practice of self-inquiry and choice-making can ensure that the choices offered are genuine. It is important to avoid options that imply a hierarchy of difficulty, mastery, or achievement, such as, "This way is more challenging." Even a phrase such as "if you can't do this form like this, then try that" can stymie a student's sense of competence, leaving them feeling that they cannot do it correctly.

Make allowances for choice-making in the session protocol. At the start of every class, it may be useful to remind students that they may choose where to set their mat, to not do a form, or that they are free to take breaks, to walk out, to not listen, to lie down, or to take other forms. If you are teaching in an institution where leaving the room is not possible, you can create a space in the room for non-participation or rest, or have an agreement with available staff who can come and go with students.

A trauma-informed teacher should be aware of their favorite forms, too, and avoid suggesting their positive experience with them. For example, child's form is often considered restful and is known for calming emotional flooding. However, it is a vulnerable form and may leave a student feeling insecure and unable to see their surroundings, let alone relaxed.

Unless students request this, avoid the demonstration of mastery of difficult forms. Sometimes younger students request demonstrations of challenging forms. One way to place the inquiry back onto them is to introduce a yoga deck of cards with illustrated figures of each form. See Figure 4.1.

This kind of prop – a card deck of yoga forms – gives them another way of choosing and establishing within themselves, a self-directed experience. This also supports a non-competitive environment, for the very reason that each person selects to create a different shape on the mat and lightens or deepens the pressure through the body – or selects to not do that form after all. We suggest using only illustrated decks versus pictures of real people to reduce the potential for competition with the photographed expert on the card.

Best Practice
Choose yoga forms and build sequencing with trauma awareness.

A yoga class should be crafted so that all can experience their own competence and meet their capacity for range of motion. Trauma can cause constriction in a person's body, mind, and spirit. This is often visible in the fear or caution that is expressed. It is also visible in posture. Offer arm movements that allow upper arms to remain near the torso. When offering leg movements, offer varieties that allow for large or small movements. Keeping forms simple and hold-times short, inviting curiosity and awareness in the forms, and using appropriate props, if available, can be vital ways to leveling the playing field in a classroom. Teach and model modifications of physical forms such as tree with kickstand or

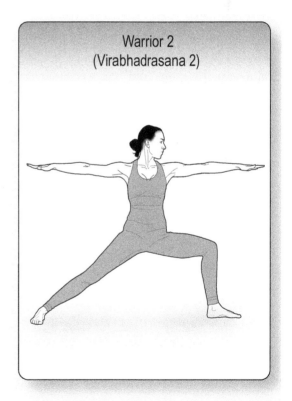

Warrior 2
(Virabhadrasana 2)

Figure 4.1
When using a yoga deck for choices, use drawn images of yoga postures versus photographs

airplane, with the back toe resting on the floor. Give options for more challenge, if indicated, but be careful to avoid suggesting that one version of a form is "better" than another.

Consider preparing modifications for each sequence or form in advance with certain contraindications and injuries in mind. Through traditional yoga teacher trainings, teachers often become familiar with physical forms that are typically difficult for survivors, forms that trigger, distress, or even retraumatize due to physical positioning or a participant's ability to see their surroundings. It is essential to create and maintain predictable and simple sequences, as students with trauma histories are often disembodied and may not know what they prefer or what is possible for them until they are in a form. A teacher's self-awareness, courage to change direction mid-class, and a regular personal yoga practice can help to cultivate a trauma-informed, accessible classroom.

When leading a class, a trauma-informed instructor practices the forms along with the students. Participants are made aware of the fact that no importance is placed on getting a form "right"; rather they are offered a chance to experience a form and to make modifications based upon what they feel or sense in their bodies. Students may choose to practice with their eyes open or closed. Letting students know what you are up to in your own practice with them can also be helpful. Through being transparent about what will happen, what is planned for class, a teacher should also let participants know that they can come out of any form at any time for any reason.

Best Practice
Allow for breath awareness; avoid breath manipulation.

Teaching breathing techniques aimed at managing the body's energy, pranayama, is part of most traditional yoga classes and a foundational aspect of yoga. But in trauma-informed yoga, consideration should be given to the potential impact of breathwork. For safety, consider using breath-awareness prompts, cues, or meditations, for example, "I invite you to notice your breath moving" or, "You're welcome to notice the pacing of your breath." Because of the intrinsic relationship between breath availability, anxiety, panic, and a fear-fueled response, a student can readily become uncomfortable and feel unsafe in some breathing exercises, for example, breath of fire or ocean-sounding breath instruction. Traditional pranayama techniques, including these examples, require the restriction, expansion, and control of the breathing muscles. A trauma-informed instructor must be aware that this can mimic or even trigger panic and hyperventilation.

It is recommended to simplify and begin to address breathing by not instructing its manipulation but by bringing attention to breath, and recognizing that even awareness may trigger someone who is actively struggling with breath. For many participants, there is utility in eventually working with deep, belly breathing as it is shown to pacify the central nervous system (Bordoni et al. 2018). However, the informed discretion of both the participant and instructor is key.

Best Practice
Use props for support.

Props are commonly used in yoga classes and, if offered with free choice in mind, students may begin to initiate a relationship with their bodies that is healthy and helpful.

Some trauma-informed classes are done solely in a chair, which provides universal stability for most people. If you do not start the class in chairs, you may leave several folded up for easy access. You can have a chair ready by your mat, for you to show them the use of the prop in a specific form.

It is helpful to have a teacher demonstrate the use of props; as well, it may be necessary for the teacher to go to a student and offer assistance with a prop. Always ask permission to come over to a student who is struggling to get into a form. Here are some ways to verbalize free-choice use of props:

"If you'd like support for sitting on the floor, you can use cushions and blocks."

See Figure 4.2.

"If you're experiencing pain or difficulty getting up and down off the floor, feel free to use a chair. I'll demonstrate the forms both in a chair and on the floor."

In this way, a person's capacity to learn how to care for themselves, support, and soothe through struggle within a form, can be improved by the careful use of props. The direct experience of physical discomfort and its relief cannot be underestimated. Less stable props such as straps, rubber bands, and poles should be eliminated from the room. They should be tucked out of sight, if possible, as they can provoke triggers of memories of being choked, bound, or memories of being trafficked, dancing, and the objectification, perversion, and sexualization of their bodies.

Best Practice

Clarify class structure and behavioral expectations.

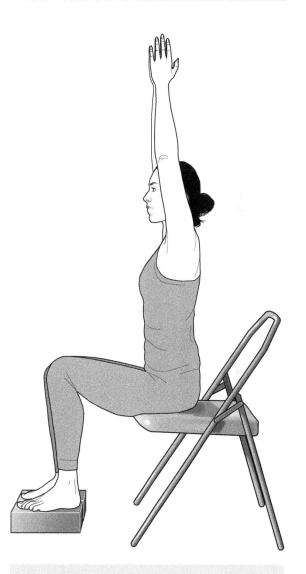

Figure 4.2

Try offering the use of blocks in chair yoga as an experiment with props, placing them under the feet. The blocks may support the spine and keep the sacrum from bearing more weight

Teachers should pay careful attention to program development and content of the class. It may be helpful to provide written material to each participant to enhance a sense of predictability, which is inherent to safety. State clearly whether the class composition is fixed or rolling, that is, whether it is a private group of participants, who are expected to attend a fixed number of sessions in a limited time, or if it is an open class for students to join in as they are able.

Teachers should explicitly address a confidentiality protocol with the students, stating that what is shared in class is private and not to be shared outside class. If this protocol is broken, it can be handled by the teacher, clinician – if present – along with the hosting studio or program. Confidentiality must be respected by teachers and modeled and upheld by them outside of class. This is the best practice for building privacy, respect, and trust.

As with teachers, students should be encouraged to wear clothing that is loose, comfortable, and non-revealing. Teachers can model this by dressing conservatively. While a teacher has little effect on what students choose to wear, it is a very personal choice, one can speak to the context of creating freedom of movement, suggesting different clothing choices in order to improve availability to yoga forms. This may have a positive effect on discernment and self-care. As well, addressing concerns over the use of perfumes, essential oils, even deodorant at the start of a series is wise. Having a "no scent" policy in writing and maybe a small reminder poster on the wall may help. Scents should be avoided at all times.

Teachers should be mindful of sticking to the schedule; having a clock, visible to teachers only, can provide a sense of predictability and control for all. It is often beneficial to set time aside for discussion and meditation, in addition to physical yoga forms. Teachers who consider leaving open periods of time for mindful transitions and explicit communication can develop a safer environment and a community of trust and responsiveness. The schedule and timing of the class is best established in advance and reviewed at the beginning of each class. Consistency and predictability in scheduling is important in a trauma-informed setting.

Best Practice
Encourage responsibility: absences, in-class behaviors, confidentiality, constructive feedback.

Cancellations and absences are inevitable. Inclement weather or illness of the teacher happen. There should be a plan in place for these events. The teacher's choice of communicating with studios, programs, and students should be made clear so that everyone knows where to get their information about the class. In the event of teacher absences, a program may have an appropriate substitute teacher to step in. Or a different plan may be used. Either way, it is important to alert students of this protocol.

Within a program, there should also be a clear protocol for when a student becomes routinely absent. In a private trauma-informed group, absences may be considered personal, self-directed choices not to continue with yoga and should not be taken personally and should not be punished. Being aware of requirements, site to site, such as those in a residential program, which will likely place a different emphasis on participation and absences, is critical. Each program or class setting will have a different set of intentions, if not goals. The teachers or programs should decide and be explicit about expectations for attendance and what happens if those expectations are not met, remembering that institutional expectations tend to differ greatly from those in a private group hosted by a facilitator.

Participants should always have an outlet for feedback, either formally or informally. A brief questionnaire given out to students after class to complete, if they want, may be helpful, with assurances that their answers will be received without harmful consequences. It is incumbent to not only elicit feedback but to actually incorporate it when feasible, so their reflections are put into effective action. Encouraging their voices and impacts on the yoga classes may not only serve the greater good of the group but may also help validate their experiences and authority over their bodies in the yoga class.

Location Considerations

Best Practice
Create a trauma-informed practice space.

When seeking a potential space to teach trauma-informed classes, consider some basic physical elements and accessibility. If you are looking to teach in an agency, residential, or institutional setting, you may need to make do with what is available. To ensure privacy and confidentiality, use shades or thick curtains in ground-level windows and close doors to the room for the class, so that those not participating will not watch the class.

It is important to consider accessibility. For students with physical disabilities and challenges, accessibility to a yoga classroom is key. A ramp and elevator are the most important modifications to hosting an inclusive class.

If a teacher would like to open a class for all abilities, then considerations about appropriate available spaces for students who may have a medical condition that makes ambulation difficult or who may use a wheelchair or crutches or who may have a service dog or an assistant must be made. This includes finding a space with restroom access. Public spaces such as the Young Men's Christian Association (YMCA), school gyms, or a veteran's administration conference room are some places to try. For a more detailed exploration of accessibility, we refer you to Chapter 11 of this book.

Privacy is optimal and particularly important for anyone hiding from an active abuser or a stalker. Understand that students may have a need to explore the safety of a room for themselves; allow them to do so. If there are closets in the room, allow students to look in them if desired. Someone who has experienced trauma or abuse may need to visually see that no one is behind a door or curtain. You can also offer to the class that you have checked all entrances and closets prior to setting up the class. Try to be explicit about the plan for heat and/or air conditioning (AC) and the need to compromise. Suggestions should be made for how to accommodate preferences, for example, placing a mat closer to the heat, or wearing layers.

Know the sounds of the building, know the room. Sounds in a room can often become distractions triggering hypervigilance or anxiety. The ticking of a clock, the constant hum of a generator, or a jarring heating system near the room can become unsettling. You may need to remove the clock for class. For sounds that cannot be controlled, you can alert people to the potential of routine sounds, such as routine fire drills, hospital announcements, and emergency alerts, or the outside sounds of police cars or fire trucks if you are located near a hospital or station.

Pictures and paintings, color and lighting should be considered. It is best to avoid pictures with mantras and words on them or portraits, as faces and eyes can bring up memories, projections of story, or emotions. In a setting with rows of fluorescent lights in the ceiling, you can shut off one or two rows to quiet the glare. Mirrors should be covered, when possible.

The room and equipment should always be kept clean; this should be communicated to the students. It should be made clear whether or not they are expected to clean the props that they use at the end of each class. This can enhance a sense of ownership, responsibility, and connection.

If you choose to play music, select something you will play each time. Playing the same track each week will become familiar and may bring focus and calm more quickly. By choosing instrumental music, you can avoid creating distraction about meaning and story-making related to lyrics. Instrumental music can be felt in the body without the mind's intrusions. Availability to embodiment is the intention of any trauma-informed yoga practice.

Arrange the room so that you are in the same place each class and preferably not right by the door. In some settings, the door is left open. In others, it is closed. Either way, allow students to come and go from class as needed, reminding them, each meeting time, that they are free to leave and to return as they need. In institutional settings, and particularly carceral settings, this permission is not always granted. A staff support person may need to leave with them or check on them, if too much time passes and they have not returned. It's helpful to know if staff or clinicians will be present, in advance of teaching; their presence and participation are strongly advisable in certain settings, as emphasized earlier in this chapter. Support staff may make for a safer trauma-informed practice space, but this may vary by context and population.

> [A] safe environment where I'm not always sort of watching ... created more of an atmosphere of being able to recognize things and feel what's inside ... the meditation aspect of the whole group situation and the whole safety situation made me sort of look at it and seeing what was in there ... instead of just trying to get rid of it.
>
> – Participant in trauma-informed yoga class
> (West 2011: 126)

Legal Considerations

Best Practice
Be clear and explicit with regard to legal issues that affect the structure of a trauma-informed yoga class.

Familiarize yourself with any laws that pertain to your state or setting that may affect your class population. Confidentiality is paramount to a sense of safety. There should be an explicit discussion regarding privacy and the sharing of information among participants. A verbal reminder before each meeting time or a written agreement should be elicited from each student.

As well, a simply written safety plan can be created for each student. Perhaps this can be co-written with a therapist, advocate, or program administrator. It should contain the name and information of an emergency contact and any other details that the student would like the teacher to know in the event of an urgent need. Both the teacher and student should retain a copy and be able to discuss and amend as needed. This information should be easily accessible; for example, by keeping it in a binder the teacher keeps the documentation portable and organized. It would be prudent to regularly remind the class to update any information as needed. A teacher who is teaching in a program such as a domestic violence shelter may not need to keep this information but should be made aware of it and any updates.

Much of the information gathered from a student falls under mandated reporting. Varying state to state, procedures for mandated reporting should be clarified. This should be discussed with each individual in an intake session and with the clinical support team or therapist. If a teacher would like to review any information with a provider or family member outside of the class, a signed Release of Information form should be obtained. The support and expertise of a clinical person or program administrator cannot be underscored enough. Address concerns and learn steps and your role in the process ahead of teaching, ahead of a crisis point.

Research and Program Evaluation

Best Practice

If data are being gathered for research, it must be done with confidentiality and participation should be voluntary.

If any aspect of the class is part of a research study this should be made clear in the initial recruitment of students. This should be reviewed once again at the onset of the initial screening process. Disclosures should be written in clear, simple language and reviewed with students. Time should be scheduled to answer any questions that may arise. All issues relating to confidentiality should be discussed. The possibility of "opting out" of being part of data collection once the class has begun should be offered and discussed. Being part of a study should always be voluntary. Participation in the class should not be contingent on participation in research. The participant should understand how the data will be collected, how confidentiality will be assured, and the purpose of the study. The student should be assured that their participation in the study, or lack thereof, will not affect their ability to be part of the class. If possible, the teacher should be blind to who is involved in the study and who is not, to avoid any unintentional bias in teaching.

Conclusion

Because sexually traumatic experiences can have lasting and broad-based impacts, the considerations in providing a trauma-informed approach to yoga may seem overwhelming. It is precisely because of trauma's far reaching impact that so much examination, preparation, and revision is required. We suggest that all instructors and/or studio owners and program administrators consider trauma-informed training to help provide a predictable and responsive environment. All teachers and organizations can assume that yoga sessions rooted in a trauma-informed approach are more inclusive of survivors. So prevalent in our society, trauma should be routinely considered in all yoga classes, not solely those classes labeled "trauma-informed."

Chapter 4

The desire to provide trauma-informed yoga must be followed by active learning and organizational adjustments as needed. For example, it is not uncommon for yoga studios to generate income and pay their teachers based on how many participants are in a given class. In general, a trauma-informed yoga class tends to have fewer numbers so as to reduce the likelihood of provoking anxiety and external focus. When a studio commits to offering trauma-informed yoga classes, they may need to adjust their business model to include, if not subsidize, these smaller class offerings. In the studio model, higher student numbers often equate to greater income; therefore, smaller, low-trigger classes may pose a challenge to this business model. When a studio owner decides to create a more trauma-informed space, offering skill-building training to yoga teachers, and making a fiscal plan to include smaller classes on the schedule, a more diverse population of people may begin to feel welcome. Such a studio can build a safe, inclusive building and group of classes, contributing to the healing of the greater community. Considerations for scholarships and sliding-scale fees can reduce financial barriers, too. The image of yoga studios as business-heavy enterprises, along with the image of the perfect yogi with a good income, may significantly change by becoming trauma-informed and may even invite donations and community collaborations.

The true pursuit of becoming trauma-informed is rife with considerations that have multi-layered impacts. A time-consuming endeavor, efforts to create trauma-informed experiences will likely bring challenges for many on personal and professional levels. But when we do not foster awareness of the impacts of trauma or build programming that is trauma responsive and universally inclusive, we run the risk of adverse responses and doing damage where we intend to help. The movement towards impactful inclusion in any community must have a trauma-informed approach.

Authors *Dani Harris and Amanda J.G. Napior*

Contributors *Keyona Aviles, Jacoby Ballard, Lisa Boldin, Alexis Donahue, Beth Jones, Sue Jones, Anneke Lucas, Pamela Stokes Eggleston, Rosa Vissers, Kimberleigh Weiss-Lewit, Ann Wilkinson*

Introduction

In one of his books, Zen Buddhist monk Thích Nhất Hạnh recounts a story about Saint Francis of Assisi, the thirteenth-century Christian friar. In the story, Francis comes upon an almond tree, in the dead of winter, and says, "Almond tree, tell me about God." The almond tree immediately blossoms into full flower. Here, Nhất Hạnh distinguishes between daily life, in which "the almond tree does not yet have flowers," and "the ultimate dimension," in which "the almond tree has had flowers for tens of thousands of years" (Nhất Hạnh 2006: 70–1). Nhất Hạnh shares this story in order to communicate his thought on the nature of time, reality, and the divine. For our purposes, this story invites us to notice how appearances can be deceiving or may tell only partial truths. With a strengths-based approach to yoga for survivors of sexual trauma, we invite practitioners to see everyone as brilliant and unbroken. Those who have experienced trauma may well know that wholeness and beauty can unfold alongside pain and suffering, even in the dead of winter. We can honor the resilience of those we serve by being clear that sexual trauma does not define anyone. The misapprehension that it does can rob students of the opportunity to access their own empowerment. At the same time, we share the burden of others' pain by recognizing it, refusing to look away, and being able to see healing and growth as ever in process.

In this chapter, we invite you to consider a range of issues that have a broad impact on one's capacity to offer yoga to people who have experienced sexual trauma, starting with an invitation to take a strengths-based approach to offering care. While we address some best practices specifically to teachers, we hope these practices will be helpful to a diverse range of service providers and agencies seeking to integrate yoga programs into their organizations. These best practices, together with those from the preceding chapter, stand as a foundation to the rest of the text. Subsequent chapters supplement our recommendations with ones tailored to working with survivors of the specific contexts of sexual trauma. Like one's own yoga practice, developing capacities and skills to better care for those impacted by sexual trauma can be a lifetime practice of ongoing learning and growth.

A Strength-based Resilience Approach

In working with survivors of trauma, it is essential to behold an individual's survival strategies as tools that are worthy of respect and celebration. Acknowledging that everyone present has carefully tailored survival skills that meet their needs as both assets and strengths allows people the opportunity to be seen. Seeing a survivor's strength creates the groundwork for increased resilience that, when accompanied by yoga, grows with an increased sense of grounding, ease, and self-trust. Strengths-based resiliency alters well-established paradigms of contemporary yoga. Seeing strengths rather than injuries shifts the view of seeing traumatized individuals as having psychological damages or hurts that need mending to individuals having a set of fine-tuned survival skills that have kept them from more significant harm. It gives voice to previously unheard or unrecognized skills one had to create in response to trauma and calls upon the skills as invaluable strengths.

There is space for traditional trauma-informed yoga to move from the premise that people who have experienced sexual trauma are at a considerable disadvantage in comparison to those who have not. As such, there is a growing need for practitioners to understand that everyone has a unique opportunity to encourage resilience based on strengths and capacity. Yoga encourages this capacity-building when it draws from an individual's successes rather than catering to perceived deficits.

We have a precious opportunity here to illuminate with vast spaciousness the inner resources that people bring to a yoga session. Shining a light on strengths connects people to the core of their resilience; when shared with a community, this resilience grows.

Readers may notice that many of the best practices that follow pertain to areas of awareness to cultivate, more so than to discrete actions to practice or to avoid. We invite you to notice how these best practices assert themselves as challenges to growth and learning edges, as well as perhaps reflect areas of strength in which you already reside.

On Language

Best Practice
Be mindful that some people who have experienced sexual violence do not like the term "survivor."

Experience is complex and particular. We use the word "survivor" in this book because many people who have experienced sexual trauma embrace the term and find it descriptive and validating of their experiences. Others, however, do not.

Best Practice
Use gender-neutral language throughout any yoga session.

Be mindful of the language you use to address students in your class. Choosing gender-neutral language not only helps to create an atmosphere of acceptance; when people feel included, they can work towards their full potential in their yoga experience.

Best Practice
Use non-coercive language and modeling.

Be aware that coercion can have many subtle forms. This subtlety can look like suggesting or illustrating ways of engaging that are acceptable or unacceptable, by affirming that among options of choices offered in a class, some are superior to others ("more advanced yogis will…"). Keep in mind that these subtle coercions can reinforce shame.

Best Practice
Be mindful of words that are likely to be triggering for many survivors of sexual trauma.

The authors of *Best Practices for Yoga with Veterans* note that "'being triggered' is part of the pattern of physiological disequilibrium produced by a traumatic experience." Yoga teachers working with people who have been impacted by trauma can minimize potential triggers by adapting standard teaching practices (Horton, et al. 2016: 20). This includes choosing not to use words that have an increased likelihood of triggering survivors of sexual trauma. For example, consider using the words *shape* or *form* instead of *pose*, which may be triggering for people who have been sex trafficked. Also consider not referring to form names with easily sexualized rhetoric, such as *downward-facing dog*.

Best Practice
Understand the contemporary and historical perpetuations of trauma for many that have been pathologized by society at large or in clinical settings.

Understand that common diagnoses of PTSD or complex post-traumatic stress disorder (C-PTSD) have definitional limitations that are too narrow to account for history. Yoga teachers might consider studying how historical trauma affects whole populations as an important aspect of their trauma-informed learning. Recognize that we often think of trauma in terms of psychological diagnoses, which are for individuals. But trauma is also collective. Further, even some individual diagnoses first developed out of gendered or racist understandings of entire populations. "Hysteria," for example, was considered women's pathology during the founding of psychoanalysis.

Teach and Learn with Trauma and Resilience in Mind

Best Practice
Foster consistency in your own practice by selecting studios and teachers wisely.

Trauma survivors can foster consistency, safety, and their own resilience, by learning about the culture of any given yoga studio, as well as by seeking out teachers who are a good fit for their needs. Consider asking the studio owner which instructors might be most appropriate, and who is trained in trauma-informed yoga. You may find that attending only one studio, rather than many, will foster this consistency. Note also that some online yoga purchasing platforms can work counter to this aim, by omitting pathways to student–teacher communication or student community. Take care not to sacrifice safety in exchange for a discounted price.

Best Practice
Teach to the resilience in people.

Teaching to people's resilience means meeting people where they are and partnering with them on their journey. Resilience is the ability to recover quickly from life's challenges. Support people in channeling the strength they cultivated in the midst and aftermath of trauma, toward healing. Listening and asking questions is one way of learning how to meet people where they are. You might ask a student how they responded to the prior class, or ask how you can work together to create the best experience for them. Remember to "teach the person, not the form." The human capacity for recovery and healing is vast. Help people cultivate this capacity by offering tools that develop the "felt sense" of embodiment, or interoception, as well as by providing choices and truly embracing their decision making, over your own.

Best Practice
Be aware of the prevalence and variety of sexual trauma.

Chapter 5

We invite you to prioritize trauma theory over yoga theory. Your classes will include both those who have experienced sexual trauma in the past, as well as those currently experiencing some form of sexual violation. Teach with this in mind, incorporating trauma-informed practices in all settings. Know also that sexual trauma takes many forms and that individual responses vary. After experiencing traumatic experiences, the body of a survivor registers a threat to survival where one may not exist. The range of impacts from such an experience depends on many factors, including an individual's circumstances before, during, and after the event occurred. Through deepening your understanding of the contexts in which sexual violence occurs, and of trauma theory and practice, your ability to encourage participant resilience will only grow.

> **Best Practice**
> Establish a firm grounding in how trauma impacts the brain and body, and how they can heal.

Resilience and trauma are directly linked. Understanding how the brain responds to traumatic experiences, the somatic imprint of trauma, and how embodied practices can support healing will help you teach with trauma and resilience in mind. In the context of a sexually traumatic event, people often experience dissociation, which can be an experience of "leaving your body." Those who have experienced abuse spanning long periods of time may be more predisposed to dissociation than others. It is a neurobiological adaptation the body creates to protect itself from the immediate psychic threat of trauma. Trauma-informed yoga is but one embodied practice that can facilitate healing. With an understanding of the process of dissociation and how somatic work can help heal trauma, one can develop programming that supports healing. See Chapter 2 for a thorough discussion of the neurobiology of trauma.

> **Best Practice**
> Insist on your own continuing education.

If you are a yoga instructor, learn about the context in which you are working, and receive appropriate training from the organizations through which you serve (such as shelters and prisons). This will increase your capacity to serve. If you are a service provider, insist that yoga instructors offering care in your setting should go through training. Having the best intentions is not necessarily enough. Ongoing learning will help you stay abreast of the growing field of trauma-informed yoga service, as well as energize you as you undertake this inherently difficult work. Seeking continuing education at the intersection of yoga, trauma, systemic violence, and the settings in which you're teaching should be a top priority.

> For years, my therapy involved only regulating my brain. I felt as though I was not making any progress because the somatic experience of simply being alive was interfering so greatly and so devastatingly in my daily life. Ultimately, for this, I was stuck in an endless cycle of some recovery followed by a crashing relapse. It wasn't until I started understanding my somatic experience, most of which happened through yoga, that I realized one part of me could not be healed separately from the other. The whole self had to be integrated, regularly for any healing to take place.
> – Trauma-informed yoga student, sexual trauma survivor

Practice Care in How You Represent and Relate to Survivors

> **Best Practice**
> Be aware that sexual trauma does not define someone.

Each of us has many identities and ways of being in the world. Sexual violence is something that has *happened* to survivors, but it does not define who they are.

> **Best Practice**
> Do not assume anything about the student, except that they deserve respect and care – it is impossible to know everyone's whole story.

These stories require time and trust. Nurture what understanding you do receive, so that other parts may be gradually recognized.

> **Best Practice**
> Recognize dominant narratives about "success" that shape your expectations for what trauma recovery looks like – reset them.

This practice is two-fold. First, we come to this work knowing that post-traumatic growth is possible, and the joy we take in our work comes in part from witnessing it. Be patient, keeping in mind that transformation takes time, may not be visible to the facilitator, and does not always reflect societal norms of success.

> **Best Practice**
> Be intentional about the degrees to which you self-disclose or share your trauma history.

Even when we share no personal information, simply interacting with others with mindful, compassionate attention is one way of sharing oneself with another. In crafting relationships with students, yoga instructors should be mindful of how greater degrees of self-disclosure may be helpful or, alternately, harmful. Keep in mind that sharing your trauma history has the potential to be troubling and confusing for students. With discretion, this could forge a powerful connection, however. This level of sharing should only happen after reflecting on the reason behind your self-disclosure, and its possible impacts on others.

Make Self-reflection an Ongoing Practice

> **Best Practice**
> Reflect upon why you want to offer yoga service to survivors of sexual trauma.

Inquiring into your reasons for doing any work can help enrich the experience for yourself and those you serve. Doing so when working with survivors of sexual violence makes this a necessity. New and experienced teachers alike can be excellent facilitators of yoga for sexual trauma survivors. For new teachers, we wish to emphasize that the *need* to build experience is *not* an acceptable reason to offer survivors yoga. New teachers with a clear motivation can, however, be among the best equipped to do this work.

> **Best Practice**
> Consider how privilege has shaped your life.

We all come from somewhere, with various access to resources. What kind of privileges have your life circumstances afforded you or withheld? We bring our experiences with us into our encounters with others and they, into their encounters with us. Making an honest assessment of your relation to privilege can help you to recognize inherent power dynamics and to navigate (or diffuse) them in ways that are not harmful. This best practice is closely related to the next.

Recommendations for Further Reading on Intersectionality and Privilege

Developing awareness of our own social location is an ongoing practice. Consider the following readings as possible companions in the journey.

Alexander M (2012) The new Jim Crow: Mass incarceration in the time of colorblindness, New York, NY: The New Press.

Baptist EE (2014) The half has never been told: Slavery and the making of American capitalism, New York, NY: Basic Books.

Crenshaw K (1991) Mapping the margins: Intersectionality, identity politics, and violence against women of color. Stanford Law Review 43 (6) 1, 241–1299.

DiAngelo R (2018) White fragility: Why it's so hard for white people to talk about racism, Boston, MA: Beacon Press.

Flaherty J (2016) No more heroes: Grassroots challenges to the savior mentality, Chico, CA: AK Press.

hooks b (2015) Feminist theory from margin to center, New York, NY: Routledge.

Johnson M (2017) Skill in action: Radicalizing your yoga practice to create a just world, Portland, OR: Radical Transformation Media.

Magee R (2019) The inner work of racial justice: Healing ourselves and transforming our communities through mindfulness, New York, NY: TarcherPerigee.

Margolin M (1997) The Ohlone way: Indian life in the San Francisco – Monterey Bay area, Berkeley, CA: Heyday.

Moraga C and Anzaldua G (2015) This bridge called my back: Writings by radical women of color, 4th edn, Albany, NY: SUNY Press.

Oluo I (2018) So you want to talk about race? New York, NY: Basic Books.

Peacock J (2018) Practice showing up: A guidebook for White people working for racial justice, Louisville, KY: Jardana Peacock.

Thompson BW (2001) A promise and a way of life: White antiracist activisim, Minneapolis, MN: University of Minnesota Press.

Best Practice
Recognize how we are interconnected and each of us, multiple.

Legal theorist Kimberlé Crenshaw coined the term "intersectionality" in the late 1980s to name how each of us sits at a crossroads of identities and embodiments (race, gender, class, and so on). This does not only mean that we are luminously complicated (although that's true, too). It also means that systemic oppression hits some much harder than others. Even sexual trauma advocacy work has often spoken for one group at the expense of others. Recognize the various identities or embodiments you inhabit. How are the people you serve similarly or differently constituted? What do these similarities and differences mean for how others perceive you and you, them? Ideally, the person offering the yoga service, in any setting, is the one who shares multiple kinds of context and identity with the students. Where this is not possible, a person who brings honesty and self-awareness about their motivations for serving can be an asset.

Making Spaces

> ### Best Practice
> Go for brave spaces rather than safe ones.

It is not always possible to create, let alone promise, a completely safe space. But we can do our best. We can allow people to choose their own location to practice, when possible. We can cover windows or door openings when appropriate and requested. Knowing that we cannot impede all possible threats or triggers, we still have an obligation to do what we can. In addition to making spaces as safe as possible, we can intend to create *braver* spaces. You can implicitly or explicitly acknowledge the risks, precarity, and vulnerability of being human and possibly the dangers of the setting in which you are teaching. Emphasize choice, in spite of these. Emphasizing the bravery of a space may allow the meaning of *safe space* to change, from one about the inviolable nature of a room or one's body, to a growing bodily capacity for interoception and choice, as well, perhaps, of a growing sense of oneself as more than a physical body. Discovering that

one's own locus of control is not bound by other people happens on the margin of bravery and safety.

> ### Best Practice
> Consider that your classroom could become a refuge; craft it.

Your classroom may become a place where survivors of sexual trauma experience feelings of safety for the first time. With conscientiousness and care, you can help craft this experience. Real-time, felt experiences of safety can be deeply transformational for survivors, especially when the experience recurs. Aim to keep your own behavior and your classes as consistent and predictable as possible. Consistency and predictability help survivors feel safer in their bodies. When repeated, these experiences help create positive associations and embodied experience that can be built upon.

> ### Best Practice
> Learn to hold space.

Holding space is a practice of acceptance, non-judgment, non-attachment to outcome, and selective action. You can learn acceptance and non-judgment with yourself by witnessing, embracing, and releasing emotions and thoughts that arise. Likewise, you can listen to and witness how others show up. In a group setting, you let go of attachment to outcome by allowing people to feel what they are feeling and to adjust their own behavior as needed, as well as by taking action selectively. One of us has a colleague who taught a group class in which one person violated a physical boundary of another, by moving their chair too close. The facilitator had to make an adjustment in order to address the violation, while not coming across as a power figure. Holding space for everyone involved a delicate and dynamic balancing act. Your inner resources will only deepen as you develop these skills, in which we all have much room to grow. Creating and holding space for survivors of trauma can help them become comfortable and to reconnect with their bodies.

> **Best Practice**
> Understand that there is a process to having someone trust the process.

For many survivors of sexual trauma, the very person(s) they trusted most were the ones who violated them. *Not* trusting people may have become an adaptive strategy. Recognize that someone not trusting you is not personal. Rather, practice mindful acceptance (as above). Do not try to rush a sense of comfort or connection with students. Keep in mind that this foundation of trust builds over time and that you cannot always see it happening.

Be Accountable to Your Students and a Community of Practitioners

> **Best Practice**
> Have mentors and mentorship programming.

The importance of mentorship keeps teacher mentors and teacher mentees on top of their original intentions for sharing yoga.

If a teacher lives in an isolated area with little to no support or local organizations, they can work to develop partnerships with local mental health providers, human service agencies, or behavioral health organizations. Joining an organization in a different location as an affiliate for support and consultations can bring an isolated teacher to a larger network of teachers doing the same work and exposure to a variety of models. It is important to have a support system in place – peers, therapist, if needed, a yoga community. No one can or should do this work in isolation.

> **Best Practice**
> Develop community and self-management through peer supervision, professional conscious relationship, and mentorship.

We create strong communities when there are high levels of transparency and professional conscious relationships. First, seek out ways to receive feedback on your teaching (peer review, peer supervision, and so forth), and, if necessary, find opportunities for mentorship within the field of trauma-informed yoga. Second, to create safer yoga spaces and offerings, yoga teachers need to be transparent with one another, creating professional conscious relationships. We all have blind spots. A community that holds space for open and honest communication will thrive. We need to be able to check in with one another when it comes to breaches, horizontally and honestly, without judgment. Yoga is shared through community; we cannot work in isolation. Developing community not only keeps our spaces as safe as possible but also creates safety for our practitioners and our teachers.

> **Best Practice**
> Know both your own scope of practice, as well as the scope of your offering.

Be clear about the scope of the service you're offering. If you are a yoga instructor, remember that your role is to teach yoga. The focus on your role allows you, as a trauma-informed yoga instructor, to help students build upon their strengths and gain tools in the context of the yoga practice. You can refer out when you feel another's input and service would be in the best interests of the person you are serving. Build relationships with other professionals in and beyond the setting of your practice, so that you can refer out when needed. Do not take on more than what you are offering.

Best Practice
Recognize the value of collaboration.

Be in community with others doing similar work. Fellow practitioners and service providers are an accountability network whose support can help you take care of yourself and others. If you are a teacher, consider team-teaching. This collaboration can be fun and supportive, as well as an opportunity to model conscious relationship (please refer to Chapter 1). Identify people in your service setting who also serve your students/clients and consider working as a team. Individual teachers and small yoga organizations should seek out other organizations doing similar work in the same geographic area. Aligning and working with others inside and beyond your setting of service can help you focus your resources in the interest of providing the best possible teaching. Further, this community of support will introduce you to colleagues willing to help you identify your strengths and blind spots. Together, you can support one another in your growth and self-awareness.

Best Practice
Develop consistent and reliable systems of checks and balances to ensure minimal power imbalances.

Consider the components of your programming and whether they are going to support current power imbalances or take control away from your students and relinquish control from your practitioners. Regularly take time to evaluate your teaching practices through the lens of power. Consider whether or not there are ways that power dynamics and imbalances can be lessened or shifted.

Best Practice
Develop and maintain self-care practices.

Working with survivors of sexual violence affects everyone differently; having practices that support one's own needs is necessary to remain grounded and present in this work. For further discussion of self-care in the context of boundaries, or *relational wisdom*, see Chapter 6.

Create a Responsive, Collaborative Classroom

Best Practice
Reexamine student–teacher dynamics that emphasize deference, in order to minimize the power disparity between facilitator and participants.

While this may be a general best practice for working with those impacted by trauma, consider it especially pertinent to those who have experienced sexual violence. Opt for a model of teaching that cultivates self-empowerment rather than one of deference to the teacher. You can do this by providing frequent opportunities for students to engage in conversations about their practices and by letting them be the experts in their own experience. Doing so will help create spaces of transparency, co-created safety, and collaboration.

Best Practice
Offer an orientation for participants before the program, when possible.

Use an orientation as an opportunity to introduce people to the practices you will be offering and what participants can expect from classes. Do not assume that people in the contexts where you work have any understanding whatsoever of yoga. Consider explaining even the little things. For example, will your classes use music? Why or why not? Offer context for what will happen in class, and ensure that elements can be changed or omitted if students find things unhelpful or uncomfortable.

Best Practice
Make good on your promise to co-create a responsive classroom.

If someone is feeling triggered in class and voices their discomfort, the teacher needs to follow through on the promise for a responsive classroom. See how you can find a creative solution, together, or simply meet their request if it is reasonable. If the lights are too dim, brighten the room. When beginning yoga programs with consistent membership, you can use the beginning of the first session to frame your time together more deliberately. Even in drop-in classes, however, teachers can explain what they mean by a responsive classroom and invite students to create it with them.

Best Practice
Forecast sensation and normalize diverse experiences.

Yoga instructors should use language that normalizes new sensations or the absence of sensation. Name sensations that might arise from certain practices, while leaving room for students to experience any number of different things. Assure that all feelings are valuable while leaving space for students to have their experience. Refrain from assuming students' experiences. For example, meditation is not always peaceful, a stretch is not always pleasant, the body and emotions are not always full of vim and vigor but rather may feel heavy, angry, and sad.

Best Practice
Build in opportunities to debrief at the end of class for reflection and feedback.

Yoga students practicing in studios will usually have a chance to ask questions or voice feedback after class – especially if the instructor makes such an invitation known. Some settings, like youth residences or prisons, however, may not allow for this kind of access to a teacher. In such a context, consider designating the last segment of class for discussion and feedback. Debriefing enables students to ask questions that may not have come up earlier and reinforces the reciprocity of the student–teacher relationship. Debriefing also gives the teacher the opportunity to ask questions or make observations.

Feedback goes both ways. If you are teaching in a facility where being in touch with students outside of class is not possible, ask the organization hosting you about appropriate ways for you to be available. Abide by all rules of confidentiality prescribed by the facility. Be clear on what your availability entails.

Best Practice

Learn the skills to decrease activation in students and gain the skills to help individuals navigate through the experience of activation with a sense of agency.

Learning to navigate feelings of being activated by a traumatic memory is key to recovery. Embed in your curriculum frequent inflection points where students are redirected to predictable practices that support grounding, breath, and orientation to the present moment.

Conclusion

As discussed above, there is a greater need for all spaces where yoga is practiced to be trauma-informed. Undoubtedly, every class will have someone impacted by sexual trauma. As such, it is our collective responsibility to ensure our spaces are as safe as possible. Trauma-informed teaching practices that offer a sense of orientation, containment, predictability, and flexibility gives voice to survivors of trauma, and can reconnect them to themselves and community. Lastly, teaching to people's strengths offers all participants the chance to build capacity for greater groundedness, self-understanding, self-trust, and increasing resilience, on and off the mat.

Relational Wisdom: Self-care, Boundaries, Compassionate Leadership, and Cultural Humility

6

Author *Kimberleigh Weiss-Lewit*

Contributors *Keyona Aviles, Maya Breuer, Regine Clermont, Dani Harris, Diana Hoscheit, Mark A. Lilly, Jana Long, Amanda J.G. Napior, Austin Sanderson, Nicole Steward, Rosa Vissers, Ann Wilkinson*

Compassion is not a relationship between the healer and the wounded. It's a relationship between equals.

(Chödrön 2007: 64).

Introduction

The project of this chapter is to address how to cultivate self-care practices, appropriate teacher–student boundaries, and cultural humility in the context of supporting survivors of sexual trauma through yoga. Here, we suggest that the cultivation of *relational wisdom* may support our learning process of how to be in these right relationships with self and others. *Relational wisdom* is a term that Rev. Dr Emily Click, Harvard Divinity School, professor and United Church of Christ pastor, uses to express how to develop self-awareness and discernment while navigating complex power dynamics and multiple kinds of relationships. She often uses this term instead of the word *boundary*, in order to express a more capacious, and, at times, flexible, understanding of that separation between you and me (Click 2014). While the authors of this book find the word *boundary* helpful and

often indispensable to our discussion, we also find Click's insight important: sometimes the image of a boundary – as in a wall or impassable barrier – is not the most helpful way to imagine our relationships with others. For this reason, we frame our discussion with Click's term, in order to recognize that cultivating self-care, appropriate boundaries, and cultural humility is an endeavor in *wisdom*.

We find it imperative to explore a relational idea of the self, as at once contained and interconnected. Today, the human person is often regarded as a neatly bound entity, self-sufficient and independent. In a culture that holds up this kind of person as a paragon of success, we ask: might we strive to encompass diverse configurations of family and community in our notion of self-care? At the same time, can we insist on a kind of self-care that supports the self that so cares for others, with practices of self-love, nourishment, and the willingness to know one's limits (like saying "no")?

A student of yoga and contributor to this project who wishes to remain anonymous generously offered a window into her experience:

Case study

These days, I have a strong sense of my own boundaries. I did not use to. This growth has come about from a variety of factors. But at the top of the list is my yoga practice, without which I would not be

the person I am today. Developing a clear sense of boundaries – in relationship to others; to time commitments; to my creaturely needs for nourishment and sleep; to my desires for connection, for pleasure,

continued

and belonging; to the causes I am willing to struggle for; and to the struggles in which I only need permission to stop – is not a finished endeavor nor one in which I have always taken a straight path. But in the process, I have grown and become wiser.

I remember a certain evening, twelve years ago, as if it were yesterday. Class had just come to a close, in a studio where I only took my first class, a month before. People were rolling up their mats, filing out. What was going on, in my head, was the weirdest thing: nothing in particular. I was so accustomed to anxiety. Loud, vocal anxiety. Thoughts somersaulting over one another to vie for my attention. Instead, nothing. This "nothing" was not a dull absence. I could feel a palpable aliveness in my entire being. The moment sang, softly, with a hopeful sense of the possible. That evening was the beginning of my yoga journey and the beginning of healing from debilitating anxiety that I had not yet recognized partially stemmed from multiple sexual assaults.

This moment is a key one, for me, as I reflect upon how yoga has helped me construct a healthy sense of boundaries – or, in the language of this chapter, how yoga has helped me become more relationally wise.

First starting in high school with one boy and then with a number of men in college (I stopped counting the number), my use of the word "no" was repeatedly ignored and my physical actions to deny someone's advances, denied. I never left an encounter with bruises or had what I could identify as a "fight," and so I did not recognize my encounters as assault. That would take years. What I recognized instead (or, rather, what I mistook for the truth) was that my own desires, for careful, loving touch or for threatening advances to stop, were unreliable, at best, and, at worst, invalid. This perverse learning resulted mentally in the tendency to second-guess myself, nonstop (hence, anxiety); it manifested relationally and physically as losing a sense of integrity to my being. I lost a sense of where I ended and others began, which often meant both over-extending myself to help others while simultaneously being unable to take responsibility for myself. Spiritually, these experiences hindered my capacity to trust: myself, others, or the very unfolding process of my life. Who I belonged to, what I owed others, what they owed me, the validity of my hopes and aspirations, were all a confusion. The parts that made me up were constantly tumbling in the wind.

Sexual trauma results from boundary violation. We yoga providers must keep this awareness central, in considering appropriate teacher–student boundaries, and remembering that, at all times, people have a right to refuse consent, withhold their story, and step back from this work. Some boundaries need to be clear, hard lines, in order to affirm a practitioner's and survivors' integrity. Sometimes, the boundaries in question are not protective enough for survivors or people at risk of victimization. Other times they are too restrictive, inhibiting a process of healing. In any case, we may notice how the boundaries we set can directly relate to the creation of power dynamics, in facilitating both group and individual yoga experiences. Through our work, we must ask: What are appropriate boundaries in *this* context and in *this* relationship? How can we recognize when supporting someone calls for firmer boundaries? How can we ensure that we listen in ways that recognize and respect when others are creating boundaries for *us*? We have a tremendous opportunity and a responsibility to model and guide boundaries for our students, as well as to learn them from our students.

In these challenging times, we are also wrestling with fatigue in connection to issues of human rights and abuses of power. We need spaces for ourselves and others that are safe and healing. We may ask: "How can we create local and intimate communities as a refuge from stress while refusing to deny larger systemic trauma?" The very act of re-learning how to be in community with one another takes work, practice, and guidance. Much of the dysfunction that we are trying to address through trauma-informed yoga is the breakdown of healthy community, which has been created by systemic and structural components of the societies in which we live – like hegemonic capitalism, patriarchy, whiteness, and racism. Together, these structures have created isolation – as well as this idea of the person as an independent, bound self – that move us away from relational wisdom, cultural humility, and care of self and others. Perhaps we can consider that community is who is in front of us at the moment. Can this approach make space to care for yourself and them in that moment? This best practices book is a statement in itself. We strive to explore and shine light on how we show up in the world, how to do deep and challenging work, and how to continue to return to resilience and love for ourselves and the people we serve. *It takes a village to heal a village.*

Best Practices
In Pursuit of Cultural Humility

Best Practice

Shift focus from cultural competency to cultural humility.

We are asking if we might shift from a goal of "cultural competency" to a process of cultural humility. The term "cultural competence" implies an unattainable ideal; it can be a red herring, as no one can claim full competence in a culture, especially one that is different from their own (Lee 2011). Cultural humility, on the other hand, speaks to the fluidity and evolution of one's understanding of a particular culture/subculture or cultures/subcultures (Fisher-Borne, et al. 2014).

How we engage with the ways we are different from one another can be fundamental in creating possibilities for authentic relationship. Cultural humility and awareness is a practice – one that requires ongoing personal accountability and an inquiry approach to connection and understanding. Every human culture is unique and multifaceted. For those who have survived sexual trauma, the experience of surviving can become part of their self-defined culture – they may identify as a *survivor* and with other *survivors*. For those who have faced or are facing institutional – and often dehumanizing – trauma and for providers working with institutional barriers, cultural humility creates possibilities for human-to-human connection and healing focused on true inclusion and respect for diversity.

Best Practice

Wait for invitation into the communities you seek to serve.

One should understand that the first step to service in any community is to establish yourself in the community before doing work. Genuine, authentic, mutual relationship is primary. Different settings, such as a prison setting, may make invitation directly by the community to be served impossible, but invitation can also be subtle – how are the people you are serving receiving you and your offering? Have you connected with and made yourself open to learning from genuine, local leadership within the community to understand how you might serve this community? When communicating with a community and its local leadership/elders, seek to understand the communication manner that suits their needs and preferences. For example, one contributor to the project reminded us that their Indigenous elders do not appreciate being emailed; rather a face-to-face discussion is culturally appropriate.

Best Practice
Seek to create programming that is sustainable within the community and brings students back to their culture.

We have a responsibility to educate ourselves on cultural understandings, totems, teachings, and ceremony. Especially for youth who are generational survivors of historical trauma, this can support them in connecting to their heritage. For example, in an Indigenous culture that centers teachings around a medicine wheel one might co-create a practice that takes into account the significance of the four directions (north, south, east, west) and the teachings related to each compass point (Katzman 2018).

Best Practice
Recognize that yoga may not be the first or most appropriate trauma-informed offering in the community you are in relationship with – the community may have their own healing practices that can be uplifted.

We believe in the power of trauma-informed yoga to heal; however, we also recognize there are *many* healing practices. As you build relationships in communities you are serving look for opportunities to use your power to seek funding and support for healing practices and healers within the community. Be willing to invite figures from the community to work with you in the capacity that suits them and pay them for their knowledge accordingly. You may also create a resource list of people, organizations, and healing modalities in the community you serve and seek to make connections with those on your list.

Best Practice
Recognize when you are not the right person to serve and respect the wisdom of the elders, teachers, and mentors both serving the community and within the community.

Through honest self-assessment and feedback from those you serve, consider if another person or organization can better serve the individual or community. If so seek to support and lift up leaders who are better suited. Recognize that sometimes you may need to serve while building new leadership and supporting emerging leaders to take over from you when the time is right. Always use your position and power to open doors for others and more effective providers. How can you close gaps on leadership?

One might:

- Support students to lead portions of the practices and look to offer training (yoga and otherwise) to those within the community.

- Build leadership within the class, through giving everyone agency and choice.

- See what and who is already there – every community has leaders/healers but they may not have your access or resources. Please look in the community, see who is already doing work, and use your power to support them.

- Consult cultural leaders about co-creating practices that both acknowledge and relate to its members in the wake of historical/intergenerational trauma.

- Consider that recent graduates of Yoga Teacher Training (YTT) are often encouraged to offer yoga service while gaining teaching experience. Instead of going into an unfamiliar community, and offering novice skill for free, new teachers may need to practice in their own/familiar community. It is not acceptable to experiment with novice skill on an underserved population.

Best Practice
Be aware of the cycles of systemic oppression that you may be replicating in your efforts to serve.

When working with people who have been systematically oppressed and taken advantage of, be mindful you do not do the same. In our work, we are mindful of any dynamic that appropriates people or focuses on the "exotic other." See each person who attends or supports your class or program as an individual, one who is likely making sacrifices to attend. Consider how to best recognize class participants, community leaders, and staff appropriately.

Consider opportunities to change the system through intentional action:

- How can people be compensated for their time either with money or creative, culturally sensitive currency? For some sexual abuse

survivors, cash may be triggering – consider giving another currency/gift (subway cards, gift cards, services, and so on).

- Give space for people to say "no" and listen to their refusal (both verbal and nonverbal).

- Women are historically paid less, as are "women's work"/service and caregiver roles. Push back against objectification of women.

- Consider hiring practices. Representation matters as does diversity but do not over-tap the same people for all tasks – it can be taxing on the individual. Expect that all people need adequate time and resources for self-care.

- Know where your funding comes from and what you are required to do to obtain or keep the money given. Does the funder align with your mission? Does the funder want access to participants or their stories? What kind of data will they ask you to collect?

Best Practice
Let the people you serve define the words used to describe themselves, their experiences, and their culture(s).

You may ask people, "How do you identify?" It is key to know when it is appropriate to ask and to know your motivation for asking – ask out of need to understand for the support and services you are providing, not out of your personal curiosity.

Consider that race is a "social fiction. But it is also, for now at least, a social fact" (Biss 2009: 17). Seek to understand the history of oppression and colonialism and know that within communities there are many subcultures. Levels of oppression or access to resources and opportunities can vary widely within cultures/communities.

Leading with Compassion

> **Best Practice**
> Recognize that lived experience is an important source of knowledge and expertise for both teachers and students.

In our work, we are survivor-focused. We do not place the credentialed professional's knowledge above that of the survivor. We come from a place of "*I believe you.*" We take the person's experience and needs seriously in the moment. We understand that perceptions of past experiences can change over time. We also know that the legal definitions of sexual abuse may be very different from a person's victimization and as yoga providers our focus is on the individual's needs not the details of their story or case.

> **Best Practice**
> Allow survivors to choose when and how to share their stories.

Just because someone is on your panel/book/such like – they owe no one their stories. Their experience is their own. Every time a story or any information about an individual is shared there needs to be explicit consent. Do not commercialize survivors or their stories – ever. If you ask a survivor to represent your organization/work, then there needs to be fair compensation. We know that so much work in the yoga community is uncompensated; plan accordingly to

always compensate survivors for their time and wisdom shared.

Understand that by asking one member of a (diverse) community to represent everyone you may be exploiting them and their story. By relying on one person or a small group of people, we may place tremendous pressure on them that works against the goals of inclusion and service and asks them to take on the labor of an entire project or group – labor that may unfairly tax their time, resources and emotional well-being (Stephens 2018).

> **Best Practice**
> Know your scope of practice as a yoga teacher and the limits of yoga as a trauma-informed modality.

As a caring yoga teacher, you may earn people's trust and they may share information and needs with you. It is imperative to know and develop relationships with community resources (legal, physical health, mental health, social services) that you can direct survivors to with a goal of fully meeting their needs. Your relationships with other professionals can allow for a "warm hand off' for someone you are serving – rather than simply giving them an address or phone number. Those relationships can also allow for referrals to your programs and classes. It may be possible to join task forces or agency gatherings in your community or to set up meetings to learn more about what is available for survivors.

Knowing your scope of practice also includes knowing your own limitations or bias as well as patterns of your teaching/practice that may not be best suited for all people. Most importantly, remember that as yoga teachers we cannot diagnose any condition as we are not clinical health professionals. Harm can happen to yourself, your profession, and those you are serving when you are outside of your role (even if you are well-meaning in your actions). For additional discussion on scope of practice, refer back to Chapter 4.

> **Best Practice**
>
> Practitioners of trauma-informed yoga need to utilize mindful communication.

One may consider using trauma-informed language in all communication knowing that the impact of words and communication trump intention. During verbal and nonverbal communication, be mindful of your actions and the reactions and responses of your students – learn to listen well and consider using active listening techniques. Be prepared to take responsibility when your words harm another person and allow those harmed to set the conditions for forgiveness (if and when they are ready).

When we strive to make our classes trauma-informed spaces, communication will be a key component in our effort. Both the words we use (and those we do not) and the tone in which we deliver our words, especially while guiding a practice, can make a huge difference in a survivor's feeling of safety. The current yoga culture is strife with body-shaming language and images. Actively counter this in your classes and pledge to be body positive for all bodies.

> **Best Practice**
>
> Seek to understand spiritual bypassing so you can avoid and reject it in your work.

Spiritual bypassing, a term first coined by psychologist John Welwood (1984), is incredibly common and may occur even more so when those aiming to serve are showing up with spiritual or quasi-spiritual objectives. When one uses their own practices or beliefs to avoid taking responsibility for doing their own emotional work (which can be the hardest work) they can intentionally or unintentionally ask those they are serving to do their work for them (Masters 2015). In addition to the importance of practitioners taking responsibility for their own emotional, spiritual, and developmental needs, concepts like "being in the present moment" or "practicing peace" do not absolve someone of knowing the cultural and historical context and the implications of trauma. We strongly encourage you to be mindful not to use yoga or spirituality to turn a blind eye to suffering and your potential role in suffering, oppression, and re-traumatizing behavior.

> **Best Practice**
>
> Be mindful of trends and big names in the yoga and service communities.

Be aware that the large organizations may not always be the best vehicle for serving those most impacted by trauma. By looking at who and what gets funds, support, and attention, we may notice trends that actually create barriers and/or create a culture of "this trauma trumps that trauma." Vu Le, Executive Director of Rainier Valley Corps, calls this Trickle Down Community Engagement: "This is when we bypass the people who are most affected by issues, engage and fund larger organizations to tackle these issues, and hope that miraculously the people most affected will help out in the effort, usually for free" (Le 2015).

> **Best Practice**
> Be prepared to hold space for conversations about privilege, oppression, and intersectionality and know when you are taking up too much space in these conversations.

> **Best Practice**
> Practitioners of trauma-informed yoga and those serving people who have experienced sexual trauma will need to seek additional training and keep an openness to learning.

Many privileged people operate under a false scarcity argument that says that more rights for others means less rights/space for them. You may unconsciously hold similar beliefs or attempt to keep power or privilege over others (perhaps by coming in as an "expert"). Be aware that your position of power comes with a responsibility to call out disparity in all forms and for all people. Rather than thinking of this work as a win–lose proposition, consider that we are trying to create a win–win world where everyone gets their needs met.

We should be prepared that during this deep work of healing in community many emotions, including mourning, anger, and sorrow, may surface – plan to care for yourself and others in the wake of these emotions so you do not shut down or discourage other people's emotions for your own comfort. Knowing, recognizing, and embodying moving through your own defense mechanisms is an important place to start and return. Working on your own emotional health and well-being is key as privileged guilt and shame are not end destinations and you will need to find ways to work through them without asking the people you serve (in this case survivors of sexual abuse and communities who have experience of historical trauma) to do your emotional work for you. There is discomfort in looking at your own privilege – seek to change your tolerance to the discomfort rather than changing what we are doing that is causing the discomfort. Recognize that discomfort can be part of the growth, understanding, and healing needed for you to best serve.

As the fields of trauma, trauma research, and trauma-informed practices grow and evolve there will be opportunities to learn and adjust your work. Expect to change your mind about things and expand your framework. Additionally, it is important to be aware that powerful and meaningful leadership will look different based on culture and can vary by group. Clear and culturally appropriate facilitation is a skill to learn, practice, and hone (Lawrence & Tatum 1999).

You may also need to seek out training related to the population you are serving. Social justice training and training around diversity in all forms can be invaluable in preparing you and maintaining your ability to serve your students well and without further harming them and their communities.

> **Best Practice**
> Work to identify your own limitations and bias.

It can be easy to make assumptions about people. Our brains are designed to make quick judgments; we are wired to make shortcuts in order to process large amounts of information. However, this can lead us astray and even cause grave harm if we do not engage in ongoing work and reflection to make these biases conscious.

Can you commit to not assuming you know someone and remember that humans are complex and multifaceted? By seeking to challenge yours and others pre-existing stereotypes versus what is really happening you may gain awareness of unconscious/implicit bias and learn to notice when you are uncomfortable and what this discomfort can teach you about your own *blind bias spot* (Scopelliti, et al. 2015).

> The Harvard University Project Implicit bias tests offer a readily-available online tool to consider your own biases and offers a jumping-off point to dive deeper into subconscious biases that can affect our work and ability to serve.
>
> (Implicit.harvard.edu 2019)

Discomfort is not the same as lack of safety. You will find that staying rigidly within one's perceived role (often based on status, or title) can feed into limitations and bias. You might ask: how can I find flexibility and openness in my work? How can I move toward my biases, rather than turn away from them? (Myers 2014).

A group or community may ask for their own yoga programs with facilitators who mirror their own identity and/or culture. This can be an opportunity to lift up other teachers and leaders while honoring what the participants are asking for.

Best Practice
Consider how and where you share your work and recognize your unique voice as a yoga practitioner.

When you are in a position to share your work, use your power to elevate the people you serve rather than yourself. Be aware of media portrayal of service providers as saviors – this narrative perpetuates the myth that those we serve need to be fixed or saved. We can remind people of their humanity by understanding their wholeness. It is our job, particularly as yoga practitioners, to show up and be present for people just as they are and without judgment. This is rooted in mindfulness work and can be deeply healing – a practice of radical acceptance. How can we be with our students, rather than create a relationship based on hierarchy? When we share about our work, how can we use our power as a protective force and as an opportunity to humanize and bring acceptance to the communities we serve?

It is important to acknowledge that when sharing with the media or supporting survivors who have chosen to share, you cannot control how the message is received or portrayed. Choose your media outlets and platforms wisely and ask to review anything before it is printed/broadcasted.

Best Practice
Commit to not doing this work alone – this is a best practice for both you and the people you serve.

It is not sustainable or wise for one person to be hyper-responsible or hyper-accountable. For many empathic people, saying "no" can be a huge challenge. Practice saying it. Partners or a team of yoga practitioners can cover one another so every client/survivor is cared for while also allowing breaks. This may look like having qualified back-up and substitute teachers when you are a "small shop," or, if you have multiple programs, it means being part of an established organization or agency. This allows the person on break to know (and hopefully feel good) that the work is supported in their absence and moves away from the unhealthy feeling of "if not me – who?" It also prevents clients/survivors losing access to a program they have come to rely on when the sole provider has to step away temporarily or permanently.

While we acknowledge that many of the systems we work in are designed to oppress people and do not prioritize self-care, we must strive to open up conversations on how we can create structural support, or to call attention to the need for it. We must notice when we have thoughts concerning being all-important (*if I leave everything will fall apart*) and resist the "badge of honor" for overworking and not taking a break. We may be cast into the martyr, hero, or savior roles. Remember that these roles are not healthy for us or the people we serve – no role exists in isolation and embracing such roles implies that those you serve are in need of saving. (They are not.) How can we as wellness professionals steward the transitions to more sustainable practices?

You may consider time-limited offerings (for example, an eight-week series) while cultivating leadership and training others to offer the class or program. Time-limited offerings give both you and those you serve structure and help to manage expectations.

Best Practice
Give people the tools and respect to be in control of their own process and their healing.

In addition to supporting survivors with additional resources and services, how can the practices we offer build resilience so that survivors can take ownership over their own healing? They do not *need* you to heal. Allowing you on their journey is their choice and we should strive to work ourselves out of our positions. Dependency is not healthy for any yoga student, but autonomy takes on special importance for survivors – it breaks the abuse cycle. Give away the tools of yoga and mindfulness freely so people can decide how they want to use them for their own healing.

Best Practice
Connect with others doing this work and intentionally create organizations that prioritize sustainability and care of providers.

We know from experience that people doing this work often feel isolated. Service work, especially with communities who have been systematically oppressed and shamed, can be challenging to discuss with those not doing similar work. Our society has long avoided conversations about sexual trauma and the power dynamics that allow cycles of violence and sexual violence to continue.

Even when we have supportive people willing to hold space for us, the intensity and exhaustion of this work can create distance. Being part of an organization or seeking out others in this field can break the isolation and allow honest and real exchanges about the challenges of this work. Connection is fundamental.

For longevity of the field of service yoga, we all need to fully support the people who do the work and strive to create organizations that holistically care for providers with support, adequate compensation, access to self-care, and opportunities for community and connection.

Best Practice
Allow yourself to be human.

Being honest, human, humble, and real in this work is everything. This includes giving yourself permission to not know everything, to make mistakes, and to acknowledge that you have real feelings. You cannot do this work well if you are disconnected and in connection you will have your own feelings.

Consider also your own levels of trauma. Many of us can be drawn to this work because of our own stories and survival from deeply traumatic experiences. These experiences can closely mirror that of our students and their experiences can trigger us. You may plan ahead for how you will deal with these possibilities – how will you take care of yourself? There is also, of course, the stress and trauma of everyday life – how do you prepare to enter into service with the inevitable challenges you will face throughout your life? Be compassionate toward yourself and recognize that you too are in a continual process of healing.

Additionally, it is important to allow the full spectrum of your experience in the work (and the experience of our students) to be valid. Look for joy in the work, the small or big wins, and find what you can lift up. This means you can also acknowledge what is challenging, hard, heartbreaking, and frustrating. Your scope as a yoga teacher can feel very narrow and there will be many things that are outside your job and role. Celebrate and focus on what you *can* do rather than what you cannot.

Fostering Healthy Boundaries

Best Practice
Consider and respect issues around trust for the people you serve.

Trust can be challenging for many people and especially survivors who many times have had their trust betrayed by not only those who abused them but also other people who were unwilling to believe, hear, or support them. While we want our students to trust, it is incredibly important to remember that survivors have learned not to trust and that building trust with them will take considerable time and grace.

Best Practice
Consider and respect issues connected to trust for yourself.

You may find in this work that you struggle to trust others and attempt to "do it all." Many of us have found that this work is simply not sustainable in isolation and have had to develop trusting relationships with colleagues in order to best serve our students. You may also have to let go of a desire to do everything and trust that what you can give is enough.

Best Practice
You and your students have a right to safety.

Learning to trust your instinct or "gut" is important both for your safety and the safety of your students. Understand that really any space is a space a perpetrator can come in to. If something or someone does not feel right in your space or class, pay attention to your instincts and keep yourself safe. It is also important to know the people and procedures to keep your students safe both physically and emotionally. Do not feel that you need to sacrifice safety (yours or your students) to "follow through" or keep the space open to all. Sometimes it can feel like a delicate balance between doing the work and maintaining safety and other times you will feel the need for a very clear boundary. In many places, there are safety measures in place to keep you safe. Lean on them as you need to and know you have a right to safety – just like your students do.

In the yoga teacher role, you may or may not be a mandated reporter in your jurisdiction, but we feel it is important to be an ethical mandated reporter even if you are not required. This means that you would report to the proper authorities, supervisor, or a state-run hotline if you know or suspect a person is being abused. We acknowledge that our current law, legal and social support systems are imperfect but calling or involving the authorities can interrupt an abusive situation and, it is hoped, open doors or resources to care. In order to build trust, you should be transparent with those you serve that you need to report abusive situations.

Depending on where you offer classes, you may also know that your students will be going back to potentially violent situations. Many victims of domestic abuse, for example, stay with their abusers out of fear of worse abuse if they leave or because they do not have the resources to leave yet. When you know people are returning to violence or potential violence structure your practice to give time for students to prepare themselves to return. For classes in prisons, for example, leaving students vulnerable can put

them at risk – take care to properly close your class with a predictable routine.

> ### Best Practice
> Open communication and a thoughtful approach is key when considering friendships with colleagues.

We must be aware of the power dynamics that may be in play in all of our relationships. While you may develop true and lasting friends with colleagues it is important to name and speak about any possible power dynamics. You will also need to be aware of the perceptions of your relationships and how they may affect your work environment – this includes how your relationship exists both in person and online. There will be many times when staying professional will be imperative even if you have a close relationship with someone outside of work. When developing relationships think ahead on how you will handle conflict. Romantic and/or sexual relationships should be avoided and only taken on when true consent and equal power are possible – this is *not* possible in student–teacher or boss–employee relationships.

> ### Best Practice
> Take extreme care when considering friendship with adult students.

We caution you to be very mindful with relationships with survivors. Many survivors are relying on you to have strong boundaries that keep them safe and allow them to begin to heal. Consider how you are seen by the student – as a "guru," leader, parent-figure, friend? First and foremost, you will need to follow the rules and regulations of the facility. There is a difference between being friendly and warm and "friends" with someone. You can be very clear upfront with the student – this relationship can feel like friendship, but it is a different dynamic. Most importantly, your student's needs are cared for in the relationship and yours are cared for elsewhere. It is a professional relationship that can feel very intimate. When you live in the community where you work, you may want to bring up the dynamics from the beginning – how will we handle seeing each other at the grocery store? To maintain confidentiality, allow students to choose to initiate contact or not. You will need to be particularly careful with social media. Friendship with children or teens is always inappropriate – you can love and serve your students best when you hold boundaries for them.

Best Practice
Survivors have had their boundaries violated and may present with overtly or overly sexualized behavior – know that this is part of their trauma and their process.

For both adult and child survivors, anticipate that they may present with overtly or overly sexualized behavior. They may have developed a distorted view of love, attention, kindness, and sex. While they are healing, they may be exploring and figuring out new boundaries concerning sex and intimacy. Withhold judgment about appearances, clothing, or behavior, while mirroring back qualities and values you see in the person outside of their sexuality and appearance. You might acknowledge their bravery or curiosity in coming to class, or their intelligence in group discussions. Know that the person may "show up" the only way they know how and that it is healing for you to see them as a whole person and not as a sexual object or victim.

By holding strong boundaries, in particular about any sexualized behavior, you have the opportunity to show your student that there can be intimacy and connection without sexualized behavior or power-driven control. It is important to remember that survivors have a right to have self-defined, healthy sexual lives just like anyone else. They get to define for themselves and with mutual consent from their partners what that looks like.

Be incredibly mindful of the words you use for people who have been abused or exploited. Words like "provocative" and "prostitute" and phrases like "she's asking for it" severely undermine the healing of survivors. They are used to shift the blame away from the power-driven dynamics that lead to the abuse and to place the blame on the victim. Refuse to be part of any victim shaming and blaming. Educate yourself on language best practices (for example, use terms such as *sexual assault survivor, sex trafficking survivor,* and *sex worker*). Know that guides for language are available and recognize that appropriate terminology may shift over time. Ask the populations you work with how they identify.

Best Practice
Show up ready to support someone as long as it serves them and be prepared to meet them where they are.

Some people will come into your life for a short time and others much longer. By being present, grounded, and whole in each interaction, you will do what is needed in the time that you have. It may be helpful to have faith that there is a higher power at play in their and our lives.

Remember you are simply "walking alongside" someone on their journey; the healing is theirs and on their timeline. You are not in control of their life, and it is imperative to know when to let it go. It can be a hard lesson for any provider to learn but the truth is you cannot work harder on recovery than the person recovering; all you can do is support them right where they are without judgment. Make it a practice to leave the door open whenever possible; often a student will return to class when they feel ready for the work.

Best Practice
Honesty and humility prepares us for connection.

We must seek to counter the cult of personality. Anything that disconnects us from our communities and from the people we serve stands to do more harm than good. Ultimately, we are with our students to have an empathic connection human-to-human. We should seek to interact with transparency, honesty, and realness. There is a beautiful uniqueness in each of us and in our relationship to one another. Acknowledge your students' power by giving value to their knowledge, experience, and intuition. By showing up humble you make space for true reciprocity and with it comes the possibility of authentic connection.

You can share with students that you may not have the same experiences but that you can recognize and relate the emotions they are sharing. You will find your points of connection and acknowledge the ways you are different. If you do decide to share personally, only share as far as is needed for rapport and trust.

Best Practice
Check your own abuse of power as it mirrors sexual abuse and make yourself knowledgeable about sexual abuse within the yoga industry.

The cult of personality, which unfortunately is ubiquitous in the mainstream yoga world, puts a person on a pedestal and does not allow them to be human. This can lead to serious harm, as leaders' behavior is not questioned or is blindly accepted. We have to counter the blind-faith guru system, even as we recognize that much of the yoga lineage derives from this approach. We have to acknowledge that when people put their trust in authority figures (in this case yoga instructors), doing so can leave them vulnerable to power abuse. Be aware that often times, in mainstream yoga, the leader/guru can take on the persona of a hero, saint, or savior. The dynamic created can be harmful for authentic connection, and can work to counteract your own ability to engage in meaningful self-care and self-reflection. In your own work, how can you actively reject this idea of yourself as perfect, all-knowing, or above the human experience?

Sadly, there have been many cases of sexual and other abuse in the yoga community, both in recent years and throughout history. The majority of yoga classes involve a teacher seeking control (either verbally or physically through "adjustments") over another person's body, and this dynamic can prove both triggering and potentially abusive. For his *I am my own guru* campaign in response to sexual abuse in the yoga community, Lucas Rockwood (2013) states: "There are no ethics committees or watchdog groups for yoga students, and yet teachers with huge power and influence are clearly taking advantage, and in some cases, even assaulting their students who came to class to get fit or relieve stress." Often people are shamed for speaking out; they risk losing their community, their social standing, and even employment. Abuse in the yoga community is addressed further in Chapter 17.

Self-care and Community-care as Imperative

> **Best Practice**
> Understand vicarious trauma and its effects on you and your colleagues.

It is imperative that those working with survivors understand and are given care (ideally self-care space *and* professional help) in connection to vicarious trauma. Often times when we talk about burnout we may really be encountering vicarious trauma. For the individual experiencing it, vicarious, or second-hand, trauma can feel like being overwhelmed, hopeless, triggered, and physically/mentally stressed or unwell. You may struggle with intrusive thoughts and have difficulty sleeping. Vicarious trauma can affect your ability to concentrate, to connect with others, and your relationships in and outside of your work (Pearlman & McKay 2008).

In her book, *Trauma Stewardship: An Everyday Guide to Caring for Self While Caring for Others*, Laura van Dernoot Lipsky introduces the concept of *trauma stewardship*. In sharing her own experience, she implores the reader to "respond to even the most urgent human and environmental conditions in a sustainable and intentional way. By developing the deep sense of awareness needed to care for ourselves while caring for others and the world around us, we

can greatly enhance our potential to work for change, ethically and with integrity, for generations to come" (Lipsky & Burk 2009: 39). Oftentimes those suffering from vicarious trauma need time away from the work, significant time to reconnect with things that bring them joy, and a support system that understands what they are going through. For some providers, it may be possible to shift to less-triggering work or to vary their work. Prevention of vicarious trauma, with the goal of healthy trauma stewardship, is a key reason this work should not be done in isolation – a support system is critical to make work with survivors sustainable. See Chapter 2 for additional discussion of vicarious trauma.

> **Best Practice**
> Recognize systemic barriers to self-care.

We believe that often times it is not the work you are doing that causes self-harm or "burnout" but rather it is how we are doing the work or are expected to do the work. We cannot do the work well when we ourselves are depleted. Most of us live and work within systems that are hierarchical, capitalist, and patriarchal and not designed to give time for self-care. We have to ask (for ourselves and for all people): how can our work be more sustainable?

There is an unequal distribution to access to a variety of self-care practices. In some circles, self-care is seen as luxury and in truth many self-care practices come at an expense (cost or time wise) that the majority of people cannot afford. Even after thorough self-assessment, you or your colleagues may not have access to the care you need to stay present, healthy, and whole in the work. Part of our work in this field is to shine light on *this* inequality as it is critical to opening doors for yoga practitioners from all backgrounds to do this work. Understand that self-care is about meeting our foundational needs, and this is fundamental to doing the work of yoga service.

> **Best Practice**
> Be open to what self-care can look like and plan it into your work and life.

Many trauma-informed yoga teachers find it critical to maintain their own yoga and mindfulness practices both to maintain their own health and well-being and to best offer the practices to their students. While yoga can have a powerful healing force in our lives, be aware that the performances of enlightened wellness and magical thinking can be misleading and harmful. Even as dedicated yoga practitioners, recognize that you may need resources for yourself outside of yoga.

Self-care can be formal or informal. It can be steady (*I do this practice every morning*) as well as dynamic and flexible (*some days I need or have access to deeper self-care and other times my self-care is brief*). This list is by no means exhaustive but can serve as inspiration or as a reminder and is based on our own self-care practices as active teachers in this field:

- drinking adequate and clean water
- eating healthy food
- getting enough sleep
- taking bubble baths/salt baths
- creating or seeking "safe" shelter

- spending time with friends and/or family
- exercising (*you may consider home videos, walks at the park, community gyms/studios, and other low/no-cost options*)
- attending yoga and meditation classes (*you may consider practicing in a separate space from your work*)
- attending support groups away from your colleagues and clients
- participating in psychotherapy
- practicing the art of "letting go"
- giving yourself time to do nothing
- finding a spiritual community and incorporating spiritual practices into your life
- staying involved in your community
- considering simple forms of self-care, such as positive self-talk or affirmations
- being spacious in the work – giving yourself enough time to complete your work and understanding how urgency affects your nervous system
- writing and journaling
- making art, dancing, and creating music
- allowing yourself time to play and have fun.

> **Best Practice**
> Embrace the idea of radical self-care.

Working with those healing from trauma is intense and challenging work on many levels. In order to meet this work with equally intense stores of energy and courage, we must adopt a practice of radical self-care. The word *radical* can be defined as getting to the underlying/root cause or fundamental nature of a thing or idea (Merriam-Webster Online 2018). By embracing radical self-care, we acknowledge the need for regular, intentional support to balance and sustain us in the deeply courageous work with at-risk and high-trauma populations.

In addition to maintaining our own health and well-being, taking care of our basic needs, we must go deeper and assess from where our burnout symptoms are truly coming. Part of this deeper assessment work is being aware of and acknowledging our own past traumas and our exposure to the trauma of others, or vicarious trauma. The reality is that when we work with those recovering from trauma, are exposed to the details of others' trauma stories, and must work on behalf of survivors of trauma within systems that may be traumatizing themselves, we are absorbing vicarious trauma.

The inevitable impacts of vicarious trauma exposure are real and must be met with equal intensity in the form of our radical self-care. We must continue to take care of our basic needs (food, water, sleep, exercise, and connection with others) and we must also dive a little deeper to find out what in our own past is being triggered by what is happening in our current environment. This requires being grounded, centered, and present with ourselves and with those for whom we hold space while finding practical, experiential tools (like yoga, mindfulness, and meditation) to keep our mind and body fully engaged in this work with the goal of sustainability and longevity.

We can do this by checking in regularly with ourselves as we do the work:

- How is it in my mind?

- How is it in my body?

- How is it in my heart?

The answers to each inquiry will lead us to our next action of radical self-care. This inquiry gives us information on how we are showing up for those we serve (on and off the mat), and allows us an opportunity to begin again and move toward grounding. Working with trauma requires that we dive deep and take care of ourselves in the most basic, "root," radical way. This is radical self-care.

Best Practice
Plant seeds for the future.

While this work is at times exhausting, overwhelming, and seemingly impossible there are also times and experiences of unbelievable joy, healing, and profound connection. We will spend much of our time in this work preparing, proposing, and implementing classes and programs. We will strive to be fully present while with our students and practice mindfulness throughout our interactions. Taking time to think about the future as an individual and in collaboration with your colleagues in the field of yoga service allows you to strategize for the future of our collective work and the individual needs of your students and their communities. All relationships and connections have the potential to build bridges on the most basic level for your student and on the highest level for our society. We dare to imagine a world free from sexual abuse and filled with healing practices for all.

Conclusion

We return to the village and the need for all people to be seen, heard, and understood. Author David W. Augsburger implores us: "Being heard is so close to being loved that for the average person, they are almost indistinguishable" (1982: 12). And so we listen. Not just to the people and communities we serve but also to our own needs. We learn to say, "Yes!" with an open and non-judging heart but also to say, "No!" with the same level of compassion for ourselves and others. No amount of yoga, meditation, and mindfulness will make any of us invincible. Rather, with *relational wisdom* and in community we have an opportunity to apply the tools of yoga in our efforts to build resiliency and connection (both with ourselves and others).

In closing, with honesty and hope, the person we met at the opening of this chapter offers us this:

Case study

That first post-yoga moment of clarity, of stillness – its sigh of hope – was a taste of the parts of myself, re-collected. My recollected self is not confused about who she is, what she wants, where she ends and others begin, even though those boundaries were denied in the past. Over time, I have become really very excited about reclaiming the word "no," as well as more elaborate ways of expressing the same. (I have had plenty of opportunities, such as in standing up for myself or others when the situation requires. This moment has seemed to present quite a few such opportunities – and for years, I was the silent one.) Perhaps most paradoxically, as my sense of boundaries has become clearer, the experience of extending myself in service – whether spontaneously, or as a planned event – has become less encumbered and decisions around it, freer.

Right now, I am lingering at a learning edge pertaining to trust. So far, this requires a deeper unfolding of what I have described, above. I am paying attention and holding what arises, lightly. My yoga practice is essential, in that process.

PART 3

Development and Sexual Trauma

Pregnancy and Postpartum

Author *Amanda J.G. Napior*

Contributors *Lisa Boldin, Anneke Lucas, Rosa Vissers, Kimberleigh Weiss-Lewit, Ann Wilkinson*

Introduction

In her reflections on the existential, relational, and embodied experience of pregnancy, Kimberleigh Weiss-Lewit reminds us that no amount of training and expertise can rightfully empower the instructor to make decisions for the pregnant person. Rather, there is really only one person who can:

> Well of course they are guarded, I remind myself. I know the inevitable vulnerability of pregnancy so well – it doesn't matter how strong you may feel, and oftentimes you may not feel strong at all. You are viewed differently as soon as someone knows you are pregnant. Hopefully you are surrounded with respect, autonomy and love, but so often there is judgement and even violence at the hands of those you are supposed to trust. So, as yoga teachers we can't expect a free pass. It isn't all sunshine and rainbows. We should expect to have to earn trust again and again by offering choice rather than control, space and time for people to decide how and if they would like to participate, and personal freedom rather than whatever we "think" is best for anyone else. It doesn't matter how much I may know about pregnancy, birth, new parenthood or yoga. There is a health crisis in the United States, especially for black and brown birthing people and babies. Informed consent can't and won't
>
> start in a hospital during labor. I can offer it from the first moment I offer a yoga practice. Over time it has become simpler for me (after I realized it wasn't about "me" at all!): the pregnant or parenting person is the expert on their body, birth and baby. I can offer tools and resources and empathic presence. They decide how and what they would like to receive.
>
> (Weiss-Lewit 2019)

Pregnancy and labor and delivery may not necessarily overlap with trauma experience. For survivors of childhood or adult sexual abuse, however, pregnancy, birth, and postpartum can be especially challenging. This section offers best practices for trauma-informed prenatal yoga with pregnant survivors, and postnatal yoga for postpartum survivors. Trauma-informed prenatal and postnatal yoga are but one kind of tool to provide both preparation for labor and delivery, as well as healing from past trauma. In this brief introduction, we also provide some context for birth trauma and obstetrics abuse – two forms of trauma that may impact postpartum people. Birth trauma and obstetrics abuse are intertwined, although birth trauma may occur without abuse. Some definitions will help ground this distinction.

Birth Trauma and Obstetrics Abuse

Birth trauma is post-traumatic stress disorder (PTSD) that occurs after childbirth, as well as something experienced by persons "who may not meet the clinical criteria for PTSD but who have some of the symptoms of the disorder." Studies report that postpartum PTSD impacts from 1 to 30 percent of postpartum women (Grekin and O'Hara 2014). Since PTSD can arise from "any experience involving the threat of death or serious injury to an individual or another person close to them" (such as their baby), PTSD can arise from a traumatic birth (The Birth Trauma Association 2018).

This understanding of birth trauma highlights that birth can become a context of trauma when injury or a threat of death occurs for the birthing person or their baby. These circumstances might also be precursor to postpartum depression, which is distinct from birth trauma. Something as commonplace as perineal tearing could be an impetus for birth trauma, as well as the heartbreaking experience of one's baby not surviving birth. Whether or not someone feels traumatized after birth can depend, in part, upon how much choice the birthing person was given: did they make choices that others honored? Or, were their choices overridden by someone who, in that moment, had more control?

Such questions point to our second topic: obstetric abuse. Obstetric abuse is itself a form of sexual violence (whereas birth trauma can happen without abuse). It is a relatively new legal term introduced in Venezuela, by obstetrician and gynecologist Rogelio Pérez-D'Gregorio. He defines obstetric violence as

> any sexist act that is likely to result in harm or physical, sexual, psychological, emotional, occupational, economic or patrimonial suffering; coercion or arbitrary deprivation of freedom, and the threat of executing such acts, whether

> occurring in public or private practice ... [It may involve] the appropriation of the body and reproductive processes of women by health personnel, which is expressed as dehumanized treatment, an abuse of medication, and to convert the natural processes into pathological ones, bringing with it loss of autonomy and the ability to decide freely about their bodies and sexuality, negatively impacting the quality of life of women.
> (Pérez-D'Gregorio 2010: 201–2)

Obstetric violence, therefore, is a term recognizing the inherent and extreme vulnerability of a birthing person, the inherent authority of those in a position to serve them, and how both subtle and explicit coercions on the part of those authorities are forms of violence. The terms obstetric violence and obstetric abuse can helpfully illuminate a dimension of some birthing people's experiences: that when a birth experience goes badly, many people may assume going into birth comes with a loss of voice. "Whatever happens, happens." These legal terms give language to the reality that such birthing mishaps were not the birthing person's "fault."

Legal scholar Farah Diaz-Tello notes that while discerning the prevalence of obstetrics abuse from case reports is difficult, research in the United States points to "significant pressure and loss of autonomy in maternity care." Diaz-Tello recounts a study by Roth, et al. (2014), in which a survey of "doulas, childbirth educators, and labour and delivery nurses ... found that more than half had witnessed a physician engage in a procedure explicitly against a woman's will, and nearly two-thirds had witnessed providers engage in procedures, 'occasionally' or 'often,' without giving the birthing person a choice or time to consider the procedure" (Diaz-Tello 2016: 57). These findings point to a disconcerting frequency that may put bad birthing experiences in new perspective. The growing recognition of instances of obstetric abuse may allow postpartum people to uncouple personal responsibility with turns-for-the-worse. The onus is on medical professionals, to use their power with care.

In this section on best practices for pregnant and postpartum survivors of sexual violence, we emphasize both that pregnancy, birth, and postpartum can be experiences of remarkable joy, as well as ones that resurface past trauma or introduce new ones. Accordingly, this section offers best practices for trauma-informed prenatal yoga with pregnant survivors as well as postnatal yoga with postpartum survivors. Note that postpartum survivors may have additionally (or only) experienced birth trauma and/or obstetric abuse. A number of the following best practices also apply not only to working with survivors of sexual trauma but also to working with pregnant and postpartum people who have *not* experienced sexual trauma. Because pregnancy and birthing *can* be times of extreme vulnerability – physically, relationally, and socially – it is important to emphasize a few basics that would be appropriate for working with prenatal or postpartum people, in general.

Best Practices

> **Best Practice**
> Pursue training in prenatal and postnatal yoga and postpartum education, if you intend to work in these areas.

Receive training in areas you do not know, and do not teach in them until you do. Training in prenatal yoga, for example, does not qualify someone to offer education about postpartum depression. Facilities seeking teachers in these areas should verify that they have training.

> **Best Practice**
> Be mindful that not all pregnant people identify as women.

Use gender-inclusive language, as not everyone who is pregnant identifies as a woman. The language "birthing person," or "person with a uterus" are some examples. Consider checking out helpful reference guides like Tynan Rhea's article, "8 Gender-Neutral Birth Terms and How to Use Them," or the *BirthRoot Online Childbirth Class Blog* (2019) post on "LGBTQIA Inclusive Pregnancy and Birth Care."

> **Best Practice**
> Normalize the full range of human experience.

Pregnancy can be a joyful time, a confusing or harrowing one, and potentially some combination of these. Service providers and instructors should be mindful to embody presence, support, and affirmation for the pregnant person, no matter what their experience is. Not everyone is excited, curious, or accepting about the changes happening in their body and life (although some are). Use language that embraces the human experience in front of you. Celebrate someone's excitement to bring a new life into the world. Likewise, hold space for someone's grief, if pregnancy is either not what they wanted, expected, or both.

Best Practice
Develop the student–teacher relationship before going deep.

Pregnancy and birth can be an opportunity for healing, for the person who has experienced sexual trauma. However, it is also potentially retraumatizing because of the violation that has occurred. Yoga instructors should keep this paradox in mind. If pregnant survivors want to have a vaginal birth, they need to be able to access the pelvis. Therefore, developing a strong student–teacher relationship before taking the practice to deeper places – energetically, emotionally, or physically – is integral. This relationship is central even if a vaginal birth is not desired. Surgical birth may be very challenging for survivors. Continually offer education and transparency about the "why" of certain shapes, and then reinforce that the choice is the student's. Practicing in this way can offer the potential for transformation and healing.

Best Practice
Designate special class time for conversation and sharing.

Opportunities for sharing are important in both prenatal and postnatal classes and are ways of fostering community that might not otherwise form, as well as for continuing education. In prenatal yoga, class discussion is an especially ripe opportunity for social change because students may feel inclined to form community for the sake of their children and families. (By contrast, this is less likely to happen in other yoga classes in which students do not have community-based reasons for staying in touch.) Justice starts with community and new community starts with friendship.

Make room for stories

Hold space for birth stories, and prepare for loss stories. Loss of an infant or child may result from natural causes in an otherwise healthy or materially well-supported birthing situation, but may also result from systemic or physical violence. If you are teaching prenatal yoga in prisons, be aware that some people in women's facilities will have been pregnant a high number of times, and potentially due to sex trafficking. Many people will keep their pregnancies, and others may elect to terminate them or may have experienced coercive pressure to abort. Research findings suggest that pregnant prisoners are often functionally denied abortions, due to institutional and legal restrictions (Sufrin, et al. 2017; see text box below). Allow people to opt-out from hearing stories. Some may not be ready to hear others' glowing ones. Give permission for people to leave the room, when that is possible (it may not be, in a prison).

A study by Caroline Sufrin and colleagues indicates that incarcerated women do retain their legal rights to abortion, but institutional restrictions can result in pregnant people being denied access to it. "Only half of prisons [in the U.S.] allow abortion in both the first and second trimesters, 15% do not allow abortion at all, and 65% require the woman to pay".
(Sufrin, et al. 2017: 265)

Reframe postnatal yoga as an opportunity for healing rather than for weight loss or shaping

Many postpartum yoga students come to yoga with the desire to "get their bodies back." Use class discussions as a way to frame healing time, as well as to *re*frame postnatal yoga practice as being about healing, rather than erasing the physical effects of pregnancy and birth. Physical fitness goals can be a positive and motivating source of self-empowerment. But they can also encourage body-shaming. Hold space for this experience (do not silence it). But use language that encourages empowerment fueled by love, curiosity, and patience, rather than by shame.

Best Practice
Create a space of empowerment and education.

Establishing a context of consent by giving back power at every turn is an important best practice in every context. It insists upon student choice, modifications, opt-outs (and opt-ins), and advocates student leadership. This best practice is especially important to emphasize here, as many people harbor the misconception that prenatal yoga is the place where the expert on their experience is someone other than themselves, and that this person – the yoga teacher – can give them knowledge. However, pregnant bodies are already imbued with embodied knowledge. They know how to grow and nurture a fetus and how to birth. The aim of prenatal yoga teacher and birthing educator is to offer practices and information that makes embodied and informed decision making more accessible than it was before.

Enable empowerment amid vulnerability

Childbirth can be one of the most vulnerability-inducing experiences in a person's life. Yoga practice likewise creates a vulnerability and openness in a person, however differently. Teachers can mirror choice and decision making amid the vulnerability of yoga, which can have benefits for the birthing experience itself. Give the power to make choices back to the student again, and again, and again, so that the birthing person is more likely to be able to assert choices in the extreme vulnerability of labor and delivery. If we can experience our own power when we are in a more vulnerable place (such as in yoga), we may learn that being vulnerable does not mean we suddenly have no voice.

Establish a foundation for choice through education

Educate toward empowerment. Offer strength-based childbirth education, education about reproductive system and anatomy, and education about the pregnant and birthing person's legal rights in medical settings. These foci provide pregnant people with the information they need to make their own informed decisions, which will enable a person to look to others for support and guidance, rather than for decisions.

Best Practice
Seek continuity of support through the birth process if possible.

Yoga instructors should connect postpartum students with the next level of care, when continuity in the student–prenatal yoga teacher relationship is not appropriate or possible. If you have training in postnatal yoga, you might offer a student or community such a class. If you are working at a community center, you may be able to connect them with support connected to breastfeeding, chest feeding, bottle feeding, postpartum care and adjustment, and more. If you are connecting students to care beyond the setting in which you have worked with them, explore ways in which you can thoughtfully close the relationship. Establishing continuity of care is important for all postpartum survivor students. However, know that domestic violence statistically increases after birth due to increased vulnerability. Establishing continuity of care can therefore be of urgent importance.

> **Best Practice**
> Do not tell pregnant people not to do what they are doing.

You can't ... you can't ... you can't ... you can't! How many pregnant people have been told not to do this or that? Offer classes that are strength based, rather than fear based. If you are teaching prenatal yoga, you learned in your prenatal yoga teacher training about contraindications for pregnancy; therefore, you are already teaching in ways appropriate for the pregnant body in a given trimester. Allow contraindications to inform your teaching implicitly rather than explicitly. Focusing *only* on contraindications for pregnancy can pathologize the whole experience and reinforces societal patterns of taking power away from pregnant people, rather than giving it back.

> Fear and control of women is more of an issue than pregnant women doing twists!

> **Best Practice**
> Keep the focus on the pregnant person, not on their baby.

Remember the aphorism about the oxygen mask: put your own mask on first, before helping another. When working with a pregnant person, direct your attention to supporting them, and their baby will be supported, too.

> **Best Practice**
> Stay in breath, without retaining breath.

Remember that breath is your most powerful tool for self-regulation. See the best practice, "Keep in mind that being told how or when to breathe can be triggering," in our section on sex trafficking, for recommendations on how to offer breath guidance without coercion, and while being sensitive to likely triggers. Also keep in mind that survivors may find breath retention triggering. We suggest avoiding this practice. Guiding people in a free-flow of breath without retention is particularly important when working with pregnant people. Breath retention can temporarily interfere with oxygen flow to the baby.

> **Best Practice**
> Be aware that pregnancy can become a free-for-all, for judgment, unwelcome touch, and advice.

Pregnant people may be accustomed to a funny phenomenon: relatives and strangers reaching out and touching their pregnant belly (as if this part of their body has suddenly become communal or public). Likewise, pregnant people may be accustomed to receiving advice they did not solicit and that may not feel particularly appropriate to them. So, too, they may be the object of judgments, regarding their relationship choices or circumstances, as well as what they could be doing better to care for themselves or their baby. Allow yoga for a prenatal survivor to be free from such unwelcome advances – physical, verbal, and psychic. Notice your own judgments, if they arise, with loving kindness and self-inquiry. Notice the well-intending urge to give unsolicited advice and let that pass, unless someone requests it. In accordance with our best practices on instruction and curriculum development, consider the use of touch carefully. If you do use touch, ensure it happens in a context of consent, with permission to opt-out at any time.

Conclusion

Eleven best practices can only scratch the surface of an area of specialization that calls for such depth of awareness, training, and care. And yet, the contributors to this chapter have hoped that these practices will serve as guideposts for your service, whether you are a service provider or instructor who is new to offering yoga to pregnant and postpartum survivors, or someone who knows such work, well. Working with pregnant and postpartum survivors is work that can be incredibly challenging as well as life-giving, and that will continue to teach a person for as long as they are a practitioner. Surely, the same can be said of working with children and adolescents, the topic of our next chapter.

Children and Adolescents

Author *Lidia Snyder*

Contributors *Jennifer Cohen Harper, Dani Harris, Nan Herron, Mark A. Lilly, Nicole Steward*

Introduction

The effects of childhood sexual trauma are numerous, and persist over a lifetime. Survivors face statistics such as being 400 percent more likely than the general population to experience drug abuse, and 300 percent more likely to experience a major depressive episode as adults. What statistics do not always capture is the toll of childhood sexual trauma on relationships and on a child's essential experience of who they are, what their body is for, and what they have the right to as human beings. As we offer practices to support healing in this context, there is much to keep in mind and we should proceed slowly, with continuous reflection on both our offerings and their impact.

While working with children can at times seem like a journey into the land of "anything is possible," there is general agreement that human development is marked by milestones. While variation can be expected, it can be useful to frame expectations on recognized developmental stages that address four main components of development: social/emotional, language/communication, cognition (learning and problem solving), and movement/physical. Having a familiarity with recognized developmental stages and associated milestones is useful in gauging expectations and interactions.

It is important to keep in mind that there is a wide range of normal development, and factors outside of the trauma experience will play a role in each child's developmental trajectory. As we seek to support childhood survivors, it is essential that we recognize, and remind ourselves of, their primary identity as children, with all the needs, worries, and opportunities of all children. We can do serious work, in difficult situations, with joyful engagement and the playfulness of spirit that our children, all of them, need and deserve.

> When working with people who have survived sexual violence of any kind, it is fundamental to take into account not only the age of the person at the time of your collaboration, but the age at which the hurtful things happened.
>
> One of the hallmarks of post traumatic disorders for people who have endured sexual trauma is that oftentimes, ordinary developmental steps and milestones will have been missed, especially with violence endured during childhood. Instead of learning to play cooperatively at age 4, a child with a history of victimhood may spend all of his or her time in terrified survival mode. If they first come to breathing and yoga at age 8, their need, for example, to learn how to collaborate with their peers remains, but so too remains the shadow of cooperation that was never learned at age 4.
>
> A brief glimpse at working with two different aged young people can illustrate this.

When working with a 3-year-old, for example, you are also working with a caregiver. To a three year old the need for a strong basis of attachment is primary so that explorations of motor skills and cooperative play can occur. It is important to note that it might be the caregiver who has abused the child, so it is imperative that scrupulous care be given to ensure that only vetted caregivers are present. At all times our task is to show up grounded, whole, centered, present and regulated, and in so doing we the yoga teacher can give that child some semblance of safety that maybe a caregiver cannot.

When sharing yoga with such young people, the relationship between the young person and their caregiver will be central. Yoga and breathing sessions can be focused on establishing and building trust between child and caregiver, and from there creating opportunities for playful exploration of the practices, and of bodies in healthy ways.

This focus with a 3-year-old can allow that child to feel a semblance of safety and connection. Once that support of helpful grown-ups is established, the work can become more spacious and exploratory, allowing their natural curiosity a chance to flourish.

Alternately sessions with older participants will have a different approach, focus, and content. It should be noted that no age group is more or less challenging or intense. No matter the age of injury or the age of coming to breathing, the work is demanding and requires we be at our finest.

Many 15-year-olds have been hurt, but few seem to wish to focus on the hurt.

Developmentally, they have a deep need to grow up; this need is accelerated because childhood, in the cases of teens who have been abused, has not been a safe, secure, or joyful experience. These young people will want to know – whether they ask for it or not – how to survive as an adult. At the same time, they have the age-old need to still be vulnerable like a teen, to make mistakes, to see themselves as the center of the world.

In working with teens such as these, helping gain mastery of skills such as growing stronger, understanding themselves better, and relating to peers are as important as giving them the chance to simply explore, to play, to be goofy, to fail, and to succeed. This helps meet their urgent need for adult skill-building without sacrificing developmental exploration.

For example, with teens in these sessions you might say "come to standing, and press your feet into the ground." Then ask, "Okay, a question, what is this 'ground' I'm talking about? How does it help us right now to feel grounded?" And we discuss, and they guide the conversation, because that allows them to articulate their needs and feel in control.

In terms of specifics, a core principle is to understand what developmental steps are most common for any given age group, and then to understand that due to the trauma and its aftermath, many of these milestones will go unmet. For example, a 3-year-old without a history of safe and present attachment will have that huge need unmet, with potentially devastating lifelong consequences. Trying to provide safe as possible space for some of that growth to occur in the presence of breathing and resilience building is primary.

Thinking then of 15-year-old, they could have been forced into parenting younger siblings, and may have missed out on the freedom to try new things and risk making mistakes. Creating opportunities within a yoga practice for experimentation is a way to address this in a manner that doesn't feel condescending. A challenge with teens is that the missed developmental milestones add up and reinforce and trigger each other. Respect coupled with new challenges plus you being the safest possible container go together to help meet myriad teenage needs.

Each age, and each individual set of circumstances deserve our attention and our care. This is all part of our job as those who share these practices, part of our own practice and preparation.

All young people who have been harmed are impacted on the developmental level and their behaviors and needs may vary based on the developmental stage at which the trauma occurred. There are times when working with 18-year-olds who were harmed as 3-year-olds and their behavior is not dissimilar to an actual 3-year-old.

– Mark A. Lilly, Rebel Breath, symposium contributor

Best Practices

The following best practices are organized by age range. With each section, developmental milestones and contextual backgrounds are offered. Best practices are then shared, with an understanding that many recommendations are applicable across age ranges. In conclusion we offer more specific considerations that apply in contexts where a trauma history is known or in settings where high percentages of children have experienced sexual trauma.

Infancy

In interacting with caregivers and infants, it is useful to recognize that the first year of life involves the general task of building trust. Work at this stage should always include a caregiver, and the focus of any yoga offering should involve supporting the caregiver in attuning to and co-regulating the child.

Developmental Milestones of Infancy

By year one, most children will meet the following developmental milestones:

Social/Emotional

- repeat sounds/actions
- have favorite people and things
- show fear of strangers
- engage in interactive play

Language/Communication

- make sounds, mimicking words
- respond to simple one-word requests
- wave bye, shake head indicating "yes" and "no"

Cognitive

- identify objects if given verbal cue
- follows simple directions, that is, "drink your milk"
- mimic speech with varied tones

Movement/Physical

- can come to a sitting position without help

- might be "cruising" – walking while holding on to furniture

- may take a few steps or stand alone.

In acknowledging that yoga has the capacity to improve mental and physical health it is not surprising to note the ever-growing offerings of "Baby and Me" or "Parent and Baby" yoga sessions globally. Providing or participating in yoga sessions involving infants and caregivers creates an incredible opportunity to begin establishing bodily autonomy and healthy physical boundaries. Working with caregivers and infants can be a rewarding and joyous opportunity, but it is not without challenges, especially when approaching this work with an eye toward healing sexual trauma.

When working with this age range, opportunities exist for caregivers to learn about and practice attunement — establishing a harmonious and sympathetic relationship in which the caregiver recognizes and respects the infant's experience including level of tiredness, comfort, displeasure, or fear. For some caregivers with a sexual trauma history, establishing a sense of safety (either for themselves, or for the child) may, at times, preclude attunement. Yoga instructors have a unique opportunity to foster and support a caregiver's own self-awareness in relation to the child.

Many caregivers' struggle with their new role, and this struggle can be exacerbated by a history of sexual trauma. Gentle and consistent reminders of the importance of attending to *their own* needs while (and prior to if possible) attuning with their child is vital. Yoga can provide

a space for practicing this skill. Extending the opportunity to check in with themselves first, to know their own feelings and sensations, allows for a more stable and effective response to the child. Caregivers will be better equipped to meet their child's needs if they take a few moments to breathe and assess.

It is incumbent upon instructors to consider parents or caregivers in a session who may be grappling with trauma specific to the pregnancy or birth (that is, pregnancy that was a result of sexual assault, violation during pregnancy or birthing). For some with a history of sexual trauma, pregnancy, birth, or taking on the role of parent/caregiver can be triggering experiences that bring added layers of challenge to their new role as parents. Postpartum depression and anxiety are correlated with prior sexual trauma. A history of sexual abuse in women who become depressed postpartum may have long-term implications for the woman's mental health, her relationship with her child, as well as the emotional development of her child (Buistand and Janson 2001). Yoga sessions that adhere to a trauma-informed approach can be part of recovery and resilience building for both caregiver and infant.

Infants and Caregivers

Best Practice

Familiarize yourself with human developmental stages, while recognizing that trauma can be one cause of significant developmental delays.

As discussed prior, becoming familiar with the emotional, physical, cognitive, and social components of human development will give you a way to orient expectations and set goals. Traumatic events, whether chronic or sudden, can significantly delay onset of normal developmental stages, or result in developmental regressions. Sensitivity to both the child and the caregiver involves creating experiences that will support the child within their current developmental trajectory.

At the end of the chapter you will find a variety of resources ranging from websites to peer-reviewed journals; you might find these helpful in expanding your understanding of human development.

Best Practice
Offer sessions that are developmentally appropriate.

Understanding that a primary task for newborns and infants is to establish a sense of trust will be informative in designing yoga sessions. Trust is built through caregiver–infant interaction. The pursuit and establishment of trust when working with this age group can be facilitated by utilizing and *repeating* forms that build an opportunity for trustful interaction between adult and child participants. This might include opportunities for eye-to-eye contact between adult and infant/child participants, simple shared belly breathing, and caregivers practicing letting the infant know what is about to happen prior to movement. More important than variety is the use of repetition to aid in building memory and self-regulation for this age group as they experience a yoga practice. Recognition of developmental milestones (such as rolling over or sitting up unassisted) will assist in creating the most developmentally appropriate experience.

Best Practice
Maximize opportunities for attunement between caregivers and infants.

Bearing in mind the primacy of establishing trust during this time, instructors are encouraged to prioritize attunement. Attunement lays the foundation for a securely attached relationship by establishing an emotional, non-verbal symmetry. Giving adult participants a chance to serve as reliable, trustworthy partners to their infants/children aids in the development of emotional security of both child and parents. Adult participants should be encouraged to notice and attend to the needs and responses of the infant during a yoga session.

Working with Children Aged Two to Six Years

As infants move into early childhood, the best practices above remain, with new areas of attention emerging. An ongoing commitment to safety should be balanced with offering real choices, to support the child's trust in their own body and mind.

Developmental Milestones Aged Two to Six
Social/Emotional

- shows excitement and cooperation with other children
- shows a wide range of emotions
- wants to please friends
- sometimes very demanding and uncooperative

Language/Communication

- knows names of familiar people and body parts
- can be understood by strangers
- can tell a simple story
- differentiates between past, present, and future

Cognitive

- follows two-step instructions: pick up your coat and put it on

- knows some colors and numbers

- counts to ten or higher

Movement/Physical

- kicks a ball

- walks up and down stairs one foot at a time

- can use the toilet on their own.

Teaching young children presents unique opportunities and challenges. Unlike infants, who have limited physical and cognitive capacity and expression, this age group is beginning to understand instruction and verbalize their own experiences. Because this age group is advancing their communication skills (both verbal and behavioral) instructors should carefully consider their ability to work with this age group given that sexually traumatized children can and do act out in session. Instructors who become dysregulated themselves in the presence of challenging toddler behaviors (potentially including crying, tantrums, hitting, and biting) cannot support either the child or the caregiver, and have the potential to do harm. Building the capacity to manage one's own nervous system, even when provoked, is important for working effectively with all children, but especially with toddlers.

Children in this group are learning how and when to trust their own body, their own intuition, and their own minds. The experiences they have day to day can be validated or denied by those around them, giving them valuable information about how much they should listen to and trust themselves. Instructors should cultivate a space where participants, even young ones, are encouraged to have their own relationship to the practices offered, forming their own opinions and sharing what is true for them. In this spirit, instructors should avoid assigning an experience or feeling to a particular form or exercise, that is, "It feels good to stretch" or, "This breath is so calming," instead asking participants what their own sensations were during various practices.

An opportunity exists when working with this age range to establish and/or expand protective behaviors that can serve individuals throughout their lives, far beyond the yoga mat. We can support the development of our children's self-awareness and build their confidence in themselves through practices that foster bodily awareness (proprioception) in an environment of safety and choice. Instructors and program administrators should work to establish an environment where self-agency/autonomy is prioritized over following specific movements or getting things "right." This can be challenging, and instructors are encouraged to consider their own comfort level with a session that might at times appear chaotic but is in fact building solid self-perception and regulation capacity for younger students.

Instructors can facilitate participant orientation to their own internal experiences, as well as their environment, by continually allowing for check-in through inquiry, "What do you notice/hear in the room?", "What do you notice around you?", "What do you notice in your own being/body?" Instructors may need to introduce vocabulary words connected to sensations and feelings. Even many adult participants could benefit from expanding their capacity to describe internal experiences. For example, one class session may focus on *how our feet feel* and the instructor could say that they notice "my feet feel warm, stuffy, and tingly. Does everyone know what tingly feels like?"

Ongoing trauma impacts cognitive processing and instructors should be ready and willing to deliver sessions with a pacing that is suitable for all participants. There is an increased chance for success (safety, building self-knowledge …) when sessions are short in duration. Even fifteen minutes can be a significant amount of time for young children to engage with this offering, and if sessions are longer instructors may want to break up the time with tactile activities (such as coloring) if the children seem to be struggling with sustained attention.

Best Practice
Familiarize yourself with human developmental stages.

See the previous section and developmental milestones for further detail and seek additional reading and resources.

Best Practice
Offer sessions that are developmentally appropriate.

While there are best practices that are universal, certain approaches will yield better results depending upon the age of the participants. The milestones of attaining autonomy or self-efficacy, and taking initiative, are prominent from the ages of two to six years. Giving students meaningful ways to make choices and have those choices validated supports those developmental goals.

Most children in this age range can begin to support their body weight with their hands, work on increasing balance, and generally are advancing their physical capacities. This, combined with the energy of early childhood, can lead to a natural tendency to fling themselves into shapes and lose track of their felt experience. Slowing down and bringing their awareness to *how* their bodies are doing what they do can be a valuable part of recognizing their own strength and capacity.

Best Practice
Understand that children learn through play.

In this age range, the utility of play is paramount. Participants should be given options to explore yoga forms, perhaps with the use of music or flash cards, so participants can choose which yoga forms are of interest (see the reference list for children's yoga resources). Young minds and bodies crave exploration without restriction and yoga forms are one way to facilitate this. For a further elaboration of the importance of play as part of development see the text below, which shares a best practice from *Best Practices for Yoga in Schools*.

Use play to support learning, understanding, and development

Play is the work of young children. It empowers them to learn and develop socially, emotionally, and academically.

Providing ways for children to explore that are engaging and free of judgment or evaluation activates their curiosity and natural capacity to learn. A spirit of playfulness puts value on a child's experience and reinforces the importance of practice for its own sake. Opportunities for collaborative (non-competitive) play with others supports children as they develop their capacity to exist in a social environment and see themselves as a member of a community. Successful yoga programs for young children integrate play into the curriculum and encourage a spirit of playfulness in the teachers as well.

In early childhood settings, props can be used playfully to create meaningful and accessible classroom agreements and conflict management approaches. Props such as puppets, dolls, or stuffed animals can be an effective way to engage playfully with young children and examine broader ideas around conflict management. They can also be used to further develop ideas and concepts being explored in a yoga program (e.g., kindness, self-care).

Children of a young age will frequently seek to understand their world by acting out what they do not understand. Be aware that play such as superhero or weapon play has a developmental and social context. Adhere to school policies around what is and is not allowed, but avoid using language that might make children experience shame around their attempt to understand what they may be experiencing in their lives.

(Childress & Harper 2015: 91–2)

Best Practice
Utilize sessions to practice resilience building (autonomy/self-efficacy) through choice making.

Giving participants repeated, yet contained, choices will lend itself to furthering a participant's initiative. The idea is not to have a set group of practices, but rather to allow young participants the chance to sense their own experiences and preferences. Giving choice communicates that each participant, however young, is in charge of their own body. This is a skill that can be protective. There is no "correct" way for a child to practice yoga, and as such there is no "incorrect" way, as long as everyone is safe. Helping participants understand that there is huge variation in how individuals experience practices, and encouraging them to value and attend to their own feelings and sensations, will help the participants grow both self-awareness and agency.

Best Practice
Instructors should examine their own willingness to allow for student choice, knowing it may look and sound chaotic in session.

Teaching young children generally requires letting go of preconceived expectations. Sessions with children who have survived sexual trauma may be particularly challenging in light of cognitive and behavioral impacts that can present as difficulty following instruction or acting out verbally or physically. Many survivors experience a chronic hyper-arousal of their nervous systems, leading to a fight-or-flight response that can be evident in yoga sessions.

Best Practice
Keep sessions brief and small as developmentally appropriate.

Aligning with a developmentally appropriate approach, brief exposures to yoga may be more appropriate based on developmental stage and severity of post-traumatic challenges. For example, children from two to six have limited attention spans, which can be even more reduced in the aftermath of trauma. Often, the asana (physical yoga forms) can be interspersed with art activities, snack, story time, and more, so that the yoga becomes a part of their lives rather than a singular, periodic event.

Best Practice
Offer partner forms judiciously.

The use of "partner poses" is common in many children's yoga programs. These practices can be useful in learning to establish boundaries, request and offer consent, and can potentially be community building. Being sure to offer real choice (and accepting student decisions) is especially important when we introduce close contact with another person. Participants may be developmentally inclined to seek approval, and may override their own sense of physical or emotional safety to please an instructor or a peer. Before offering the opportunity to do partner work, much time must be spent on getting to know one another and creating an increased sense of community. It is also important that students have had many experiences of choice making being honored and even celebrated, so they know unequivocally that they can say no without being pressured, diminished, or dismissed. Instructors are cautioned to *never* require any touch between participants and to allow opting out at any time. In any partner work, the instructor should offer a variation that can be explored independently, so those who opt out of partnering remain an active part of the group.

Grooming children into sexual abuse

Molly R. Wolf, LMSW, PhD

In order to make sure that children comply with sexual abuse, individuals who offend against children use a set of behaviors called "grooming". These behaviors not only establish compliance, but also trust and secrecy from the child (Bennett & O'Donohue, 2014). In general, before and during sexual abuse of a child, perpetrators have already groomed the child, their environment (such as parents and other adults in the child's life), and sometimes entire institutions (such as was seen recently with Catholic churches, or United States of America Gymnastics) (McAlinden, 2006). Grooming behaviors are pre-calculated by the offender, and are designed to ensure that once the actual sexual abuse takes place, the child will keep the abuse secret. These behaviors are also designed to ensure that the people in the child's environment maintain an air of disbelief if the child ever does disclose the abuse. Grooming behaviors run the gamut from verbal coercion (such as promising the child money/gifts/special treatment, or telling the child that it's "just a game"), to threatening the child by saying they will tell the child's parents, or hurt something/someone the child loves (Wolf, Linn, & Pruitt, 2018). Grooming can also sometimes involve the use of drugs and alcohol, or the promise of drugs and alcohol (Wolf, Linn, & Pruitt, 2018). Current research suggests that the grooming process itself can be considered an act of child sexual abuse, and is associated with trauma symptoms (Wolf, Linn, & Pruitt, 2018).

Working with School Age Children (Seven to Twelve Years Old)

Commonly referred to as "middle childhood" these years are marked by the emergence of industry or self-efficacy. Children are becoming more independent and holding friendships in higher esteem while many encounter greater peer pressure. These years are pivotal in a child's acquisition of confidence in all spheres of their lives.

Developmental Milestones Aged Seven to Twelve Years

Social/Emotional

- begin thinking of the future
- pay more attention to friendships
- desire to be liked/accepted

Language/Communication

- mental capacity increases quickly
- capacity to express emotions increases

Cognitive

- begin to see others' point of view/opinions
- have an increased attention span
- knows months of year in order
- begins to apply logic

Movement/Physical

- movement becomes more graceful
- adult teeth arrive
- secondary sex traits begin to emerge.

While the field is still emerging, there is evidence that yoga in schools has the capacity to improve physical and mental health, increase positive behaviors as well as academic performance. Research, while limited to date, suggests that yoga improves mental health and behavior in children and adolescents (Birdee, et al. 2009; Galantino, et al. 2008). Yoga was found to have significant effects on academic performance (Kauts & Sharma 2009; Butzer, et al. 2015). A randomized controlled trial examining school-based yoga programs identified a range of results from enhanced attendance to increased emotional regulation (Frank, et al. 2017). Youth in this range are particularly susceptible to feeling inferior. One of the most promising possibilities when engaging this age group is enhancing bodily autonomy, which can serve as a protective factor against future sexual traumatization. Assisting participants establish their own sense of mastery is key. An instructor's vigilance over language that allows for individual variation in ability and inclination should remain a priority.

Participants in this age range are developing the capacity to accept the truth of their own experiences (self-trust) and an awareness of others' feelings and experiences (empathy). To this point instructors will benefit from direct language relating to proprioception: a participant's sense of their own bodily placement. In doing so, instructors can aid in students recognizing that their own experience may be the same or different from those around them. When an instructor has an established relationship with students, it is then possible to incorporate practices that allow for mirroring or joining. Cultivating opportunities for industry/autonomy and empathy are especially important when working with this age group.

We encourage a "life skills" approach when interacting with this age group to further enhance autonomy off the mat. Concepts of resilience, choice making, and strength are accessible for many students in this age range. Discussions become more appropriate in this age range and the establishment of "community agreements" is strongly encouraged prior to commencing sessions. These agreements are effective in establishing norms and can provide much needed boundaries and an accompanying sense of safety and predictability for participants. Instructors and other involved adults are encouraged to give voice to students so they can help shape sessions including but not limited to lighting, use of music, and arrangement of mats.

Of particular importance for session instructors is their own presentation, including choice of clothing and personal adornment. A best practice is to present in a manner devoid of extensive accessories or clothing with messages (brand name insignias can be suggestive to students). For further detail, see Chapter 4.

In a yoga session, there is often much to be gained by having smaller age ranges within middle childhood. For example, grouping seven to nine year olds together, and ten to twelve year olds together can often make the session run more smoothly, as some of the precocious behaviors that might be presented by a twelve year old are developmentally very far removed from the needs of a seven year old. This is especially true when the participants have any history of sexual trauma, because perpetrators may be older siblings, cousins, or students.

In offering best practices for school-age students within the current context, we acknowledge that our engagement of the topic cannot be comprehensive. If you plan to offer yoga in schools, we recommend that you seek further education, including the Yoga Service Council's *Best Practices for Yoga in Schools* (Childress & Cohen Harper 2015). This text is a valuable resource for working with this population in intentional and trauma-informed ways.

Best Practice
Offer choices based on invitational language.

Invitational language is a key component of a trauma-informed yoga approach. Examples of invitational language include phrases such as, "at your own pace...", "when/or if you're ready ...", "you're welcome to ...", "one option is ..." Instructors can offer students opportunities to choose movement or stillness, varying heights/angles for arms and legs, eyes opened or closed. Using invitational language conveys an acknowledgment that each participant is in charge of their own body and avoids establishing expectations for "success" in a yoga practice.

Invitational language leaves space for students to make choices. They can choose if they want to move, how they move, and for how long. It is important that the session leader is 100 percent comfortable in the choices being offered to ensure that a participant's choice is not met with resistance.

Offer choices that are accessible to participants, recalling that participants in this age range are working on building confidence, and they desire peer approval and belonging. An instructor may want to consider doing forms to less than capacity when demonstrating in order to avoid the impression that the more physically challenging or "advanced" version is the right one. Finally, clearly communicate that no particular choice is "better" than any other and that our needs are different at different times. Whatever is chosen will be the correct one and builds success (as long as it does not include acting out against another student).

> **Best Practice**
> Understand that the physical forms are secondary to establishing personal safety and autonomy.

As yoga has become more popular in the West, many of the more well-known formats involve rigorous physical exertion along with ongoing stimulation of the nervous system. While these classes are geared toward adults, it is not surprising that many young people's impressions of yoga involve extreme forms (that is, handstands) and the notion of "being good at yoga." It is vitally important for those considering offering yoga to children in this age range to establish an environment that is not competitive and allows each participant to notice and make choices about how or if they position their bodies. Instructors will want to safeguard against injury (which begins with choosing forms to introduce to the group) while also allowing individuals the freedom to position themselves in a way that makes sense to them based on how they are feeling in a given session.

Oftentimes participants will ask, "Am I doing this right?" and if an instructor is operating from a trauma-informed perspective the answer might be something like, "The only right way is how you decide to do the practice while listening to your own body." Offering yoga to this age range provides an excellent opportunity for students to safely experiment with noticing their bodies and making choices. Instructors are encouraged to repeatedly state that there is no "right" way to participate.

Having a participant suffering physically or mentally while trying to "master" a physical form negates the positive impact of establishing and strengthening decision making and autonomy as part of a trauma-informed yoga practice. The idea is not to discourage physical exploration but to remind participants that each person will have their own practice and because we are all different shapes and sizes, our forms will look different as well.

Another way that instructors can maximize the opportunities for participants developing personal safety and autonomy is to refrain from making comments on student participation. A seemingly harmless "nice" or "beautiful" while well intentioned can set the stage for participants to identify with an external voice or measure of themselves.

Working with Adolescents (Aged Thirteen to Eighteen)

Adolescence is a time of significant change; simultaneous social, physical, emotional, and cognitive milestones are being met, requiring elasticity.

Developmental Milestones Aged Thirteen to Eighteen

Social/Emotional

- separation from parents becomes more pronounced

- peer approval and desires for popularity dominates

Language/Communication

- use longer sentences; usually seven to twelve words or more.

- know how to use sarcasm and recognize sarcasm

- understand and use slang terms with friends and differentiate from the more formal language used with adults

Cognitive

- develop abstract thinking

- logic is more readily applied in schoolwork as compared to personal, emotional situations

- authority is questioned

- individual worldview is established

Movement/Physical

- increased need for sleep

- increased need for food; may always be hungry due to growth spurts.

Teaching yoga with adolescents comes with many challenges in general and more pronounced issues in the wake of sexual trauma. Of all reported sexual trauma victims, two out of three are aged twelve to seventeen. One in nine girls and one in fifty-three boys under the age of eighteen experience sexual trauma by an adult. Females aged sixteen to nineteen are four times more likely than the general population to be victimized by sexual assault (Finkelhor, et al. 2014).

According to the National Intimate Partner and Sexual Violence Survey Report:

- Being raped as a minor increases a woman's likelihood of being raped as an adult by 15 percent.

- One in five females and one in seven males who ever experienced rape, physical violence, and/or stalking by an intimate partner, first experienced some form of intimate partner violence from eleven to seventeen years of age.

- More than half of all rapes of females occur before age eighteen; 22 percent occur before the age of twelve.

- Adolescent girls who experience dating violence are more likely to exhibit other serious behaviors, such as substance abuse, increased suicide attempts, unhealthy weight control, and risky sexual behavior (Black, et al. 2011).

Adolescence is naturally a time of experimentation, testing boundaries, and furthering self-concept. Young people are solidifying their ego identity and typically experience role confusion under the best of circumstances. If you are interested in working with this age group you are encouraged to celebrate the chaos of adolescence while offering all students opportunities to experience feeling as safe as possible.

Instructors can be instrumental in supporting a healthy identity formation provided there is an awareness of some key realities: sexual explorations, issues of consent, peer pressure, intimate partner violence, social media shaming, and revenge pornography can all be part of adolescents' lives. Attempts for peer status can promote destructive behaviors without any consideration of consequences. Because the prefrontal cortex is not fully developed, adolescents can have less access to executive functioning, including memory, cognitive flexibility, and inhibitory control. This may play out in yoga sessions.

While adolescence can be a time of tumult, yoga sessions have the capacity to help participants navigate accompanying emotions and experiences. As stated previously, the skills gained in yoga sessions are ideally those that can positively impact life off the mat, including personal safety, self-agency, and efficacy. Promoting community agreements set at the beginning of sessions is one way to encourage this in allowing for collaboration by establishing a shared purpose for sessions. This is also aligned with a strengths-based approach.

It is not uncommon for programs in schools or residential settings to mandate student attendance, which can present a conflict when operating from a trauma-informed perspective. As part of the self-inquiry process, instructors might consider how to allow for choice once students are in the physical yoga space. For example, allowing students to participate to whatever level they choose on a given day including modifications or simply sitting or lying down.

If you are a clinician wishing to use body-based modalities, including yoga, you should complete specialized training before engaging in this work or seek proper referral. Bearing in mind that many yoga classes are highly arousing to the nervous system and prior to referring clients, clinicians should make themselves aware of the class particulars, that is, level of intensity or duration of silent meditation. For further recommendations on referral to yoga in consideration of a sexual trauma history see Rousseau, Weiss-Lewit, and Lilly (2019).

At the beginning of our 4 week session, the instructors asked us what our needs were to feel safe enough to access yoga with the group for the month. After we shared our needs, as a group we created a set of guidelines. These rules, or "agreements" made each of us feel a sense of agency and predictability. I was able to practice yoga knowing the rules so I knew what was appropriate to do or not do.

– Yoga student

Our clinical experience with this population over the past several years has demonstrated that the potential for yoga to play an important role in helping shift chronically traumatized adolescents' relationship to their bodies from negligence, gross indulgence, numbing or self-harm toward capacity to feel safe in and accepting of their bodies, to increase tolerance and regulation of painful affect states and behavior impulses and begin to identify, cultivate, and possibly appraise physical competencies.

(Spinazzola, et al. 2011: 432)

This section that follows shares practices that support work in settings where trauma histories are common, including shelters or residential treatment centers, or in circumstances that a sexual trauma history is known. While these recommendations apply to working with adolescent survivors, they are certainly appropriate for survivors of different ages.

Best Practice
Complete trauma-specific training and education.

While this recommendation has been discussed elsewhere and is of fundamental importance in working with survivors of sexual trauma more generally, the importance of seeking trauma-specific and more specifically age-appropriate, trauma-specific training is worth noting. This is especially salient for residential facilities where the likelihood of residents having survived sexual trauma is greater than in the general population. A report by Georgetown Law Center on Poverty and Inequality found that 35 percent of girls in residential and corrections facilities reported a history of sexual abuse (Epstein, et al. 2017). The desire to offer yoga as part of a wellness program can be co-opted by well-intentioned, but undertrained, instructors offering sessions that are overly stimulating and triggering for participants. Offering yoga to those who are known to have survived sexual trauma is not merely a recreational activity and should be approached with care so as to not re-traumatize participants.

Best Practice
Establish and respect agreed upon protocol for sessions – recalling the importance of community agreements and predictability.

Following the tenets of a trauma-informed approach, transparency is key. While it is unrealistic to cover everything, a community agreement is an opportunity for participants and the session instructor to arrive at agreed upon conduct or conditions while exemplifying the notion of shared power across the group. It can also limit the chances that one or some will "police" others in the group, recalling that autonomy is being practiced.

Participants deserve to know what the expectations are for a session, that is, are they free to set a mat up anywhere in the space, do they need to face the instructor, is it OK to lie down instead of choosing to move, is talking allowed, can they come in late, will the instructor be stationary, will the instructor participate alongside participant(s), will lights be adjusted at any time, can they chew gum. Each instructor is encouraged to set time aside for setting up community agreements as a road map for the yoga experience. These agreements may need to be revisited if the composition of the group changes or just as participants or the instructor deems useful. Regarding predictability, it is also important that a consistent, fully trained instructor is identified who can begin and end sessions on time. Without this, the instructor will be deemed untrustworthy.

Best Practice
Instructors are encouraged to be intentional in relation to decisions around touch.

As a general rule, the best practice is to avoid touch and hands-on adjustments. Considerations around the use of touch are discussed further in Chapter 4. The text that follows discusses these considerations in further detail as they specifically apply to working with children and adolescents.

Considerations around touch and consent in children's yoga

The role of touch and consent is complicated in any field that involves human contact. Teaching yoga to children generates many opportunities to consider this complexity, and work towards creating safe and meaningful experiences for all involved.

In yoga touch may be used for a variety of reasons – to adjust or assist a posture, to support relaxation, to offer connection – but it is possible that the way a student receives touch may differ from the intention of the teacher offering it. Most notably when a student has experienced interpersonal trauma, touch can easily be experienced as invasive, overwhelming, or aggressive. Because we rarely know the prior trauma history of our students, this possibility for doing harm must be considered.

Beyond this potential for harm is the subtler but significant message that adjustments might send to any students, even those who welcome touch. One of the goals of sharing yoga with young people should involve increasing awareness of one's own body, both its needs and capacity. When the body is adjusted by an instructor, students can receive the message that they are doing something wrong, that they are not good at the practice, or that they need an external source to adequately assess and control their body.

All yoga instructors, but especially those working with children, should carefully consider the implication of adjustments to postures, as well as our intention in offering them. If our intention is to make the posture "better" we should consider if that goal is the one that is most important in the moment. Verbally cuing adjustments to postures, in cases where there is a safety concern, or if we are offering an opportunity to explore another aspect of an experience, is a safer choice than physically adjusting in most circumstances.

While touch can be problematic, human contact is an essential part of healthy emotional and physical development. Touch, such as an optional high five, can support relationship and the child feeling valued. Touch that is student directed (such as inviting a student to reach for an instructor's hand) can help with the understanding of body positioning in a posture, but such touch should be carefully considered and always have an easy "out" for the student if they'd rather not make contact.

Consider that true consent to be touched can be difficult, if not impossible, to confirm when working with children given the inherent power dynamics. Young people are vulnerable. As they are developing awareness around their body, and around consent in their lives, they may struggle to articulate what they are comfortable with. There may be social pressures to either be touched or not be touched that play into their decisions in a yoga space. If they feel that the instructor will be offended or hurt, or that their participation in class will be questioned by their decision not to be touched, it may contribute to their decision making. Students that have experienced sexual abuse may not feel they have the right to make such decisions for themselves, and compliance with perceived "want" of the adult may be engaged as a safety mechanism.

Often in a yoga studio environment, students are given the chance to opt out of being touched. I don't recommend this strategy with children. Consider that a student might not hear the invitation to opt out, might be self-conscious making a decision that is different from the group, might assume that physically being adjusted is the default and that by opting out they are doing something less than the full practice, or might even feel that they don't have the right to make decisions for their own body. If you choose to include any kind of touch in your classes, students should be actively opting in, with a clear and easy way to communicate a change of mind.

In the vast majority of situations, refraining from touch will allow students to better connect with their own experience and develop a greater sense of agency. If we find ourselves reaching out to touch our students, it's important that we ask ourselves why. If it's to connect, we can challenge ourselves to find other ways of building relationship that don't risk harm or reduce autonomy.

– Jennifer Cohen Harper, Little Flower Yoga, project contributor

Best Practice
Realize that the details of any particular trauma are never part of a yoga session.

Aside from the respect and trust-building of strict confidentiality, any focus on particular traumatic events in a yoga session makes it more challenging to build resilience and strength, which are broad-based powers, useful for all manner of needs-meeting and life goal attainment.

Best Practice
Respect people's survival strategies.

Remember that in order for participants to be in a yoga session resilience is present. The traumatic experience does not define a survivor. Survivors bring with them a range of survival strategies. Be open to the many ways that survivors present and honor the resilience in the room.

While yoga is known to support physical and mental well-being, as well as contribute to the building of resilience, we do not want to push people to change their behavior – for example, to stop smoking, eat more organic food, or leave their abuser. People do what they do in order to survive, and survivors of sexual violence often expend enormous amounts of energy on the tasks of getting through each day. By not trying to "correct" people's behavior, but instead focusing on helping them be as strong, capable, and clear-minded as possible, we honor their agency and individuality, while at the same time giving them tools to address needs in a sustainable way.

Chapter 8

> **Best Practice**
> Be aware that survivors may have a destructive relationship with themselves, including ongoing self-loathing, blame, fear, and guilt, and much of this might arise in a yoga session.

Coming into a yoga session can be an unnerving experience for some and takes great courage for many participants. If you have space that includes mirrors, be aware that catching one's reflection can be a triggering experience for trauma survivors. Consider using shades or curtains to obscure mirrors in your practice space. Students may feel inadequate, uncoordinated, or scared in a new environment such as a yoga session. Be sure to offer opportunities for participants to feel "successful," which is related to developmentally appropriate content as well as physical "asks." Instructors will benefit from teaching to the most physically restricted member of a session to facilitate befriending one's self in the aftermath of trauma.

> **Best Practice**
> Know your community resources and recognize when and how to refer students for additional attention beyond your scope of practice when warranted.

Keep in mind the scope of your work as a yoga instructor, studio owner, or program manager. Familiarize yourself with your local Crisis Service provider and behavioral and mental health providers and have their contact information on hand to share as appropriate. Many communities have a 211 system that is available by phone and online that directs users to local services for a host of needs (www.211.org).

> **Best Practice**
> Have a safety plan in place (some students may still be experiencing ongoing trauma) both during and after sessions.

We truly have no way of knowing how safe participants are or feel outside or even during yoga sessions. Participants might be at risk of continued trauma at the hands of another or they may experience episodic suicidal ideation or attempts in the aftermath of trauma, or a host of other dangerous or less than safe behaviors. Consider use of a safety plan or work with partner organizations to ensure a plan is in place. An example of a safety plan follows (Figure 8.1).

> **Best Practice**
> When possible engage and work collaboratively with non-offending caregivers, social supports, and other service providers so they can be partners.

As stated previously, knowing one's scope of practice or area of expertise is key to this work. There may be a worker who the participant trusts who might be able to participate alongside the youth. Additional supportive team members can reinforce the participant's developing autonomy as well as gain an understanding of how the body can be incorporated into healing sexual trauma.

If there is a supportive, safe caregiver consider inviting that person to be part of your sessions with a youth. Depending upon circumstances, the supportive caregiver may be healing from their own trauma as well. Bear in mind that the decision to participate in sessions is individual and no one should be pressured or convinced to participate.

Safety plan		
Step 1 Warning signs		
1		
2		
3		
Step 2 Internal coping strategies – things I can do to take my mind off my problems without contacting another person		
1		
2		
3		
Step 3 People and social settings that provide distraction		
1	Name	Phone
2	Name	Phone
3	Place	
4	Place	
Step 4 People whom I can ask for help		
1	Name	Phone
2	Name	Phone
3	Name	Phone
Step 5 Professionals or agencies I can contact during a crisis		
1	Clinician name Clinician pager or emergency contact number	Phone
2	Clinician name Clinician pager or emergency contact number	Phone
3	Suicide Prevention Lifeline	1-800-273-TALK (8255)
4	Local emergency service	Phone Address
Making the environment safe		
1		
2		

Figure 8.1

Sample safety plan. From Stanley B and Brown GK (2011) Safety planning intervention: A brief intervention to mitigate suicide risk. Cognitive and Behavioral Practice 19 256–264.

Source: Sample safety plan. From Stanley B and Brown GK (2011) Safety planning intervention: A brief intervention to mitigate suicide risk. Cognitive and Behavioral Practice 19 256–264 – see PDF.

Another option that is sometimes more effective is to offer parallel classes, one series for the children, and one for the caregivers. As each group has differing needs, this method allows each group to grow stronger, calmer, and more capable in ways that are appropriate to their needs. This approach often concludes with one or two "celebration" sessions where young people and caregivers practice together, and can share all that they have learned, and celebrate the yoga knowledge they both now have in common.

> **Best Practice**
> Practice should focus on proprioception and interception as developmentally appropriate, and individual bodily safety, not posture "mastery."

As stated previously, the physical representations will vary and should not be prioritized. In a trauma-informed session there is no "full expression" of a form as exists in other types of yoga. Repeated invitations and opportunities to notice their bodies in relation to the world around them are key to moving the focus off the physical representation and into the felt experience. Many participants, regardless of age, will not recognize words such as "proprioception" or "interoception" so instructors must understand these concepts and be ready to explain them in the most basic way.

Proprioception senses the position, location, orientation, and movement of the body's muscles and joints (STAR 2018). Proprioception provides us with the sense of the relative position of neighboring parts of the body and effort used to move body parts. The invitation to notice their bodies may take time as many survivors experience disembodiment in the wake of sexual trauma. Instructors are cautioned to never suggest

a sensation or an attached meaning. Allowing exploration of the experience of having one's leg bent or straight, or crossing one arm over the other, are examples of how proprioception can be addressed.

Interoception adds onto proprioception to include the *emotional* component to sensory experience. More than just recognizing a physical sensation, interoception encompasses any and all emotions that accompany a physical sensation. As Barrett and Simmons (2015: 419) point out, "Interoception is a fundamental feature of the human nervous system that has relevance for many biological, as well as psychological, phenomena, such as eating, craving and decision making."

> **Best Practice**
> Consider yoga as just one piece of a larger healing picture that might include equine or art therapy, photography, or other activities that promote a sense of industry/autonomy.

The intent of utilizing trauma-informed yoga in the aftermath of sexual trauma is not to be a standalone intervention. We know there are multiple approaches that can augment recovery ranging from art therapy to dance. In offering trauma-informed yoga there needs to be an allowance for participants to decline after trying a session or two. There is no "right" way to process and heal from sexual trauma and some youth may not wish to utilize a yoga practice in any way. Recalling that the intention is to provide access to sensations while building autonomy, other options should be considered either in addition to or in place of a yoga practice.

> **Best Practice**
> Work in conjunction with therapeutic/clinical service providers.

Prior to offering sessions, a list of qualified mental health professionals should be compiled and made available to all instructors. This list should include emergency/crisis service providers who may need to be called upon during a session as well as resources for participants who might seek or be in need of additional therapeutic counsel. For those working in a residential setting, in-house clinical staff are ideal partners. Instructors can offer session notes relative to the treatment goals and progress of individual participants. In some instances, participants might be encouraged to journal about their experience with yoga as they heal from sexual trauma.

> **Best Practice**
> Create empowering opportunities for participants to celebrate their wholeness.

To the best of your ability, and utilizing a community agreement, sessions should be enjoyed by all (please see prior section on community agreements). Giving participants the chance to feel capable, potent, and whole paves the way for them to extend empathy to others. One idea is to give participants the option to choose a form that they find particularly useful/enjoyable/positive about. This can be done simply by using the name of a form or by using pre-made or self-made yoga cards. Depending on class size, some might use a rotating approach whereby one student picks a card each week or if working individually offering the option each time to

the student. Again, this reinforces a balancing of the power differential between a typical "teacher–student" relationship. In allowing students choice, you will gain access to what brings them a sense of accomplishment. There is always room in a session for light-heartedness, celebration, and maybe even laughter and joy.

Conclusion

While human development varies, becoming familiar with generally recognized stages, domains, and milestones is an important undertaking. Perhaps the greatest takeaway from this section on working with survivors of sexual trauma from birth through adolescence is that human development is an intricate process involving genetics, environment, and experience. The interplay of these factors can alter cognitive, emotional, social, and physical development, especially during the first four years of life when the vast majority of structural brain development and organization is happening. Sexual trauma that takes place during this window of organization has a greater potential to influence the brain, including problems with attention, memory, and learning challenges. As such, sexual trauma should be considered in relation to human development.

We know that relationship to perpetrator (known or stranger), availability of social supports and the age(s) at which the trauma occurs impact survivors' experiences. And while sexual trauma can impact the progression of human development it is equally important to note that not all who experience sexual trauma experience a developmental impact. For example, a child living within a supportive family context who experiences one episode of sexual trauma perpetrated by a stranger may have a vastly different outcome than a child whose caregiver is neglectful and experiences sexual trauma at the hands of another family member.

Readers are reminded of the pivotal role that attachment plays in facilitating human development, including an individual's sense of personal power, trust, self-worth, and capacity for intimacy. Sexual trauma perpetrated by an individual who holds an otherwise nurturing role, that is, parent, sibling, teacher, coach, pastor, or priest, can have an especially detrimental impact.

Developmental domains and milestones are only to be used as a guide: there is tremendous variation and overlap. It is not uncommon for an individual to struggle reaching an emotional milestone while readily mastering a cognitive one or vice versa. Our recommendations should be understood as guideposts or markers as opposed to step-by-step directions.

In teaching yoga it is critical to understand that predictability in sessions allows a sense of safety to emerge and this sense of safety is the foundation of healing in the aftermath of sexual trauma. Once safety has been experienced, participants can explore attunement – a sense of their own being as well as others around them. Consider the teenage survivor of childhood sexual trauma who is consumed with watching the entrance to the room and is therefore unable to notice how they are feeling or follow the instructor: a sense of safety precedes all else.

Lastly, despite the potential for sexual trauma to begin a cascade of struggles, encompassing physical, mental, and emotional health, survivors rally on to find a sense of wholeness in their lives. Surviving sexual trauma does not eliminate the possibility for joy, laughter, fulfilling relationships, and general success. For some it impedes or delays these life-enriching experiences, and our hope is that trauma-informed yoga can be one piece of the puzzle in putting a rewarding, enriched, joyful life together.

Recommended Resources

American Psychological Association (2014) Child sexual abuse: What parents should know [pdf] [Online] Available: http://www.apa.org/pi/families/resources/child-sexual-abuse.aspx [10 December 2018].

Anderson-McNamee JK and Bailey SJ (2010) The importance of play in early childhood development, Montana: Montana State University.

Childress T and Harper JC (2015) Best practices for yoga in schools, Atlanta, GA: YSC/Omega Publications.

Copeland WE, Keeler G, Angold A, and Costello EJ (2007) Traumatic events and post traumatic stress in childhood. Archives of General Psychiatry 64 (5) 577–584.

Cruise K and Ford J (2011) Trauma exposure and PTSD in justice-involved youth. Child and Youth Care Forum 40 (50) 337–343.

Flynn L (2013) Yoga for children: 200+ yoga poses, breathing exercises, and meditations for healthier, happier, more resilient children, New York, NY: Adams Media.

Fromberg DP and Bergen D (2006) Play from birth to twelve: Contexts, perspectives, and meanings, 2nd edn, New York, NY: Routledge.

Goldberg L (2004) Creative relaxation: A yoga-based program for regular and exceptional student education. International Journal for Yoga Therapy 14 68–78.

Hagen I and Nayar US (2014) Yoga for children and young people's mental health and well-being: Research review and reflections on the mental health potentials of yoga. Front Psychiatry 5 35. 10.3389/fpsyt.2014.00035.

Jensen FE and Nutt AE (2015) The teenage brain: A neuroscientist's survival guide to raising adolescents and young adults, New York, NY: Harper-Collins Publishers.

Kaley-Isley LC, Peterson J, Fischer C, and Peterson E (2010) Yoga as a complementary therapy for children and adolescents: A guide for clinicians. Psychiatry (Edgemont) [e-journal] 7 (8) 20–32.

Kauts A and Sharma N (2009) Effect of yoga on academic performance in relation to stress. International Journal of Yoga 2 (1) 39–43. 10.4103/0973-6131.53860.

Kraag G, Zeegers MP, Kok G, Hossman C, and Abu-Saad HH (2006) School programs targeting stress management in children and adolescents: A meta-analysis. Database of Abstracts of Reviews of Effects (DARE): Quality-assessed Reviews [Internet]. York (UK): Centre for Reviews and Dissemination (UK) [Online] Available: https://www.ncbi.nlm.nih.gov/books/NBK73326/ [1 March 2019].

Meggitt C (2012) Understand child development, London: Hodder Education.

Nunez N, Warren A and Poole D (2008) The story of human development, New Jersey: Prentice Hall.

Putnam FW (2003) Ten-year research update review: Child sexual abuse. Journal of the American Academy of Child and Adolescent Psychiatry 42 269–278.

Siegel DJ (2013) Brainstorm: The power and purpose of the teenage brain, New York, NY: Penguin Group.

Solter AJ (2013) Attachment play. How to solve children's behavior problems with play, laughter, and connection, Goleta, CA: Shining Star Press.

STAR Institute for Sensory Processing Disorder (STAR) (2018) Your Eight Sensory Systems [Online] Available: www.spdstar.org/ /basic/ your-8-senses/ [15 November 2018].

Sternberg EC (2017) The effects of daily yoga practice on the academic engagement and achievement of middle school students in a special education classroom. Theses and Dissertations. 2411.http://rdw.rowan.edu/etd/2411 [15 January 2019].

Thomas RM (2001) Recent theories of human development, California: Sage Publications.

Trickett P, Noll J, and Putnam F (2011) The impact of sexual abuse on female development: Lessons from a multigenerational, longitudinal research study. Development and Psychopathology 23 (2) 453–476. https://doi.org/10.1017/S0954579411000174.

Identities and Intersectional
Perspectives

Gender and Sexual Minorities Community

Author *Dani Harris*

Contributors *Jacoby Ballard, Nan Herron, Diana Hoscheit, James Jurgensen*

Introduction

For the purposes of respectful inclusivity and honoring the spectrum of diversity within this population as well as its past and contemporary history, this book will use the term Gender and Sexual Minorities (GSM) to address those who identify within the gay, lesbian, bisexual, transgender, queer or questioning, intersex, asexual or allied community.

When considering sharing yoga with vulnerable young people who have identified as being part of the GSM community, in the context of helping recovery from sexual violence, there are many subtle things to consider. The following narrative example serves to highlight some of those.

Note: all the names, ages, and other potentially identifying information have been changed to protect privacy and anonymity.

Case study

Jay and Kyra are fourteen and nineteen years old respectively, and both will be living in the same specialty medium-term group for the next four weeks. At that time, Kyra will age out of the system and face life as an adult. She does not feel ready. Kyra was raised as a boy by her fundamentalist parents, and when she decided to live more authentically as a girl, and then woman, her parents screamed invective hatred at her for four hours, and then kicked her out for good. She has not seen them since.

Jay has been living at Golden Tree Youth Home for two weeks (Kyra for three years), and is still terrified. He lived with his mom and sisters until he was six, and then with his grandmother until he was nine when she died. He then lived with various "relatives" for five years, suffering terrors he's never spoken of to anyone, and finally the courts, advocates, and cops intervened and took him to Golden Tree.

Kyra and Jay will be participating in a weekly yoga session in the day room, making space between the very old couches, tilting bookshelves, and the oft unworking video game console and controller. They participate for different reasons: Jay because he has to attend self-care and well-being sessions as a new member of the group home, and Kyra because she's terrified of aging out and being alone again.

As session time comes, everyone gets mats out of the ripped cardboard box in the corner, moves the coffee table, and, usually, chat constantly. Well, of the seven young people five talk a lot and two almost never.

When the furniture is moved the staff on duty comes in to explain the rules of the space, which everyone is familiar with, and one of the talkers

continued

asks if it's time for crow and Jay stares like he knows he's going to screw up and Kyra is breathing fast but slower than usual.

The doors remain open due to regulations, and it is not uncommon for staff, other young people, or even police officers to walk by in the hallway and look in. One officer three weeks ago commented that "you ladies look great, keep it up!" that was not well received and led to a twenty-minute discussion in the middle of warrior. The class was scattered the whole rest of the session.

Before you even begin teaching, what sort of needs are you identifying with the people you're sharing yoga with today? How might you adjust your language, pacing, and verbal cuing to help out as much as possible?

Background

Recognizing that history is also experienced in the present tense, these words are a mere beginning for conversations and learning that will come. We further acknowledge that there are gaps in our understanding, given the scale of the GSM community. We can say, however, that the GSM community is, without question, skillfully resilient. There is a vibrancy and joy in this willingness to stay connected and grounded to a sense of self that has been demonized and criticized for years. It is simply strong and brilliant.

Understanding the often dark and always vibrant history of the GSM community is paramount to teaching yoga to GSM students. Through the Stonewall protests in 1969, the sexual revolution of the 1970s, the acquired immune deficiency syndrome (AIDS) epidemic of the 1980s and 1990s, the fight for attaining marriage and adoption rights, as well as current issues of trans rights, like most histories, the history of the GSM community is tremendously rich, complex, and ever developing.

The Impact of Yoga for the GSM Community

We have the greatest opportunity, right now, well researched and with heart, to create communities built on existing strengths with these best practices. With great preparation, yoga can be instrumental in reconnecting the GSM community with themselves and one another. With safety for the most vulnerable people in the room at the forefront and with deep introspection and care, change can happen, literally from the inside out. For communities that are still thriving despite their wounds, the loving practice of yoga will always win.

Yoga helps people deal with loss. The practices we share have the opportunity to help participants cope with loss, helping them to accept their grief for what it is and mourn.

While research on sexual violence in the general population is extensive, research on the same in the GSM community is still lacking (although growing), and when present is more generalized, not accounting for the wide range of gender and sexual expressions present within the GSM community. Lack of access to language connected to reporting, laws that do not incorporate same sex or trans language, and other societal factors influence both the lack of research and the willingness or capacity of GSM people to report instances of sexual violence.

In one review of existing research, Brown and Herman (2015) note that while approximately 15 percent of heterosexual women reported intimate partner sexual violence, the numbers rose to 40 percent for bisexual women reporting in the same category. Additionally, they discern that while research is sparse and ongoing, current figures suggest that transgender people may have similar or increased rates of violence to those who identify as gay, lesbian, or bisexual (Brown & Herman 2015).

Outside of sexual violence GSM people experience greater risk of losing people in their community, their personal and professional relationships, connections to their religious and cultural communities, their professions and their roles within their families during and after the coming-out process.

In addition to concerns about sexual violence, mental health considerations have been researched. Kessler et al. (2012) note that 10 percent of GSM youth present with characteristics of a mood disorder, 25 percent present with anxiety disorders, and 8.3 percent meet the criteria for substance abuse.

Further, studies over the past two decades highlight the elevated risk for both attempted and completed suicide by GSM people. These studies are also limited because death certificates do not identify a deceased's gender (other than biological) or sexual orientation. A 2008 multi-country analysis indicated that GSM males were four times more likely to attempt suicide than their heterosexual peers; females were twice as likely to exhibit the same than their heterosexual peers (King et al. 2008). The same study reports that 12 to 19 percent of GSM adults are reported to have attempted suicide. This is compared with less than five percent of non-GSM identifying people.

Yoga can help remediate the loss of self by offering levels of acceptance and places to grieve and to find joy again in being the curious, free people we were meant to be, all of us.

For many, there are multiple layers of events that have happened over time and are often still happening. This understanding goes a long way when teaching those in the GSM community who have experienced sexual trauma. It is best to go slowly because yoga can connect people to an intimacy with themselves that perhaps they have never had a chance to develop in the face of sexual and minority discrimination. This is an invitation to use your own yoga to become aware of and then challenge core beliefs and affirm the ways in which we need to rewrite those core beliefs in relationship with the GSM community.

We know the greatest risk is losing oneself in the aftermath of sexual violence. We have the responsibility to offer practices that engender strength and capacity building rather than ones that focus on victimization.

Yoga can help. It will just take time.

Sexualized Settings

For most of its history, the GSM community has had few places to authentically connect with other people outside of dark, often sexualized bars and clubs. Further, the messages concerned with developing an innocent intimacy with self and others at younger ages is often mired in confusion, doubt, mistrust, and hate perpetuated by others and internalized by self.

When one comes of age and enters the social scene, long-established power dynamics and hierarchies are present. Navigating these dynamics as well as trying to establish and learn about yourself sexually is challenging. The primal desires to be sexual and intimate, often for the first time in one's life, coupled with the norms at social events such as the availability of alcohol and drugs and the expectation of sexual behavior have the potential to increase instances of unwanted, non-consensual sexualization and sex acts. The media has normalized this behavior, and there are circles in the GSM community that have internalized this. Therefore, in some subcultures, the potential for harm increases. If you had no innocent sexual experiences growing up, you are thrown into this community that believes in its own hyper-sexualization, and the risk of assault increases exponentially.

The emergence of dating apps has created opportunities for people in every community to connect instantly with people. This is especially useful for people within the GSM community. While these meetings are becoming socially common, they too are not without risk. Many of these connections that started out online, end up as momentary, short, in person encounters. This is problematic if one is in the acutely vulnerable developmental stage of just learning about their body and learning about how intimacy works for them. The risk is that this type of sex can easily become normalized and commonplace. This works for some people and can easily leave others with a false sense of intimacy and feeling revictimized, integrating ideas that their only worth is in their bodies for sex.

It is important to recognize that while many instances of sexual violence are perpetrated by those outside of the GSM community, sexual violence is also present in GSM identified spaces advertised as "safe." This has the capacity to leave one wondering "when the community I belong to hurts me, where can I go?"

> One of my most profound moments was at a trans group of yoga, we ended it by saying, "Let's just all take a deep breath" – one person said, "I didn't realize how long it had been since I had felt safe enough to take a full breath"
>
> – Trans yoga participant

Issues of Sexual Violence in the GSM Community

Issues of sexual violence in the GSM community are automatically complex due to their intersections with culture, race, religion, and historic and systemic oppression. The traumatic complexity here is four-fold:

1. The sexual trauma can ambush the whole self.

2. The assaults by mainstream culture's phobias and hate cause intense disconnection to self and community.

3. The systems of oppression and their intersections can impact a person's understanding of their value and worth in the world.

4. Instances of sexual violence in the GSM community can happen, which further devastates a person's connection to safety and community.

These four complications create both internal and external beliefs that most, if not the entire world, is a hostile, threatening, unsafe place, and that there are no safe spaces left at all.

Barriers to Accessing and Practicing Yoga

It is important to understand that for many people in the GSM community there are immediate barriers to both accessing and practicing yoga. These barriers are compounded when experiences of sexual violence are present. As such, this is not an exhaustive list, but serves to inform your own teaching knowing that you will have students in your classes from this community who have also experienced sexual violence.

Lack of Access to Spaces to Feel Comfortable In

Depending on where one lives and what one's history is, GSM, specifically "trans only spaces" and classes are very rare for a variety of reasons. Posting that a class is GSM population specific, even in larger cities, runs the risk of becoming a target. These feelings reside deeply in the body and have the potential to increase an already present hypervigilance in students, which can prevent them from accessing many of the benefits of yoga.

If the Classes are Available, They are Often Held in Secret

This safety-informed practice is usually "advertised" through a change of connection. From a survivor's point of view, being in a concealed space where no one out of the class knows where you are can be triggering.

Feelings of Being Uncomfortable in One's Own Body

This can occur as a result of pre-transitioning, transitioning, and sexual violence.

Lack of Trust in Systems Created to Protect People

GSM people's rights are currently transitory in nature. Officials that other people would go to for help might not have a legal obligation to do anything about concerns a person from the GSM might have. The absence of GSM affirming regulatory services increases instances of self-blame and non-reporting.

Sexual violence against GSM people is highly underreported. There are three main reasons for this:

1. To report you must re-identify yourself as part of the GSM community, and others can take the instances less seriously when you do so. This is further complicated if drugs or alcohol have been a factor in the assault, as one would have to disclose that as well.

2. There are high levels of shame and minimization. Because there is often a lack of understanding from people hearing the report, there is a great risk to the survivor. GSM people who do report sexual violence are generally met with a highly nuanced response of judgment as compared to their straight peers.

3. There is an awareness that movements like #MeToo have failed to include the GSM community. Movements aimed at decreasing sexual violence have come from a place of unacknowledged privilege, where assaults are being taken seriously simply because someone identifies in the accepted majority.

This experience is in contrast to the voicing and reporting for GSM people where assaults are often met with dismissal and blame. It is not uncommon for a person identifying with the GSM community to hear phrases indicating that the assault was a result of the "choices that you made." This tends to make people respond to reports in a way that forces the blame and responsibility onto the survivor.

Being Tokenized

The commoditizing and tokenizing of GSM people by the media has had adverse effects on the community, perpetuating stereotypes and myths regarding the experience of GSM people. We simply ask that when you think you are celebrating someone ("I'm so happy that you felt you could come here; I have a trans nephew"), you are not contributing to the emotional labor many GSM people experience.

Safe Spaces

The term "safe space" is one that originated in the late 1960s, at about the time of the Stonewall riots, and was created as a way to identify GSM bars and clubs where one could experiment and learn while experiencing being exactly who they are in the company of like-minded people. What we have learned since then is that "safe spaces" have to be named as conditional. The bars and clubs of the 1960s and 1970s were only "safe spaces" until the police arrived with weapons and tear gas. Contemporary events of violence in GSM positive spaces also prove that safety can never be completely guaranteed.

Many of us still use the phrase "safe space" in our yoga classrooms. Phrases like "you are safe here" and "you are safe in your body" are common and reiterated in studios and yoga spaces around the world. Much of this is said with no maligned intent, of course. However, it is worth being aware that participants from certain communities and background have an acute and often visceral sense of what the word "safe" means. By denoting a space as "safe," at best, we risk having students who are unable to let down and move through their practices being less guarded. At worst, we risk activating their traumas and losing their trust, choosing instead to not practice at all.

One idea, which can be revisited in other sections of this book, was to consider using "brave spaces." You may find yourself having to study your own communities to see which works best given the historical foundation for this word within the GSM community.

Best Practices
Self-inquiry

> **Best Practice**
> Question why you want to work with this population in particular.

Come back to this question again and again because everything matters when dealing with a specific population; discerning your personal motivation for working with this population regardless of whether or not you identify with the community is fundamental. If you do identify with the community, you need to consider how being a part of it in the role of a yoga teacher will impact personal, professional, and community lives. You also need to consider whether or not you have the skills required to teach within your own community. Be very honest about this. The GSM community has many different subgroups; it is important to know your limits.

If you are not a part of the GSM community, this question is equally important. Consider whether you have blind spots in your teaching practices that need to be more inclusive, knowledgeable, and well rounded. Examine all personal beliefs and assumptions you have about this community. Gaps in your knowledge without examining your beliefs and assumptions will have both subtle and conspicuous impacts. If this is true for you, seek further education as a safety measure.

In both cases, create professional relationships that can keep your knowledge current, diverse, and relevant to your population. This community evolves quickly; you need a personal and professional readiness in order to engage in high-quality, resilience-focused, and sustainable teaching practices and programs.

When you have the answer, and it comes from a place of knowledge, respect, and great care, teach with the gifts of awe, curiosity, grace, and inclusivity. Everything else will follow, if you are well prepared. Commit also to ongoing self-inquiry and reflection.

Best Practice
Identify the pros and cons of self-disclosure in the context of your class and understand the impact it could have on those present.

If it is important to you to self-disclose the way you identify or what community you are a part of, please question why. Recognize that this self-disclosure could confuse participants and have them question what your motive is in teaching them. Some may see this as a way to advertise your relationship availability, as in the early years of the GSM rights movement this is how people met. However, if speaking to the way you identify within the community will bring a sense of comfort, then it may be beneficial, as representation from leaders in communities can be very powerful. Whatever your disclosure is, you are encouraged to make the disclosure at a group level rather than disclosing to just one person. This is suggested as a way to lessen the pressure the disclosure might have and to make the intention behind the disclosure clear.

Language

Best Practice
Choose language that demonstrates current knowledge and sensitivity of GSM culture.

The volume of people who fall along the gender and sexual minorities spectrum is vast in a general sense. In a community sense, there are social norms and behaviors that change depending on location, history, and safety.

For example, you may be working in a community that has experienced a lot of personal violence from within the community, by police and/or by government. You would teach to this population differently than you would a community that has established a greater sense of freedom, has police forces with self-identified members of the GSM community, or within a government that is supportive. These factors will inherently change the language you use and the references you may make in class.

Best Practice
Avoid cues that draw attention to gender-loaded areas of the body, such as "chest," "hip creases," and "pelvis."

This best practice is multifaceted, impacting both survivors of sexual violence and not. Know that you will have participants who identify on a gender spectrum and that there will be a variety of associations and responses to gendering areas of the body. This is naturally fundamental to teaching trans people, however, it is also important to recognize that cis gendered people can identify on a spectrum as well (that is, women identifying as "butch" or men identifying as "femme"). This group may encounter also a discomfort in using gendered language when referring to one's body. It is best to choose language when referencing the body that is as neutral as possible for all genders.

> **Best Practice**
> Be very specific in the language you use to address the way the body is moving.

It is important to understand that suggesting, leading, or dictating the participant's experience of their body should be avoided. Use language that promotes and allows participants to have their own experience, accepting whatever it is. For example, saying "notice how your arm is moving" is different than saying "pay attention to the way your body fluidly moves with each form." The latter is too prescriptive. This is particularly important for communities where everything its members have seen and experienced about their bodies has been regulated by others.

Likewise, be conservative in your language concerning how a form or shape should feel. As the teacher, you should not assume that their body will feel a certain way or behave a certain way. For the GSM community, there have been and still are many conflicting and confusing messages that come from both inside oneself and outside oneself about how a body should be, should behave, should respond, and so forth. The antidote here is not to add to the confusion.

> **Best Practice**
> Provide opportunities for agency and capacity building when addressing the way that a body works or encouraging the body to follow a particular cue.

Be aware that GSM participants with a past history of sexual trauma may not feel comfortable in or could even "hate" their physical bodies. Meet them where they are, offering them alternative ways to come to the present moment. For example, use the simple awareness of breath to enter a practice. Give agency, ground foundational forms, invite people to notice what each form does for them.

> **Best Practice**
> Take care not to misgender participants; if you do, adjust.

It is courageous for a participant to disclose their preferred personal references to gender; the sharing here is an honor. If you do misgender someone, do not make it their job to correct you or affirm your feelings. Phrases like "I'm trying really hard, but sometimes I forget" or "I'm normally really good at pronouns, sorry" create a tone that indicates that someone's existence is a challenge for you.

If you do misgender someone, the following suggestions take the toll of emotional labor off the participant:

1. correct it by making sure you quickly say it in the next interaction

2. quickly (but sincerely) apologize and then move on.

Practice Care in How You Relate to GSM Students

> **Best Practice**
> Meet students where they are, offering them options.

Consider what your goals are when teaching yoga to the GSM community knowing that sexual violence, because of its widespread tenure, will be present. Offer them alternative ways to come to the present moment (that is, awareness of breath versus immediate awareness of body).

Meeting GSM students where they are, every single class, creates an atmosphere where offering options becomes the standard in yoga thereby creating spaces of integrity and acceptance. This is key to teaching in a population where students may have been promised acceptance, but once they spoke their truths, experienced a loss of acceptance by friends, family, clergy, and those they have professional relationships with.

Options encourage brave agency.

Best Practice
Consider utilizing a curriculum that promotes resilience.

Tailor the curriculum within the context of challenges specific to the GSM experience, including shame, blame, and the minimization of violence and discrimination. Seek out opportunities to understand trauma in the context of resilience and resilience in the context of the GSM community.

Best Practice
Set the tone of inclusivity for the class.

You can set a tone of inclusivity by:

- Not assuming anyone's identity based on their appearance.

- Not using language that is subversively aimed at extracting information from students to confirm your assumptions about their identity.

- Remembering that just because something is "new" to you, that is, someone's identity, that does not mean it is novel and remember that it is not any participant's responsibility to educate you.

Creating Spaces of Agency

Best Practice
Let participants decide what the boundaries are for their practice and bodies.

Let the students be the expert of their own bodies and experiences. Remember that everyone has a unique experience of and connection or disconnection to their own bodies. Those who have experienced sexual violence have had those boundaries shifted for them; they often have to learn how to integrate the regrowth of their boundaries, while establishing a sense of their identity within the contexts of safety. Additionally, people in the GSM community have been systematically raised on other's perceptions of how their bodies should be, act, and respond. Create classes where students can be 100 percent guaranteed that they are able to do what they see best for their own bodies.

Best Practice
Offer statements of affirmation to promote resilience.

Orient people to choices connected to their belief systems while doing affirmations. Be mindful of when in class affirmations are offered. Some examples include:

- "I am courageous."

- "My body is strong and resilient."

- "I am strong and powerful."

- "I am valuable."

- "I allow others to support me."

- "I am worthy of love and acceptance."

- "I have the right to set limits and the courage to do so."

- "I trust I am capable."

- "I am aware of my limits and I honor them."

- "I have the courage to be present in this moment."

- "I'm learning to stand up for myself."

Best Practice
Consider the emotional impact that specific postures might have; choose and sequence wisely.

For example:

- Sequence an entire class around strength forms, being aware that certain categories of forms may be intense for some.

- Encourage agency by speaking to the feelings that might be coming up for participants as they engage in certain forms that relate to bodily shame and provide them guidance on how they can notice those feelings as well as how they can handle them.

- Remind people throughout the practice to notice what is happening and to not push themselves to a point of discomfort that is unsafe for them. Give examples of what "unsafe" means.

- Give participants guidance on what bodily experiences indicate that you are pushing your body too far (for example, you started to hold your breath or have quickened your breathing).

Best Practice
Do not force change; change will happen over time.

Remember that change is slow and happens over time. Trying to force that change can alienate students from their personal purpose for practicing.

> Yoga helped me find some level of acceptance, and a place to grieve the losses. And to find joy again.
> – Trauma-informed yoga participant

Best Practices for Removing Barriers to Practicing

Best Practice
Recognize your own barriers to teaching.

Even if you are identified as in the GSM community, you do not necessarily have the education that you need to teach this class or these concepts. You will have your own prejudices and your experience does not cover everyone.

> Just because someone shares one part of your identity doesn't mean they're a safe person.
> – YSC symposium contributor

> **Best Practice**
> Carefully discern whether or not your classes will be privately or publicly advertised and held.

Classes held in secret have the potential to conflict with a participant's already existing survival skills. Carefully word your advertising of these classes, and hold them in spaces where there is easier access to community support, while also recognizing the lack of trust in certain systems (medical, police, government and so forth) that has historically been present.

> **Best Practice**
> Mindfully incorporate themes that are empowering to community members.

It is important for this community that you be extremely precise in language and detail when describing your offering. People with experience of sexual violence have a keen sense of language and what it means, or *could* mean for them. This vigilance around safety is increased when working within the GSM community where language became a tool of oppression as well as rising up. Incorporate themes of empowerment in the context of community so people who have been marginalized or victimized feel represented and strong.

Best Practices to Creating Environments Where a Sexualized Setting is Reduced

> **Best Practice**
> Understand that perpetuating sexualized settings in your yoga class is highly detrimental for GSM yoga students.

Recognize that there is sexualization in the social culture of the GSM community, and that your teaching is an opportunity to create commonality and community in ways that does not objectify or sexualize a person.

> **Best Practice**
> Be mindful that there could be people in your classes within the community looking to make sexual connections with students. Also, be aware that people may be attending to get away from a sexualized context.

Specifically, if the group is GSM focused know that there will likely be people who attend the class to hit on other participants. This is the root of how yoga can become a very sexualized experience. As a safety measure, be aware that these same sexual dynamics could be playing out in the room and insist that your class is an opportunity for people just to exist as they are, right now.

> **Best Practice**
> Recognize that consent dynamics are taught through a heterosexual lens. Consider what are you teaching in class that may be perpetuating such dynamics.

In order to avoid, consider the following:

- use inclusive language

- give examples that are multifaceted

- use gender-neutral language as much as possible

- when you are talking about consent in the context of your yoga classes, be direct without basing the dialogue in the gender binary.

Best Practices around "Safe Spaces"

> **Best Practice**
> Acknowledge your power and the weight the phrase "safe space" holds.

As a teacher realize your power in saying "safe space." Because the origin of this term is derived specifically from conflict between mainstream sexuality and GSM communities, many see this term as valid and useful. However, recent past and current events suggest that the term "safe space" holds much greater weight now. The community has seen from time immemorial the flighty nature or imperfect practices associated with "safe space." As such you should do your best to understand all facets of safety presented in the introduction to this book as a starting place for determining the language you identify your yoga space as. Do not promise something you cannot bring reliable and consistent truth to.

> **Best Practice**
> If you do use the phrase "safe space," clearly identify what you mean by "safe space."

Be clear about what you can and cannot guarantee. Be clear that you cannot guarantee a space that is non-triggering with no threat of violence or feeling uncomfortable, but you can do your best. Outline what that "best" looks like.

Concurrent Issues

> **Best Practice**
> Be accountable.

If you designate your class a "safe space" then hold yourself accountable for ensuring containment, predictability, community relevance, inclusive language, and a lack of assumptions. Admit when you have mis-stepped and ask for anonymous class feedback.

Conclusion

With careful planning and conscious self-study, yoga for people in the Gender and Sexual Minorities community who have experienced sexual trauma can have the potential for increasing well-being. At the same time, without educating yourself on the unique issues that the GSM community faces or teaching without trauma-informed practices can bring unintentional potential harm.

The Gender and Sexual Minorities community is deeply connected, resilient, and brave. Yoga, working on both individual and collective levels, can lead to a profound change in ensuring that communities continue to be grounded, circles of healing that are well supported by its members for generations to come.

Celebrating this well-documented historical resilience and pride, honoring the strength born of that community struggle is essential. Honoring the individual strengths people bring to our yoga classes increases the entire community's capacity for greater self-knowledge, healing, and joy.

Men

10

Author *Daniel Hickman*

Contributors *Mark A. Lilly, Emanuel Salazar, Austin Sanderson*

Introduction

The formulation of this Chapter was supported by five men from North America, who were culturally, vocationally, and ethnically diverse in scope. Among them: one cisgendered straight man married with children, one cisgendered straight man divorced with children, two cisgendered straight single men without children, and one cis-gendered gay man single without children. The racial identities of the group included African American, Latinx, and White. The combined histories of the individuals had experiences in military and law enforcement, the medical field, theatrical arts, performing arts, athletics, outdoor recreation, academia, education, community outreach, and myriad yoga and meditation lineages.

> The beginning of cultivating yourself is right in yourself; on a thousand mile journey, the first step is the most important. If you can do both of these well, the infinite sublime meanings of hundreds of thousands of teachings will be fulfilled.
>
> – Zen master Ying-An

In many societal expectations, boys and men are taught to deny or suppress feelings rather than explore or express them. This being the case, many boys and men view yoga as being "boring," "wimpy," "touchy-feely," "pseudospiritual/religious," or "overly feminized." In North America most marketing and advertising of yoga prioritizes the female form, thus most boys and men view it as unmasculine. According to the "Yoga in America" study, yoga practitioners are 82.2 percent women and 17.8 percent men (YJ Editors 2017).

A portion of men might take their first yoga class to help tend an injury or mend their body after surgery. Some men might come to their first yoga class after the suggestion of a counselor, therapist, physician, or friend. They could also take yoga class from an awareness of a body–mind psychological understanding. Other men who take yoga class might already have experience with movement culture. This could be from martial arts, performing arts, dance, boarding (skate, snow, or surf), or even calisthenics.

All this being said, a number of men do take yoga classes and yoga teacher trainings. Even in some of the most brawny of environments, such as in professional league sports and the armed forces, there are men who take yoga classes utilized as "cross training." Boys and men find myriad benefits in yoga such as improved VO_2 max (maximal oxygen intake), stress relief, improved balance, strengthened stabilizer muscles, and increased range of motion. It is known that yoga helps boys and men maintain their athletic performance and a competitive edge (Stiefel 2019).

Boys and men who experience a complete yoga practice, that includes relaxation techniques, breathing exercises, sitting meditation, and self-study, know its efficacy on mental health and well-being. Male combat veterans, first responders, incarcerated populations, and even professional fighters incorporate yoga to address their mental and emotional stress. A complete yoga practice can provide ability to self-regulate mood, behavior, and thoughts, and cultivate healthier life choices. It becomes an important part of a daily lifestyle (Niiler 2013).

Male survivors of sexual violence can develop a yoga practice that benefits their entire mind, body, spirit, and recovery. Yoga has the potential to provide a way of being that is supportive, healthy, sustainable, insightful, and life-affirming.

Healthy Masculinity

The behavioral perspective of healthy masculinity aka "masculinities" encompasses strength, assertiveness, courage, independence, and leadership, as well as unselfishness, empathy, compassion, intimacy, and being in touch with a full range of emotions. Many boys and men behave in a well-rounded and balanced way. All around the world, masculinity or masculinities are defined, experienced, and subject to change within one's lifespan. This is so even with boys and men who have different lifestyles yet exist within the same culture or society (Kimmel & Bridges 2014). Recognized as something to develop and deepen, it might be said the refinement of a healthy masculinity is to be a gentleman.

In Latino culture, there is a behavioral perspective known as *caballerismo*, which can be defined as noble, nurturing, or chivalrous. It is a positive view of masculinity. It expounds on boys and men as being protectors, providers, practical problem solvers, and at the same time being tender, sensitive, appreciative, and kind (ASU 2008).

Perhaps the underlying traits in healthy masculinity are those of respect and personal responsibility. This includes values, moral principles, generosity, and harmony that are put forth in action and disposition (Clay 2012). This also includes cultivating a greater awareness of one's own self, relationships, society, and the environment.

What are the benefits of healthy masculinity or masculinities? Psychological and emotional states are free flowing and not fixed, causing a greater sense of self-regulation and empathy for others. Boys or men are able to express moods and feelings safely without being teased or attacked. Warmth, connection, and vulnerability are experienced with ease. As a result, boys and men live with nurturing and fulfilling relationships, a sense of purpose, alongside contribution, bravery, and guardianship.

Health masculinity aka masculinities might be:

- self-reflection

- cooperation over competition

- looking and living outside of the "man rules," "male code," or "man box"

- facing the dark and "unacceptable" parts of ourselves (shadow)

- feeling, communicating, and empathizing within a full range of expression

- living virtues, such as responsibility to self, others, society, and the environment

- actively seeking out help and additional resources including counseling and communities.

Toxic Masculinity

The behavioral perspective of toxic masculinity aka traditional masculinity ideology (Barth 2019) encompasses unhealthy rearing, beliefs, and specific cultural norms and traditions that are connected to hostile attitudes and actions, detrimental to (society) women, children, as well as men themselves. It is believed that some social constructs of masculinity might affect males starting from their infancy (Holloway 2015). This might begin when some parents interact with their son. These parents either willingly or unconsciously withhold intimacy, support, and safeguarding. It is also believed that boys do not need this type of connection from others (neglect). In this ideology, more constructs are placed upon boys and men. These might be hetero-normative ideals called "man rules," a "male code," or even the "man box" (Lambert 2019).

This boxed criterion (assumptions) for boys and men contains absolutes. Some are assumed to be "normal" from birth, while others are to be "earned" in order to "become" a man. This in turn could cause some boys and men to willingly not feel and abandon a fuller spectrum of their emotions. This being so, vulnerability, being wrong, or appearing defective is to be avoided. Showing fear, weakness, or a failure to fight back is wrong. In this assumed view, there might exist only a few "normal" emotions for a boy or man, such as stern, anger, silly, boastful, and brutal.

Thus, masculinity in these constructs could be more of a measurement. It might be a level of being to be obtained via attitude, behavior, action, or ritual. Expressing or carrying out measures of aggressiveness, sexual prowess, dominance, or violence might be encouraged and accepted. This could be seen through the mythos of the "strong silent type" who "goes at it alone," with an over-emphasis on self-reliance, and one who does not ask for help (Turner 2019).

If a boy or man thinks, feels, or behaves outside of this "criterion," peers, family members, or other adults might tease, ridicule, shame, or subjugate them. This could result in a lasting impact for many boys and men, leaving them unable to understand, access, cope with, or process feelings or emotional complexity.

What is considered the fallout of toxic masculinity? Bullying, misogyny, problems with intimacy, sexual harassment, homophobia, patriarchy, violence, substance abuse, depression, and suicide. It is noted that boys and men, indoctrinated to embody this mindset and operate inside these actions, will wreak havoc on others and improperly take care of themselves physically and mentally (Fitzsimons 2019).

Toxic masculinity aka traditional masculinity ideology might be:

- suppression of emotional depth, dimension, or expression that includes concealment of distress, anxiety, or suffering aka "emotional neglect"

- anti-feminine or "anti-softness," homophobia, and the avoidance of presenting of one's self as weak or passive (perceived as failure)

- presenting of one's self as hardened, tough, rigid, impenetrable, unyielding, or totally self-reliant

- unhealthy attachment to work, unending competition, or overseeking achievement

- actions or behavior, as it relates to power, that is domineering, threatening, or violent

- inclination toward risk, adventure, or extreme activity (such as promiscuity).

Male Sexual Trauma

Male sexual trauma is often unacknowledged and carries a lot of misconceptions. One is that a "real man" is not "vulnerable," and should be able to fight off an attacker and protect himself from abuse. Another common misconception is that only gay men sexually assault or abuse men or boys, and only gay men or boys are survivors of male sexual trauma.

Men and boys are victims of sexual trauma, regardless of age, gender identification, or sexual orientation. In North America alone, it is estimated that *one out of six* males have experienced some form of sexual trauma in their lifetime (1in6.org).

There is a stigma and secrecy associated with male sexual trauma and this stigma often results in barriers to disclosure. Men are less likely to report sexual trauma than are female survivors. The most common reason for not reporting, cited by survivors of male sexual trauma, is a fear of being labeled as a homosexual (aasas.ca). If a survivor does share their story with another, it can often be met with disbelief, disgust, or rejection. Some will never disclose to anyone what happened, or, if they do, it might be many, many years after the incident.

Common Myths Regarding Men Who are Survivors of Sexual Trauma

- *Disbelief*
- A man cannot be raped.
- An adult male is too big and too strong to be overpowered and forced into sex.
- A "real" man should be able to protect himself from sexual assault.
- Men are in a constant state of readiness to accept any sexual opportunity so they cannot be raped.

- *Minimizing trauma*
- Most men who are raped are not very upset by the incident.
- Most men who are raped do not need counseling after the incident.
- Men are less negatively affected by sexual assault than women.
- *Sexuality/Masculinity*
- Men who are raped by women are "lucky."
- Men who are raped by other men are weak and emasculate.
- Men who are raped by other men must be gay.

(Source: Worthen MGF (2016) Sexual deviance and society: A sociological examination, London: Routledge.)

Perpetrators of sexual violence against men can be of any age, sexual orientation, or gender identity. The majority of perpetrators in sexual violence toward men and boys are men. Most male perpetrators of crimes against men and boys identify as a heterosexual man, who has consensual sexual relationships with women. Perpetrators can have any relationship to the victim and often use emotional, physical, or psychological tactics. Adolescent boys are the most frequently targeted victims of sexual abuse against men (ptsd.va.gov).

Women also sexually assault men or boys. These such offenses can be perceived in an unhealthy narrative that if a man or boy was abused by a female perpetrator, he was "lucky" or "initiated" (French 2014). There is also the false narrative that if a man or boy experienced an erection or ejaculation during a sexual assault, the event was "enjoyed," and thus implies consent. Further, there exists the misconception that a child survivor of male sexual trauma will grow up to be a sexual predator (sapac.umich.edu).

Men will have many of the same reactions from sexual trauma as those of other gender identities. Men can feel shame from the powerlessness of the incident. Men can have feelings and thoughts that they fear or greatly avoid. This might lead to secrecy, negative coping, and lasting deleterious effects.

Many cultural perspectives instill a common belief that men are not supposed to feel a wide variety of emotions. It is expected for men to repress many of their feelings. Men might believe it is only "okay" to show basic feelings such as boldness, anger, humor, or seriousness. It is believed that "real men" are to be self-sufficient, not show weakness, and possess the capacity to fend for themselves. Unfortunately, these views are what keep many men from seeking help regarding their trauma (Weiss 2016).

As yoga practitioners, we can help others connect to a story of *resilience* rather than victimization. We can use yoga practice as the raw material for this exploration of strength, self-awareness, and capacity, without directly focusing on any traumatic storylines, either specifically or by inference.

Helping others view themselves through this lens of strength affords them an opportunity to acknowledge they have survived what they have been through. This acknowledgment is a catalyst to build self-esteem. It creates a healthy sense of resolution, self-mastery, and empowerment. It is imperative for yoga instructors to connect their students to past successes regardless of the magnitude of said success. One can remind students that their showing up to their yoga mat is a success story essential in building their fountain of self-esteem. It constructs a foundation for post-traumatic growth. Additionally, the practice of trauma-informed yoga can effectively guide others to release the past, restore resilience, and heal from sexual abuse.

What to Do if a Man or Boy Shares His Story

- Listen and believe him.

- Do not interrupt or ask him details about the assault.

- Do not defend or make excuses for the assailant.

- Do not define his experience or tell him how to feel.

- Validate his story and his feelings.

- Support him by honoring his pace and choice of discovery and recovery. Never use statements like: "You *should* of told someone about this." "Why did you wait this long?" "Maybe the (assailant) was just/only … [justification]."

- Perhaps respond with: "It's not your fault." "I am sorry this happened to you." "I am glad you said something about this." "It takes guts/courage to share your story." "What assistance and support are you getting?" "What will help you through this?"

- Provide resources for him, that you know about, in consideration of his culture, ethnicity, gender identity, sexual orientation, and age.

- Make sure to get appropriate care for yourself; the impact of sexual violence may affect you, too. Include self-care, create healthy boundaries, and be aware of compassion fatigue. Be authentic and honest with where you are emotionally (1in6.org).

We recognize that there are laws pertaining to sexual trauma, that may vary by region. The terminology might include but not be limited to: "trauma," "harassment," "violence," "assault," or "abuse." Trauma in its most basic definition is an experience that overwhelms one's ability to cope. Regardless of gender, a traumatic event was something that was beyond a person's control. It was something unexpected, and something a person could have not prepared for. It was something a person could not stop from happening. We also recognize that the survivors of male sexual trauma, as other groups of survivors, will have unique distinctions and needs (rainn.org). For a further discussion of trauma and sexual trauma more generally see Chapters 2 and 3.

In the section that follows, we offer best practice to consider when working with men in the context of sexual trauma. While many of these recommendations also represent best practices more generally that would benefit any yoga or mindfulness student, these offerings come specifically from our group of five men in thinking about the unique experiences of men who are survivors of sexual trauma.

Best Practices
Teacher Considerations

> **Best Practice**
> As a teacher, it is necessary to dress in modest clothing when you teach.

We recognize that dress codes may change from setting to setting. Remember that one intention for the yoga teacher, when teaching to survivors of male sexual trauma, is to present themselves in an appropriate professional manner. We also keep in mind to follow what the current professional standards may be when teaching in a school, office, medical center, hospital, house of worship, shelter, retirement or assisted living community, and so forth.

It is suggested to dress in layers of loose-fitting clothes, that are conservative and cover a lot of your body. Use clothing that you are able to remove or place back on, without revealing your skin. Always wear undergarments.

It is suggested to not wear shorts above the knees, low-cut shirts, or lots of jewelry. It is also suggested to not dress in tight-fitting outfits that reveal a lot of skin on your back, shoulders, thighs, waist, or belly.

Why? See *Best Practice: As a teacher, it is necessary to understand your role is one of service*, page 149.

> **Best Practice**
> As a teacher, it is necessary to demonstrate a consistent relationship with time.

It is suggested to arrive early, fifteen to twenty minutes before class begins, to address and orient new students. There might be students, nervous about practicing yoga, who show up before class to express their concerns. One idea is to implement a "buddy system" or "peer mentor" to help explain yoga class decorum and etiquette.

It is also suggested to stay about ten to fifteen minutes after class ends, to address questions or concerns of the students. Overall, be consistently on time, which feels safe to the students, and displays that you are reliable, and a professional.

> **Best Practice**
> As a teacher, it is necessary to understand your role is one of service.

We are there to provide students the time and space to work on their meditation and yoga. We are there to lead students into a safe and accessible class that is open to their particular needs and choices. Consider that on any given day, a student might be struggling with a particular internal challenge that is unique to their recovery. As well, a student might be working with a solution to apply to their recovery. By providing a place for students to be with what they are experiencing, they might start to make connections on their own and feel empowered. It is important to remind yourself to be open, patient, and generous with these possible scenarios.

We are there to share what we know, and to express what we do not know as well. We are there as a role model, not an authority figure, show-off, or a "yoga celebrity." We are there to encourage, not to order around.

We are not there to show off our body. We are not there to behave like a "know it all." We are not there to fix anyone. We *are* there to "hold the space" and give our services to those who are in need of a calm, safe, restful space to work on their recovery and wellness. We are there for them.

> **Best Practice**
> As a teacher, it is suggested to practice non-judgmental observational awareness in your class.

When leading a class, you might observe a student who is not participating. You might observe a student who is dissociating. You might observe a student who is staring at you, or fidgeting, or one who gets on their cell phone, or one who starts crying.

Any of these moments are for you to practice non-judgmental observational awareness. If one of these moments happen, there is nothing for you to do about it (generally speaking). It is suggested for you to observe any of these, or other actions and behaviors, with kindness, gentleness, and compassion, and without interacting.

> **Best Practice**
> As a teacher, it is suggested to allow students to acquire their props and set up their own spot. Alternatively, you might "set up" a classroom in advance of the students' arrival.

You might encourage students to choose any props they like and any that suit them. You might inform the students about the different types of props available. You might describe the use of the props or demonstrate how any of them may be utilized. Alternatively, you might teach a specific focus or technique in your class, and inform students to use specific props.

Consider letting students choose where they would like to position themselves in class. Some will position as close to you as possible. Some will position as far away from you as possible. Some will want to have their back close to a wall. Some will want to be near a window. Some will want to be next to an exit. Let them choose. They have their reasons.

Alternatively, you might set up the classroom in advance for the students. This can help reduce anxiety over anyone's lack of knowledge regarding props and their purpose. Students might enter the practice space to see how much attention to detail has been used in preparation for their class. As well, they might sense the mood/atmosphere of the class and how much care has been considered regarding their comfort. It is ultimately up to the teacher to gauge what will work best for their respective target audience.

> **Best Practice**
> As a teacher, it is necessary to conduct oneself in a manner that is professional and realistic.

We remember to behave in a way that is courteous. We remember to teach within our realm of understanding and expertise. We remember, and are able to express, when we do or do not have the knowledge, information, or resources to address specific concerns.

A student who is a survivor of male sexual trauma might express specific concerns that relate to their experience. They might look to the yoga teacher as a "helper" or confidant. Some students, while in their recovery, might behave in a way that seems anxious, dependent, or codependent. As a teacher of yoga, we remember that we are not able to "fix," "cure," or "change" anyone.

If you experience a student who might behave in a manner that is anxious, dependent, or codependent, be mindful of boundaries. Refer the student to a licensed social counselor, psychologist, or psychiatrist. Refer the student to support groups, literature, educational videos, or any resources that are in your sphere of knowledge. Recognize your scope of practice, and provide resources in support of your student.

Finally, any person teaching a vulnerable population with a traumatic background must also account for their own possible triggers. Often people will want to serve in communities (consciously or subconsciously) and with people who have gone through similar experiences to their own. Often the teacher will have direct experience of comparable traumatic events, and while well along with their own healing/recovery, may still have potential trigger points and shadows.

Communication

> **Best Practice**
> As a teacher, it is necessary to utilize skilled listening.

Skilled listening employs the ears and not the mouth. This means to just listen and not talk. To interrupt, react, make sounds, facial gestures, or cross-talk is not listening. It is crucial to understand the power of skilled listening. Just listen. This is done without questioning, critiquing, characterizing, or saying that "you know" what a person "should" do.

Skilled listening starts with giving your attention, calmly and totally, to the person who is speaking to you. Skilled listening is about your basic presence of being there to hear the speaker. Skilled listening makes space for the speaker to share what is on their mind and in their heart. This space will create a moment for the speaker to be seen and heard. It offers a feeling of respect and acknowledgement, which might help with recovery.

Best Practice

Mindfully choose how you communicate and what you say.

- Skilled speech is a choice to communicate and express with sensitivity and respect.

- Skilled speech is a choice to communicate and express that is free of any agenda. Skilled speech is a choice to communicate and express ideas, information, or news using a delivery and tone that is empathetic and beneficial.

- When you speak with survivors of male sexual trauma, *do not* communicate or express:

  o sexual humor

  o derogatory language

  o absolute statements

  o competitive messages

  o authoritarian directions

  o "guru" or hero-worship

  o tall tales or glorification of the dead or living "master"

  o false claims about "powers," "magic," or "healing" from yoga and meditation

  o with the intent to define another's experience or describe how they are feeling

  o phrases or words that might be triggering, such as: "Spread your legs." "Bend over." "Squeeze your thighs." "Open your mouth." "Close your eyes." "Put your hands [...]" "Rub your [...]" "Take off your [...]," "Grab your [...]" *"Don't [...]"*

  o phrases or words that might objectify body parts, such as: "Lift *the* head." "Move *the* arm." "Open *the* chest." "Arch *the* back." "Shake your money maker." "Rock hard abs." or "Buns of steel."

  o flippant responses, reactions, or opinions, such as: "What did you do?" "Why did you do that?" "Why didn't you go [...?]" "No. Did this really happen to you?" "Was the [perpetrator] bigger than you?" "Get over it." "Get a hold of yourself." "You should be happy for all that didn't happen." "Just get therapy." "Just don't even think about it." "Just move forward and don't look back."

We recognize that most people who speak with survivors might do so with the best intentions in mind. We also recognize that most people who speak with survivors might not understand what to say and, just as importantly, what not to say. This being so, we remember to emphasize deep and respectful listening before communicating anything back to a survivor. We remember to emphasize discernment with how to speak and what to say (information, instruction, description, ideas, or news). This is for before, during, or after a yoga class when speaking directly with a survivor.

Best Practice

Consider speech that gives choices.

Choices allow people to find their own empowerment. Consider speech that is inviting, cooperative, supportive, pleasant, and respectful. Consider speech that gives a survivor a sense of their own agency and success.

Speech that is experiential in the present-tense context might give a survivor a sense of being in control. For example: "Notice while in this shape/form, how you might feel strength differently in your legs compared to your arms." Alternatively, speech that is more specific might give a survivor a sense of being oriented and secure. Consider what speech is healthy and unhealthy. Consider your tone, delivery, and inflection. Consider not just what you say, but also *how* you say it.

When you speak with survivors of male sexual trauma, *do* communicate or express:

- Skillfully.

- Free of agenda.

- From your own experience.

- With first-person singular ("I" statements).

- Wholehearted positive regard.

- Kindness, generosity, and compassion.

- Free of evaluating, insinuating, or "analyzing".

- Evidence-based information from reliable and reputable sources.

- Realistic facts about the effects and benefits of yoga and meditation.

- Descriptions and examples of workable techniques of yoga and meditation.

- Phrases or words that might encourage, support, inspire, inform, calm, and motivate.

- Phrases or words that incorporate trauma-informed language such as: "Fold forward." "Contract your muscles in your thighs." "Relax your jaw and tongue to create space between your upper and lower teeth." "If you would like to, you might keep your eyes open, half open, or fully closed." "Tilt *your* head." "Rotate *your* arm." "Relax *your* chest." and "Elongate *your* back."

- Skilled responses and reflections, such as: "I believe you." "I am sorry." "It's not your fault." "What I heard you say was [...]" "What are you doing to take care of yourself?" "What else have you looked into?" "How is that working for you?" "That sounds good." "Looks like you are good at that." "Have you considered [...?]" "What communities are you a part of?"

> **Best Practice**
> Remember to use language that is concrete, direct, and simple.

Using concrete, direct, and simple language promotes a predictability and a steadiness that might help people feel safe. As well, it might augment focus and clarity.

We consider using slogans or affirmations that encourage, support, and reassure. We could share quotes that inspire, inform, or give ideas. As well, we might describe techniques, examples, or stories from evidence-based studies, literature by renowned authors, or from our own experience.

Consider framing outcomes of a yoga practice in terms of "the long view." We remind students that throughout their lifetime, they can get better, grow, and enjoy yoga for many years. We share with students that there are many perspectives in yoga. Mostly, we reiterate the original aim of yoga, which is to experience the multifaceted versatility of one's unique self.

We also tell our students that yoga is practiced in a cooperative environment, and that elsewhere there are competitive environments. More so, we share that the cooperative environment in yoga is a place to support and respect, one's self and others, in community. This being so, we remember to be open to feedback and inquiries from our students.

> **Best Practice**
> As a teacher, be mindful of verbal and non-verbal communication (body language).

Mindful communication consists of leading with presence, intention, and attention. When a teacher leads with presence he or she shows up fully available and more intuitively attuned to others. This must be utilized in every facet of working with survivors. It is crucial for teachers to have an awareness of non-verbal information that is being transmitted from students. Some things to pay attention to might be a student's posture (slumped or up right), respect of personal space (proximity and touch), facial tone (tight or loose), eye contact (fixated, darting, or avoidant) as well as any pitch, rhythm, and volume of their speech.

Non-verbal communication/information travels in two directions in a yoga class, from the teacher to the student and from the student to the teacher. Teachers will be transmitting their inner state even before saying a word. If a teacher is not present, because of stress, resistance, or ambivalence, that will register particularly with survivors of trauma who are watchfully assessing their environment.

Remember that trauma can cause PTSD and thus heighten a survivor's sense of hyper-vigilance. Recognize that survivors will likely, as a survival mechanism if nothing else, be highly attuned and hone in on your emotional state (that is, angst, lack of confidence, frustration, mindlessness, and so forth). Survivors might recognize these signs and fixate on your emotional energy and facial expressions. It is also important to note that these feelings, caused by their hyper-arousal or hyper-vigilance, may or may not be accurate.

Intentional communication primarily focuses on having a genuine curiosity about others and seeking to empathize with another person's feelings. Intentional leadership can be associated with reflective and active listening skills. Employ your introspection to notice when you are planning a response and not listening. Remember your intent to understand what a person is sharing or experiencing. To lead with "attention" is to listen to what is most important to the student.

Practice

> **Best Practice**
> In respect and consideration to male survivors of sexual violence, focus on what is safe and accessible.

As a teacher working with this specific population, remember that you are providing a service for them and their recovery. This being so, keep things down to earth and even provide information from evidence-based studies. Being that you might teach a typical hour-long class, a complete experience would include physical training (asana/form), simple respiration cultivation (pranayama), and meditation (dhyana). Be realistic and explain the benefits and qualities of these techniques.

As the culture of yoga has been changed by modern industry, it is important to be informed of and partake in what is a *complete* yoga practice – and its original intentions. Be aware of "yoga styles" that are devoid of the full breadth and depth of *sadhana*. Sadhana can be defined as a "means of realization," "means of accomplishing," or a daily spiritual practice (discipline).

This includes: in-depth study of the "self" (svadhyaya), respiration cultivation (pranayama), meditation (dhyana), physical training (asana/form), chanting, prayer, other practices/disciplines, and working to realize (and let go of) one's ego.

Respectfully and sensitively consider how and when (if at all) to share this knowledge with this population. If so, do so without any agenda or expectation.

Best Practice

Encourage that one's experience of a form (asana), and a way to relate to it, is the deeper aim.

Let the students know that one cannot do the forms wrong, and one cannot be bad at yoga. As well, let them know that one does yoga the way one does it, because it's one's own yoga to be discovered. This is the encouraging and empowering way to share yoga.

Some students might be more interested in alignment and the "look" of the form. This is okay. You might let them know about the different techniques and myriad schools that are both ancient and contemporary. Be informed. Share what you know from your own experience. Encourage them to look into what interests them.

You might also let them know that in terms of recovery, noticing their breath while in a form and being mindful of thoughts and feelings,

will provide a deeper effect. Remind them about gentleness, non-striving, and being cooperative (with their self and others) rather than competitive. Remind them one can use the forms to tend the mind and mood, and that there are certain forms and practices that can help with anxiety and depression.

Remind them that there are three parts/actions to a form – entering, sustaining, and ending. Every part has an opportunity for introspection or sensory awareness. A form is another tool to address and tend the "self."

Best Practice

Encourage simple pranayama (respiration cultivation) – that the best way to breathe is "in and out, repeat."

Let your students know that simple pranayama can be applied in a standing, seated, or lying position. That it will provide insight into their mind, muscles, heart, lungs, and mood. You might let them know some of the benefits of simple pranayama such as it:

- strengthens the bridge between the body and the mind

- affects clarity of mind and relaxation, cultivating calmness

- brings insight into the relation of emotions and respiration

- relieves stress and negative tension

- can help with cravings, addictions, and pain management

- improves the systematic functioning of the nerves, fluid circulation, glands, digestion, and cardio-pulmonary processes.

Simple breathing practice:

- breathe through your nose

- be aware of air passing over the skin of your upper lip with each inhale and exhale

- sense the rhythm and the humidity of your breath

- notice the length of your inhale

- notice the length of your exhale.

Best Practice

Encourage a dhyana (meditation) style that is suitable to the person's personality. Remind them that meditation, like a bird, has two wings – wisdom and compassion – with the latter being more important.

Let your students know that while meditating, it is best to be gentle, kind, compassionate, spacious, and even forgiving with their self. Let them know that while meditating, realizations or insights may arise, and having thoughts and feelings are okay. One is not trying to encourage thinking and feeling, and one is not trying to stop thinking and feeling. It might be more so, that meditation includes all of this, or is the space in between or more along non-resisting and non-striving.

You might say that meditation is the befriending of one's self. You might say that meditation is when you close your eyes, go inside, and practice calm. You might say that while in meditation, there is nothing to lose and nothing to gain.

Here are some ideas about different styles of meditation that you might share:

Moving meditation might work well for those who have a hard time sitting still or who have very active minds. Some examples are walking, cycling, swimming, dance class, or even gardening. Any rhythmic form or movement pattern, with dharana (concentration), can be applied to tame the mind. Examples include: vinyasa, such as the surya namaskar (sun salute), or a martial arts kata (form) like from tai qi.

Tactile repetition such as to sense your fingers in mudras (hand gestures) or sort the beads on a mala.

Visualization of an endeavor or task is used in the medical field, athletics, psychology, and even warrior training.

Imagery also can be used like a mandala, statuette, candle, or even elements in nature.

Guided meditation can be from a person, podcast, video, or even a recording of ambient sounds.

Mantra or prayer repetition is yet another style (for example, om mani padme hum), or even an affirmation (for example, peace, peace, peace).

Sitting meditation practice places emphasis on stillness (of one's physical body) in order to observe and understand one's mind and feelings. This includes any mental, emotional, physical, and psychic phenomena that come and go.

Essentials of meditation:

- find a type of meditation that suits your personality

- have karuna (compassion), metta (loving friendliness), and dana (space) for yourself

- accept, respect, and relax.

Some mental effects of meditation are:

- an increased awareness of behavioral thought patterns

- new or hidden realizations on the subconscious level of the self

- an altered perception of time

- an increased activity in the hemisphere of the right brain

- a transcendence of the ordinary into the universal.

Some physical effects of meditation are:

- a decrease in muscle tension, blood pressure, and pulse

- a decrease in oxygen consumption and blood lactate levels

- an increase in the immune response and alpha rhythms

- an increase in the cultivation of prana (qi) aka "life force."

Conclusion

> When you have attained mental and physical peace and quiet, don't get stuck in peace and quiet. Be independent and free, like a gourd rolling and bobbing on a river.
>
> – Zen master Dahui

Working with male survivors of sexual trauma can be a profound experience. Remember that there are certain "ideals" or social constructs of masculinity that some consider "toxic." More so,

keep in mind that there are "masculinities" that are not rigid or fixed. Healthy masculinity is layered, varied, and changeable, depending on identity, culture, society, and where one is in their life. It is imperative that you are well informed about the psychological complexities of trauma and of where someone is in their stage(s) of recovery. It is equally important that you maintain healthy boundaries and know how to conduct yourself professionally. Your very own self-care as well as your active and ongoing discipline of a complete yoga practice is especially significant. Introspection, and your sadhana of self-actualization, are necessary for working in a trauma-informed environment. See Chapter 6 on relational wisdom for more detail.

Reiterated is the understanding that, as a yoga professional, you are there to provide a service. By no means are you a "savior," "know it all," or "show off." This service is to "create/hold a safe space" for a student to be with their own self, their trauma, discovery, and recovery in a community with others. You are there to provide an experience of yoga and meditation that is holistic, practical, sensitive, relaxing, and empowering.

This service, to share with others, includes a complete yoga practice of asanas (forms), simple pranayama, explanation and examples of pratyahara, implementation of dharana, and a down-to-earth and accessible dhyana (nothing wishy-washy or woo-woo). These are to be taught realistically, without grandiosity, within your realm of training, knowledge, and expertise, and open to participants' varied levels and abilities. If you are triggered by a person, story, event, or circumstance while working in this specific population, then it is significant that you search out proper assistance as needed.

Elderly and People with Disabilities

Author *Beth Jones*

Contributors *Maya Breuer, Regine Clermont, Colleen DeVirgiliis, Jana Long*

Introduction

While there is not a significant amount of written material about sexual trauma in elderly or disabled populations, reports such as *Abused and Betrayed on National Public Radio* (Shapiro 2018) suggest that victimization rates are much higher than with other groups. It is also suggested that under-reporting of cases, low data-collection, and the threat to one's shelter, food and care if abuse is disclosed may explain the lack of investigation. Because trauma is identified as an abuse of power, it is important to recognize that the elderly and those with physical and intellectual disabilities may be considered easy to victimize, because they tend to rely on others to care for them. They endure touch without permission for daily care, including bathing, toileting, and dressing. A person with special needs usually has no choice about who supports them and must build a trusting relationship with whomever is on shift that day. These are forced and reinforced relationships built to meet basic needs and often without supervision. Elderly or young, these individuals can become susceptible to harm, manipulation, lies, and bribery, and to the grooming of sexual abuse. As trauma-informed yoga teachers, we must be aware of this inherent vulnerability and work, as best we can, to promote agency and self-efficacy in our classes.

Although there are similarities between the elderly and people with disabilities, such as high victimization rates, care dependency, and medical and cognitive challenges, each requires an independent focus and approach to the teaching of yoga. And although people on mental health spectrums, particularly neurocognitive disorders and autism, share similar needs and may benefit from trauma-informed yoga, we have not included them. As with all specific diagnoses, we strongly suggest deep study of a particular mental health concern, experiential exposure to impacted individuals, and specialized embodiment training. For this chapter, we have separated Best Practices into two general sections, Older Adults and People with Disabilities.

Older Adults

Background

When using the term *senior* or *elderly*, we note a wide continuum of ages with a wide variety of health concerns that impact mobility, learning, adaptations, and cognitive awareness. But for the purposes herein, the age group we refer to is sixty and above. Within that range, a person may live wholly independent of care, in a supported living home, or in a fully dependent living situation in a housing unit, residential program, or nursing home. There are people in their final years of life and who are in palliative care, as well. Common physical and mental health issues affecting older people are dementia, cognitive impairments such as short-term memory loss, loss of mobility, depth-perception changes, visual and auditory decline, trouble with organizing, slowed coordination of the body, loss, grief, and depression. All seniors may benefit from yoga, but it is imperative to learn about this group of people and the physical, psychological, and emotional changes that impact them through the aging process until death. To reiterate, as people age, they may lose their independence. The rate of abuse is higher in dependent-living models.

According to the World Health Organization (WHO), senior or elderly abuse and neglect are defined as a "single or repeated act or *lack of action*, occurring within a relationship of trust that causes harm or distress to an older person" (WHO 2018; emphasis in the original). When a relationship of trust is broken, this can create a trauma response in anyone, especially in the elderly who have become reliant upon another person to care for them. Yoga teachers must understand the importance of developing an authentic, reliable, and consistent relationship with the elderly. Their lives may depend upon it. An elder who has been victimized may show signs of trauma, appearing isolated, frightened, or unsure.

A person may be experiencing daily abuse and neglect where they live and yet functioning in their communities as typical-seeming members of their age group. This is the "don't-tell" generation and, as any victim who lives in violence or neglect knows, an abused but functioning elder is a survivor with a skill set to endure, to avoid becoming a problem to someone, to get along and go along with whomever seems in charge.

> Sexual abuse of older persons crosses the traditional gender, cultural, and role boundaries for victims and perpetrators. There is a risk that sexual abuse against older persons is not taken seriously since they, due to ageism, may be seen as asexual. Thus, many see it as unlikely that sexual abuse may occur.
>
> (Malmedal, et al. 2015)

Generational differences in our culture, regarding disclosure of trauma and abuse, are critical to understanding the elderly. Religious, political, and sexual conservatism may encourage personal shame, blaming self or the victim, and maintaining the silence. Because of this difference, it is strongly suggested that yoga teachers maintain boundaries and practice cultural humility with acute awareness. A trauma-informed teacher will lead with awareness and respect for another's history and experiences. This acknowledgment of generational difference is taken into consideration in developing the Best Practices section.

Best Practices for Working with Older Adults

Best Practice
Become aware of the culture of aging.

By becoming aware of the culture of aging – what an aging person may be exposed to, how an aging person may be perceived, and what can happen to an aging person's physical and mental abilities – a yoga teacher is better prepared for addressing the needs of an elderly student. It is suggested that teachers obtain additional training in the anatomical, cognitive, and socioemotional aging process to better understand the impacts of isolation, depression, memory loss, dementia, limited mobility, hearing and sight loss, and grief. While it would be inappropriate to open discussions and refer to these points in a yoga class, it is important to know about the deep and dynamic changes older people endure that may coincide with sexual trauma, its silence and shame. This will help you create a supportive, relevant class. Many elders experience loss of independence, often being touched without permission in the context of daily personal care, bathing, and dressing. Therefore, a trauma-informed approach must allow for a student-centered facilitation and by permission.

Best Practice
Find teaching opportunities.

Become familiar with the requirements for teaching within institutions that serve and support the elderly. Places such as nursing homes, hospitals, public or subsidized housing, private homes, churches, the Young Men's Christian Association (YMCA), rehabilitation facilities, senior day care programs, adult or continuing education classes, community centers, cancer care centers – all are potential places for offering yoga. Learn about an institution's requirements, such as the need for federal clearances and fingerprinting. Not all programs require these, but most will require cardiopulmonary resuscitation (CPR) training, insurance, and immunizations. When meeting with administrative staff, it is best to have these steps completed, so that you are prepared to teach.

After some research, do some community outreach through in-services to targeted programs that serve the elderly. Informational meetings can bring you opportunities to meet administrators and to visit spaces. As well, they can evaluate you. This will provide prospective students and staff a chance to ask questions about your experience and yoga. You may choose to include a brief sample class, as well.

Best Practice
Use invitational language.

Invitational language *invites* rather than *commands*. As in previous chapters, we suggest that teachers use invitational language that emphasizes choice-making and agency, such as "if you like" or "you may choose to try this instead." Use of this style of language promotes a noncompetitive environment and promotes interoception, while teaching simple forms with appropriate modifications. It reduces the risk of a power dynamic relationship, too. We recognize, too, that elderly people tend to be treated as children by caregivers and family members as the aging process changes and slows cognitive integration and memory. Many appear to be compliant and easily swayed to follow perceived rules and directions. Many are on medications or may be experiencing dehydration – both factors can impede cognition, coordination, and energy. Therefore, it is important to deliver trauma-informed invitational language and facilitative content of your class with an adult tone of voice at a pace that takes into account the possibilities of the above concerns. Avoid infantilization at every turn.

Best Practice
Be intentional in your selection of forms.

Forms that are simple and taught slowly are best. With simple forms, be sure to model each one and offer modifications for each. As you get to know your students, you and they will discover what works best for them. Try to avoid hierarchical language about forms, for example, "This is simpler" or "This is harder." That can leave some students feeling less competent than another who may be able to do the more complex form. Try not to highlight one student's "achievement" – and do not single out a student. Instead, create community without competition by emphasizing ability. Rest periods or brief meditations after a movement can be as helpful as the movement itself, as they offer students a chance to notice what is happening or to notice that they cannot feel anything different. But it is in those moments that body awareness can be built and be restored, if lost. In trauma, body awareness is often not available. A pause between movements may help someone begin a rediscovery of self.

Best Practice
Utilize props.

Props may include mats, chairs, bolsters, blocks, and blankets. Heavy blankets that are soft may be better than itchy wool or lightweight cotton blankets. The weight of blankets can feel comforting and grounding and assist in embodiment through meditation. We suggest that no straps be offered, in general, as they can be triggering to sexual trauma survivors who may have been restrained or strangled, for example. Use your discretion.

Best Practice
Support elderly with hearing and vision impairments.

For the safety of elderly students who have hearing and vision impairments, yoga teachers are specifically trained to move around the room. Let the entire class know that you will move throughout the space during the yoga class. Ask permission before walking over to a student unless you have prior agreement between teacher and student. If it is important to move a student closer to you, ask the student's permission before the class begins. All these options can be done with respect and care of the student's integrity, privacy, and ability to choose. Be predictable whenever possible and set up each class the same way.

Best Practice
Take safety into consideration.

Consider teaching a small class. If not, have a co-teacher or aide who can be on-hand to assist if urgent needs arise. If a student becomes disoriented, unsteady, angry, and/or incontinent, or exhibits mental confusion, an assistant can step in to help while the rest of the class continues practicing. We suggest that teachers get acquainted with the schedule of the agency and/or the area of the town in which classes take place and come to know if/when alarms or outside sirens may occur. This knowledge can help teachers prepare students, minimizing distraction or fear responses. Knowing a building's safety plan is an excellent precaution, too. Practice universal precautions, for example, hand-washing, using sanitizer for mats, and maintain CPR certification.

Best Practice
Encourage proper hydration.

Dehydration is prevalent in elders. Encourage your students to take water breaks, perhaps incorporating these breaks into the sequence of each class so that everyone is assured of hydration. These pauses also provide ways to integrate the movements through rest and to encourage self-care and befriendment of the body.

Best Practice
Be predictable, observant, and informative.

Survivors of trauma, particularly people with cognitive challenges, young or old, do best with predictable schedules and personalities. Cultivate that predictability by arriving early, limiting substitutes for yourself, dressing similarly each visit, by remembering professionalism, and providing a schedule of when you will be there to teach. As well, when planning the structure of your class, design a sixty to seventy-five minute class or even a thirty to forty-five minute class, and make time for set up, introduction of forms, rest/hydration times, and pacing that is slow and gives adequate time for transitions and time in the form. Stay consistently consistent each time and each week with this approach.

That said, it is also important to be aware of *their* schedules so that you can have a sense of how they may be doing upon their arrival to class. Privately, if possible, screen for mobility, balance, and pain, by asking if they can get up and down without assistance, or if they need a chair nearby, or an aide. Checking in with your students individually and as a group allows you to get to know them and for them to get to know you. They may be fatigued, unfocused, or chatty and pepped up in their day. Yoga class may be the only time they have to socialize that day; allowing time for some conversation may be beneficial, too. Considering their schedule as you plan a class can bring a more responsive and informed program to them.

With regards to sharing health benefits of yoga throughout your class, it is a good, general practice towards building self-awareness and care, as well as being respectful to the intellect of your students who may be curious to know about such benefits as joint lubrication, improved sleep, lower blood pressure, and balanced mood. Stay general and avoid appearing an authority or health expert, unless this is part of your education and work. Know and adhere to your scope of practice. Learn to refer out if anything is beyond your skill set. Have a ready list of contacts for referrals and keep it updated, as best you can.

People with Physical, Developmental and Intellectual Disabilities
Background

For the purposes of this guide, this section is limited to teaching people with cognitive disabilities – intellectual (ID), developmental (DD) – and physical challenges. Excluded here are people with mental illness and DSM diagnoses such as clinical depression and the autism spectrum. For this group and those challenged by mental health issues, separate, careful, and empirically based considerations should be made – although we recognize that people may have co-occurring conditions, such as physical and intellectual disabilities, along with clinical depression and anxiety. As well, learning disabilities that may be part of a person's intellectual disability (ID), such as attentional issues, non-verbal communication styles, visual perceptual and auditory processing differences, will likely impact how they learn in a yoga class. People with ID and/or physical challenges will need adapted, accessible yoga forms and accessible locations for classes. As with seniors and elders, people on the ID spectrum may be on any number of medications, in treatment for thyroid imbalance or seizure control, for example. These drugs can impair stamina, mental attention, speech, and motoric coordination.

The culture of disabled people is uniquely marginal and uniquely tribal in that they are often getting out into the world as members of a program or residence, at the behest of a service provider or a single caregiver or family member. Individuality is often lost when activity choices are made for them by an overseeing agency or person. A lack of independence, limited opportunity for making choices, or having control of their environment and their bodies to a degree – all make up a quality of life that is more institutional than not. A trauma-informed yoga class can bring great potential for empowering choice-making and for promoting agency in their bodies, if done thoughtfully. Learning as much as you can about this group of people, your potential students and their culture is essential for your safety and for theirs. Get professional, specialty training. Our suggestions for teaching this special population strive to include a respectful and thoughtful approach for people with ID and/or physical special needs and within the context of sexual trauma and potential healing.

Sexual Assault Rates among People with Intellectual Disabilities, 2011–15

The rate of rape and sexual assault against people with intellectual disabilities is more than seven times the rate against people without disabilities. Among women with intellectual disabilities, it is about 12 times the rate.

Rate per 1,000 people

Persons with intellectual disabilities – 4.4

Persons with disabilities – 2.1

Persons with no disabilities – 0.6

Rate per 1,000 people with an intellectual disability, by gender

Women with intellectual disabilities – 7.3

Men with intellectual disabilities – 1.4

Notes

Based on the noninstitutionalized U.S. residential population aged 12 or older
Source: Bureau of Justice Statistics, National Crime Victimization Survey, Special Tabulation
Credit: Katie Park/NPR
(Shapiro 2018)

In National Public Radio's ground-breaking investigative series called *Abused and Betrayed* (Shapiro 2018), the US Justice Department's unpublished data on sexual assault and trauma against people with intellectual disabilities is revealed, and the numbers of reported cases are shockingly high. With people on the ID spectrum being seven times more likely to be sexually assaulted than non-disabled people, this group is at most risk for victimization and at all hours of the day; although more likely, they will be assaulted by someone they know and in broad daylight. For many reasons, these crimes do not appear to be taken seriously, going mostly unrecognized, unprosecuted and unpunished, with the perpetrator going free, only to abuse again. Remarkably, police and prosecutors are often reluctant to bring such cases to court because they are so hard to win (Shapiro 2018). People with special needs are thought to be easy targets, because they are often perceived as compliant with authority figures – staff, caregivers, professional or family, teachers and doctors – and do not communicate easily about their experiences. In fact, some are non-verbal. Building trust relationships between teacher and student are at the heart of best practices for people with disabilities.

Best Practices for Supporting People with Disabilities

Best Practice
Know your students.

As with the elder population, it is wise to become educated about people with intellectual and/or physical disabilities but also actively engaged before opening classes. If you can, spend some time in your community using a wheelchair, navigating traffic, entering a bank, supermarket, or school to adjust your understanding of accessibility and the stamina needed to get around. Notice how you are treated by others – invisible, avoided, gawked at, or infantilized – to build cultural humility. Notice how it feels. It is an experience that may transform your teaching for the better.

Additionally, consider volunteering in a community program and attend trainings that focus on developing safe, relevant embodiment practices for people with disabilities; or find direct service opportunities to gain experience, communicating with aides and staff of community support or residential programs. By gaining exposure to the lives people lead, you can develop a sense of abilities, restrictions, and cognitive awareness. This will help you develop opportunities in the yoga classroom that support competency and free will within the body, as well as helping you learn how to engage someone in this spectrum through movement.

Best Practice
Consider appropriate settings.

You may be aware or interested in teaching yoga to children or adults in a particular spectrum such as Down syndrome or cerebral palsy. It may or may not be possible to find a group but by contacting a non-profit associated with that spectrum, you may find educational material that helps. You may also find a source of students and a welcoming hand from the agency. People with intellectual and/or developmental disabilities typically include many spectrums. Camps and recreation programs for people with special needs such as Visions Center on Blindness, Pine Tree Camp at Pine Tree Society, YMCA, or the National Ability Center may be good resources for learning about quality of life, range of abilities, adaptive physical activities, and what is available for potential yoga classes. In-services or educational talks at a program where you would like to teach are recommended for sharing information

about yoga and for connecting more widely with the community. Special education programs in schools may be open to bringing yoga to students. As well, direct support providers, residential and day programs for people with special needs could direct you. Such programs may have excellent places for trauma-informed yoga classes. Find a contact person who can be your guide. Come prepared knowing your limitations as a yoga teacher; avoid stating that you will help people with special needs heal from trauma and practice trauma-informed teaching principles in your other classes or in your own personal practice. Try not to expound on statistics of sexual trauma or put trauma at the forefront of your teaching. Trauma-informed principles can travel with you, as part of you, within your tool kit. You will not need to defend your work.

Best Practice
Know institutional requirements.

As with teaching elders, know the requirements for working with the institutions that serve the disabled community, such as liability insurance, state and federal clearances, fingerprinting, immunizations, and the Health Insurance Portability and Accountability Act of 1996 (HIPPA). Become aware of the schedule of the program and what staff are available to support the yoga class, learn the ratio of people served and staff, and whether there is supervision. Become familiar with the different programs and sites that may be open to including yoga, providers such as an agency day program, Special Olympics, residential program, camps for adults and children with special needs such as Pine Tree Camp, daily life skills programs at schools and universities, community life programs, and some arts and leadership programs that include physical activities.

Creating a supportive teaching environment, which includes co-teaching with aides, staff, and another yoga teacher, ensures safety and the feeling of competency in your students. Remember that broken trust is one of the hallmarks of sexual trauma. To that end, maintain a low ratio of teachers/staff to participants, whether it is a small class with fewer staff or a larger group of participants with many staff members. To be trauma-informed in this setting, consider letting students know before each class that staff will be walking around to help. Reminding and teaching students that they can ask for help or say "no thank you" to an assist is to be trauma-informed. Be transparent and always let them know when you are moving off your mat and why, such as when you may need to bring a chair to someone or to close a window or to adjust the thermostat in the room. But, as a general rule, a teacher should stay on the mat to limit movement and distractibility in the room when teaching intellectually disabled students. Some students will have a one-to-one aide with them to help with mobility or personal care needs. This can be very helpful, too. Be person-centered and teach to individuals rather than grouping by diagnoses.

Best Practice
Be aware of the culture norm of infantilization.

Not only do people in the ID/DD and/or physical disability spectrum often lose their individuality and their opportunities to exercise personal choice, they are often viewed as child-like, innocent, labile, and compliant. They are also known to have strong desires for trust and friendship (Shapiro 2018), leaving them open to any sign of care and belonging. This perception of them invites the predator.

To counter this, it is best to observe students, learn their capacity as best you can, and to be self-reflective about your own assumptions. People in the ID/DD spectrums, as with many elderly people, tend to be infantilized. They are commonly treated as children. As a yoga teacher, it is imperative that this perception does not follow you or them into the classroom, if you intend to help them become more self-directed in their yoga or to find their own competency. Become aware of your body language and tone of voice with students who have intellectual and/or emotional challenges. We suggest that you practice teaching with a fellow teacher or mentor to get feedback as to your tone and body language – and your use of invitational language. While it may take time to help them build capacity for self-aware movement and choice-making, you can encourage one or two options in a form, for example, as opposed to several, at a time. Over weeks, they may discover they have other choices that you have not found. These moments of discovery are equal in power to any moment of discovery in a person's development and growth into adulthood.

Best Practice
Consider classroom layout and props.

As addressed in Chapter 4 "Best Practices for Creating a Trauma-informed Yoga Experience," follow those best practices, keeping in mind the following. Be familiar with classroom layout, locating bathroom, fire exits, and props to maximize predictability and safety. It is suggested that students should have a wall and not a door behind them, so the classroom is facing the door. With students in the intellectual or developmental disabilities spectrum, a teacher should be aware of the potential for heightened arousal or emotion. Students in the non-verbal spectrum can have very specific styles of communication, some of which may be physical. The assistance of a staff person is typically available. To be trauma-informed in this context may mean knowing and adjusting to a wide variety of physical, behavioral, mental, and emotional ranges and needs. So that as you position your mat, keep these considerations in mind. You find more success with engaging them, observing for safety, and assisting if needed. Staffing should be in the layout planning, too. Often a one-to-one aide joins a student who requires added assistance.

A simple choice of props is nice to have in the room, such as mats and blocks. Blocks may be integrated later into a series of classes, depending on mobility needs and appropriateness. They may be thrown, too. Know your students, and consult with staff about each person to discover what may trigger challenging behaviors.

Best Practice
Maintain simple choices and slow transitions.

Use simple, trauma-informed forms with the goal to reconnect with the relaxation response, interoceptive awareness, and emotion regulation. Offer one or two choices after a few classes to build up capacity for personal choice-making and the self-discovery of favorite forms. Remembering that many people on the special needs spectrum tend to travel in groups, potentially losing opportunities for individual choice and personal investigation of their world. Encouraging them to be curious in yoga also supports their individuality.

That said, there are certain forms we do not recommend, because they can trigger a trauma response such as flight, fear, freeze, or aggression, including:

- happy baby
- bound angle
- wide-legged forward folds
- cat-cow
- legs up the wall/inversions.

In general, choose just a few forms and allow for transitioning into and out of them, practicing variations, and noticing sensations. Give plenty of time to transition into and out of the classroom, setting a slow pace that takes into account body in space concerns, organizational facility, mobility, and cognitive impairments.

Best Practice
Adapt yoga forms.

For people with physical disabilities, many yoga forms can be made accessible (see Figure 11.1). By becoming familiar with adaptive yoga and restorative yoga, a teacher builds a greater capacity to meet the needs of students who may have physical challenges with the forms. Become familiar with different props such as bolsters, use of blankets to bring a neutral pelvis for sitting crossed legged or to relieve a shoulder or neck in supine form. Straps are not encouraged in a trauma-informed class due to their potential to trigger memory or behaviors that impede safety. Volunteering and mentoring with a seasoned adaptive yoga teacher who offers classes may give you experience with assisting students who may have physical differences, such as missing

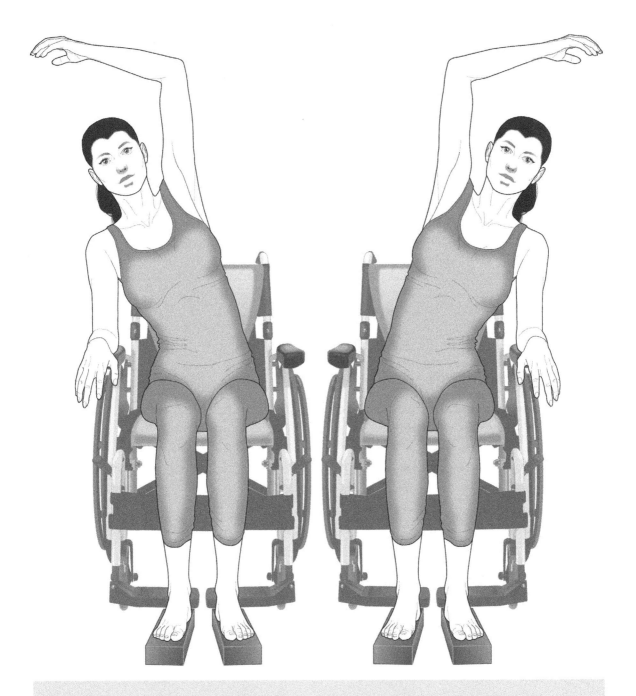

Figure 11.1

Lateral Spinal Stretch: Become familiar with the six movements of the spine to provide a predictable, safe foundational sequence for someone in a wheelchair

limbs and limited mobility. Additional training in adaptive and restorative yoga is helpful.

Best Practice
Be an advocate, observe, speak up, and follow-up.

The intellectually disabled person may be characterized as incompetent with self-care and self-directed activity, attention-seeking, child-like, and a life-long member of the *culture of dependency*. As well, there is anecdotal evidence that they are not encouraged to disclose sexual trauma, for fear of losing their home, subsidy, or a loved career. They share feelings of shame and may be threatened by an ever-present perpetrating staff member, as do the elderly who live in the culture of dependency. However, people may exhibit symptoms of having been harmed, such as chronic stomach pains, peritoneal burning or itching, and a preoccupation with scanning the room, for example. These symptoms warrant our attention and advocacy. If you are troubled by something you have noticed--and as you get to know students, you may notice differences week to week – it is best to approach the agency contact person, preferably a lead staff, and inquire, sharing your observations or a student's physical complaint or disclosure, if that happens. Abdominal pain can be symptomatic of food poisoning, flu, or a prolific yeast infection, pelvic inflammatory disease (PID), or a sexually transmitted disease (STD), requiring medical attention.

While this may uncover a sexual assault event or events, it may not. Be sure to share information with someone who can effectively help the student get proper care and be willing to let it go.

Maintain your professionalism, keep it in the classroom, and know you are doing what you can as an advocate of self-care and no harm. Yoga teachers are not mandated reporters of harm, however, following up on a student who is not feeling well is a deep act of kindness and caring.

Conclusion

Yoga provides opportunities to develop body awareness, set boundaries, make choices, and to freely express feelings about touch and/or proximity. Elder students, developmentally and physically disabled people – often referred to as our most vulnerable citizens – tend to be marginalized, infantilized, and made invisible. As a group, people with ID/DD were not even counted by the US Justice Department's data on rape and sexual victimization (Shapiro 2018). A trauma-informed teacher who is committed to showing up each week, to bringing attention to how the body moves and what effect a form may bring or not, has a front-row seat to watching people develop awareness of what is possible on their own terms. In these communities, this can be nothing short of radical, promoting better health, self-confidence, boundaries, self-awareness, and motivation. Trauma-informed yoga assumes that everyone, at any age or with any challenge, has the capacity to heal.

> Trauma-informed yoga has improved my life, both physically and mentally. It has me so aware and accepting of my body, including touches from my husband of more than 50 years. I am standing straighter. I feel more joy.
>
> – Joyce R., age 72, testimonial from a private T-I Yoga group

PART 5

Contexts of Abuse

Author *James Jurgensen*

Contributors *Nan Herron, Sue Jones*

Introduction

Demographics of the College Population

This chapter focuses on survivors of sexual trauma within the context of postsecondary institutions – such as colleges, universities, community colleges, graduate and professional schools, and trade schools. Throughout this chapter, we will use the term *colleges* to refer to these institutions and discuss the empowerment of the survivors of sexual trauma enrolled as students within such institutions through their participation in yoga and meditative programming.

Postsecondary institution demographics have shifted significantly in recent decades – particularly in terms of size and diversity. From 2000 to 2017, total undergraduate enrollment in degree-granting postsecondary institutions increased by 27 percent, growing from 13.2 million to 16.8 million students. By 2028, total undergraduate enrollment is projected to rise to 17.2 million (Integrated Postsecondary Education Data Systems, National Center for Education Statistics, & U.S. Department of Education 2019). This growing population represents a broader demographic than ever previously seen within the college population (National Center for Education Statistics, & U.S. Department of Education 2019). The college population currently includes more students of color (42 percent nonwhite), older students (40 percent of students are aged 25 years or older), employed students (62 percent of students work part- or full-time), students from low-income backgrounds (33 percent of students come from families earning $20,000 or less

per year), and those who must balance studies with parenting (28 percent of students have children) than ever before (Postsecondary Success 2019).

Although the current population of college students is increasingly diverse, the experience of vulnerability is consistent. Upon entering college, students step into an experience of complete uncertainty and unpredictability. With a change in housing, food sources, social support, and sense of identity, new college students are at their most vulnerable point in life. In her book *Daring Greatly: How the Courage to Be Vulnerable Transforms the Way We Live, Love, Parent, and Lead*, Dr Brené Brown defines vulnerability as "uncertainty, risk and emotional exposure" (Brown 2012: 175). Since vulnerability serves as "the core, the heart, the center of meaningful human experiences" (Brown 2012: 12), its presence is required for either an individual or a collective community to experience transformational change. As the center of all emotions, vulnerability is connected to difficult feelings – such as grief, shame, fear, scarcity, and disappointment – but also serves as "the birthplace of love, belonging, joy, courage, empathy and creativity" (Brown 2012: 34). Therefore, it is the college population's extreme vulnerability that both positions them to experience immense growth – as individuals and as a collective – as well as leaves them particularly susceptible to poor outcomes.

College students face a myriad of institutional and cultural power dynamics, including those labeled as "tradition." Toxic power hierarchies have become deeply ingrained in campus culture. The vulnerability of the college population – although necessary to experience significant positive growth – also leaves students at greater risk to be affected by such toxic hierarchies. The power hierarchies within institutional cultures and traditions are slow to change and thus the toxic power structure in college culture becomes normalized. This is most often seen within Greek organizations and in sports culture. Examination of cultural power structures in learning institutions is a first step in creating lasting, widespread change. Students can learn how and when their inherent vulnerability is contributing to healthy growth, and when it is exposing them to experiencing harm.

Recent estimates of sexual assault victimization among college students in the United States have reported rates of violence as high as 20 to 30 percent (Fedina, et al. 2016; Fisher, et al. 2000; Krebs, et al. 2016; Kilpatrick, et al. 2007; the Association of American Universities 2015; the Association of American Universities 2019). Data suggest that at least one in five women experience sexual assault by senior year, with the majority of those assaults occurring during freshman year (Flack 2008). Twenty-two percent of students report experiencing at least one incident of sexual assault during college. While transgender/gender nonconforming students and cisgender women report the highest rates (38 percent and 28 percent, respectively), cisgender men also experience sexual assault at a rate of 12.5 percent (Mellins, et al. 2017). Other students shown to be at increased risk for experiencing sexual assault include students of a sexual orientation other than heterosexual and those with disabilities (Mellins, et al. 2017; Cantor, et al. 2015).

In examining differences in past-year sexual assault, results from one meta-analysis (Coulter, et al. 2017) indicated that sexual assault disproportionately affects several sexual-, gender-, and racial/ethnic-minority subgroups. For instance, transgender people had higher odds of sexual assault than cisgender men and women, and Black transgender people had significantly higher odds of sexual assault than White transgender people. Predicted probabilities of sexual assault ranged from 2.6 percent (Asian Pacific Islander cisgender men) to 57.7 percent (Black transgender people). The increased diversity in the student body of college campuses can directly correlate with greater incidents of sexual assault.

Across all types of assault and gender groups, an impaired ability to consent due to alcohol and drug use was the perpetration method reported most frequently – followed by physical force and verbal coercion. Additional factors associated with increased risk for sexual assault included difficulty paying for basic necessities, fraternity/sorority membership, participation in more casual sexual encounters ("hook ups"), and a sexual assault history prior to enrolling in college. Furthermore, high rates of re-victimization – meaning the majority of sexual assault survivors report experiencing multiple sexual assaults during college – were also reported across gender groups (Griffin & Read 2012; Mellins, et al. 2017; Messman-Moore & McConnell 2018).

The culture of normalized sexual assault on college campuses has become an epidemic, and effective, sustainable cultural change requires time. Collaboration and coordination between multiple interventions, both inside and outside of postsecondary institutions, can help expedite the process. This is where trauma-informed yoga programs can have an impact. Over time, trauma-informed yoga programs can help students feel less vulnerable and more empowered and provide them with a sense of community. Through trauma-informed yoga, a sense of safety (physical and emotional), trustworthiness, and belonging can take hold. When students experience choice, a sense of control, and an awareness of the impact these things can have on their day-to-day life, a grass roots shift can take root. The practice of yoga can contribute to the creation of a healthier campus culture.

Trauma-Informed Yoga as a Resource for the College Population

The available research evaluating the effects of mindfulness programs on college campuses indicates a positive impact not only on students' psychological health outcomes (Holland 2004; Jain, et al. 2007; Gokhan, et al. 2010; Sandars 2009; Shiralkar, et al. 2013; Shirey 2007; Smith, et al. 2007; Bergen-Cico, et al. 2013; Oman, et al. 2008; Rockefeller 2006; Sears, et al. 2011), but also on their academic performance (Shapiro, et al. 2011). While studies on the impact of yoga alone (that is, without an additional component such as mindfulness-based stress reduction) among the college population are limited, the empirical evidence available indicates that yoga programming can significantly improve the health and well-being of college students. One such study with graduate health science students found associations between participation in one thirty-minute restorative yoga class (included light stretching, deep breathing, and meditation) and decreases in blood pressure and psychological stress (Rizzolo, et al. 2009). A second study of 128 college students describes yoga as effective in reducing psychological distress, state anxiety, and perceived stress (Deckro, et al. 2010). In a study of college students aged eighteen to fifty-six, results of an eight-week yoga program demonstrated significant decreases in ratings of stress, worry, and depression as well as an increase in mindfulness skills (Eastman-Mueller, et al. 2013).

A study assessing the impact of teaching solely mindfulness-based stress reduction (MBSR) practices to college students found that program participation provided students the ability to be more accepting of their limitations; to more easily identify and discuss their feelings; and to better understand their perceived-need to always be perfect as an unattainable goal that had largely been internalized. Through the MBSR program, students learned techniques to recognize and reframe negative thinking, thereby reducing the anxiety and depression that had been a contributing factor in the decrease of academic productivity and enjoyment of life (Kerrigan, et al. 2017).

Taken together, these studies demonstrate the contribution of an on-campus yoga program in helping students manage stress, promote general student well-being, and serve as a useful adjunctive to mental health services. A yoga or meditation practice can help with the difficulties caused by trauma (see Chapters 2 and 3). Traumatic experiences generate the sense that the world is no longer as understandable, predictable, or meaningful – and trauma-informed yoga intentionally creates an experience within the class that counteracts each of those notions. The instruction is ideally predicated on invitational language, emphasizing gentle exploration of bodily movements and associated physical sensations. Participation in class offers students an experience focused on individual choice, cultivation of self-awareness, healthy curiosity about one's body, and prioritization of pacing, duration, and intensity in a manner that maximizes self-care.

Best Practices

Best Practice
Be familiar with mandatory reporting, the institution's policies, the current climate of sexual violence on campus, and the most up-to-date Title IX expectations/regulations.

One notable action that has raised the national profile of sexual violence on college campuses came in 2011. Title IX – a law passed by Congress in 1972 – had been most commonly associated with gender equity in sports. More recently, it has become an effective tool for addressing sexual violence on college campuses. As stated through a Dear Colleague Letter issued by the Office of Civil Rights in 2011 reminding schools of their obligation to prevent and address sexual violence under Title IX, "Sexual harassment of students, which includes acts of sexual violence, is a form of sex discrimination prohibited by Title IX. In order to assist recipients, which include school districts, colleges, and universities (hereinafter 'schools' or 'recipients') in meeting these obligations, this letter explains that the requirements of Title IX pertaining to sexual harassment also cover sexual violence, and it lays out the specific IX requirements applicable to sexual violence" (U.S. Department of Education, Office of Civil Rights 2011).

By expanding the law's interpretation of sex discrimination to include sexual violence, Title IX became both an effective tool for reporting assault and harassment, as well as the driving force behind a push of sexual assault education aiming to help students understand the nature of sexual assault and consent (Freitas 2018). Under the new interpretation, it serves as an enforcement mechanism that requires institutions to respond to students' claims. Adding to the national attention being devoted to the issue, in 2013 President Obama signed into law the Campus Save Act, which requires institutions of higher education to teach *everyone* – students, faculty, administration, and staff – about sexual assault prevention, intimate partner violence, sexual harassment, and stalking (U.S. Department of Education, Q&A on Campus Sexual Misconduct, September 2017). If institutions hope to identify, then provide dedicated resources for groups that are at higher risk for sexual assault; all parties involved must understand the epidemic of sexual assault present in their culture.

Along with the expansion of Title IX and the Campus Save Act, increased public awareness of sexual assault on college campuses has been fueled by the #MeToo Movement, broader media coverage, and documentaries such as *The Hunting Ground*. Increased public acknowledgment is forcing university administrations to re-examine policies and procedures regarding how they handle reporting, introduce new measures aimed at prevention and intervention, and provide additional resources for victim-survivors to cope with the psychological effects of being assaulted.

In the last twenty years, federal laws have been enacted to ensure that colleges and universities develop policies, provide prevention activities, and respond to sexual assault (Office for Civil Rights 2001). Colleges are now required to collect data on the prevalence of sexual misconduct and assault, develop specific policies to address sexual assault, and implement prevention programs and support services. Efforts are being made, yet whether these efforts have made a significant impact on the rates of sexual violence remains to be seen. Sexual violence has been institutionalized on college campuses. Therefore, we must go beyond shedding light on the problem. Real solutions for addressing the problem, healing its effects, and preventing it from continuing are necessary. Institutions must work to improve their processes of reporting assaults and handling cases once they are reported, as well as ensuring that adequate resources are available for both the immediate (crisis numbers, on-call services) and long-term (physiological and psychological services) needs of victim-survivors.

An examination of the structural factors that create, enable, and perpetuate a culture of sexual violence should be ongoing.

Greek life is often a focal point of campus culture. Many institutions have identified Greek life as hotbeds of sexual violence on their campuses. Many students are drawn to Greek life – either to join fully as members or solely on their weekends for the parties – because, like all human beings, they crave connection, community, and belonging. Incoming students seek out connection, community, and belonging in their new environment, which makes them vulnerable. In some cases these vulnerable students are taken advantage of by other, more powerful individuals. This power dynamic is played out in fraternities and sororities alike, where new members are often demeaned as a "rite of passage," then encouraged to overlook morally questionable behavior out of loyalty to their new "community."

A culture of sexual violence has its roots in students' need for a sense of belonging, and their efforts to meet those needs in a toxic culture of power hierarchy and egregious behavior that has been normalized. This fact is key to why trauma-informed yoga and meditation programming is offered on college campuses: it can provide a positive, consensual experience that allows students to meet their needs for connection, community, and belonging.

Establishing a Partnership with the Postsecondary Institution

Best Practice
Be familiar with the current state of mental health wellness on college campuses and the resources currently available to meet the mental health needs of students.

By the time of reaching college, 66 to 85 percent of students have been exposed to at least one traumatic event within their lifetime (Read, et al. 2011; Smyth, et al. 2008). As they begin their college journey, students' risk of experiencing trauma only increases: as many as 50 percent of college students are exposed to a potentially traumatizing event within their first year (Galatzer-Levy, et al. 2012). To compound the risk factors associated with trauma exposure, one out of every four college students lives with a diagnosed mental illness, and that statistic does not account for students dealing with undiagnosed mental health concerns (Baker 2015).

As assessed by clinicians at campus counseling centers, anxiety and depression continue to be the most common concerns of students (Center for Collegiate Mental Health 2019). In 2018, clinician-reported rates of depression as well as average rates of student self-reported anxiety and depression continued to increase among students, and the lifetime prevalence rates of "threat-to-self" characteristics (non-suicidal self-injury, 27.8 percent; serious suicidal ideation, 35.8 percent; and suicide attempts, 10.3 percent) increased for the eighth consecutive year among students receiving counseling services. For students seeking treatment, 8.2 percent report serious suicidality in the last month, and clinicians report suicidality as a presenting concern for almost 10 percent of students (Center for Collegiate Mental Health 2019). Demographically, transfer students, upperclassmen, and those living off-campus are noted as three of the most stressed, anxious, and depressed cohorts within the general student population, and students report academic performance, pressure to succeed, and post-graduation plans as their top three sources of concern (Beiter, et al. 2015).

Given the alarming rates of mental health issues in college students, many colleges are increasing their mental health interventions

(Hindman, et al. 2015; Ramler, et al. 2016). These campus-based mental health interventions can be classified into two (non-mutually exclusive) groups: (1) traditional interventions, or (2) mindfulness-based interventions. The current traditional interventions available on campuses are not effectively meeting the scale or range of students' mental health needs. Attempting to fill this gap in mental health resources, an increasing number of college campuses are offering mindfulness-based interventions either in conjunction with traditional interventions or as a separate offering.

According to the findings of Cieslak, et al. (2016), the primary models for all outreach and prevention interventions across colleges campuses in North America are psychoeducational, with no associated costs or fees. The traditional interventions most often offered on college campuses include: prevention and outreach, support groups and workshops, individual counseling, and self-help.

Support groups and workshops across colleges focus on topics including coping skills; anxiety/depression management; eating disorders; LGBTQ; grief; support groups for different types of students (such as minority students or graduate students); and support for sexual assault survivors. Most groups available to students are scheduled during weekday regular business hours, and the bulk of group therapy sessions are co-facilitated by a combination of licensed mental health professionals and graduate students in-training. Most colleges offer roughly ten different types of groups and require a pre-consultation before attending the groups.

Therapy is provided on campuses through a variety of treatment models. Most colleges offered a limited number of counseling interventions free to their part- and full-time students. If students require further counseling, most interventions provide long-term counseling to students as needed or make appropriate outside referrals.

Although studies have shown treatment provided by campus counseling centers to be effective in reducing mental health distress, not all students who seek out their services achieve significant improvements as a result. This often occurs because some students need more extended services to experience improvements. Unfortunately, rigid policies related to session limits often prematurely terminate treatment for students who need more treatment (Center for Collegiate Mental Health 2019).

Best Practice

Be prepared to articulate how the addition of your classes on campuses could help close a gap in mental health resources available to an institution's students. Identify the established channels and relevant actors at the institution. Utilize those channels to find possible collaborators, advocates for your presence on campus, and sources of clinically based supervision.

In light of the lack of sufficient mental health resources available on college campuses and the increasing documentation of poor mental health among college students, trauma-informed yoga programs could play a significant role in bridging the gap of resources on campuses. Mindfulness-based interventions available on some college campuses include the following: mindfulness-based cognitive therapy, mindfulness-based stress reduction, guided meditations and yoga, compassion training, mindfulness-based technology, and mindful eating (Cieslak, et al. 2016). Yoga Nidra, or guided meditation, is the most common type of yoga and meditation programming offered.

While most colleges do not offer class credit for yoga and meditation programming, a variety of university departments have successfully partnered with yoga teachers to make yoga and meditation programs available to students as an on-campus resource (Cieslak, et al. 2016). When seeking out collaborators for support in bringing classes to campus, consider the following departments: physical education (PE) departments (your class could fulfill a student's required PE credit); social science departments, which may include students or professors who could be collaborators on a study on student health; student health services; student recreation departments; or student groups supported by university funding that are looking for a weekly healthy activity to participate in together.

Most universities struggle to provide enough on-campus counseling resources to meet demand. By offering yoga classes through a partnership with a campus's counseling center, you help relieve some of this burden and thereby gain the support of an important branch of the institution that has the positional power to advocate for your presence. Over time, this can help you secure more participants, a source of funding, a place to practice, and clinical support.

Often, trauma feels unspeakable. Thus, survivors can lack the language necessary to fully participate in psychotherapy and narrative therapy. Trauma-informed yoga offers a different approach to healing trauma: a pathway that is not dependent on language. By engaging with one's body in an intentional way and within a controlled environment, a victim-survivor can begin to recognize and confront the trauma that continues to live in their body

long after the traumatic experience occurred. This experience can provide the language and create the space necessary for conversation to then take place in psychotherapy. In conjunction, trauma-informed yoga and psychotherapy can offer the survivor a pathway for processing the trauma – both as narratively and somatically (the body sensations of a survivor from moment to moment). This mind and body process helps survivors gradually move from confronting the trauma to overcoming the trauma.

> **Best Practice**
> Identify your class as trauma-informed and be explicit in defining what that means. If resources permit, offer classes of different structures.

When posting flyers or sending out advertising to your classes, reach out to your contacts at the institutions to learn which organizational leaders and physical spaces on campuses tend to garner the most attention from students. In these advertisements, specify whether your classes are trauma-informed. Without specification, many students with trauma histories may not feel safe attending.

Also, be specific in the advertisement about whether your class is open-to-all, offered throughout the semester, requires sign-up at the beginning and then becomes a closed group, or follows a different structure. Open-to-all advertising could include language such as "Open to all [insert institution] students: all types of bodies, genders, and levels of experience. Free, drop-in welcome, and no sign-up required."

For a closed-group where students are self-identified as trauma-survivors, the classes should be confidential and screening potential participants may be helpful; groups should determine the specifics of confidentiality among themselves. Confidentiality can be framed in these situations as a mutual respect (for example, yoga for many is a practice for healing, and for that reason we ask to not disclose the identities of those in this room outside of this space). Discuss additional considerations with collaborators or relevant stakeholders to help with adequate and consistent attendance.

> **Best Practice**
> Choose a large, discrete, and neutral setting for classes.

Conversations about consent have begun taking place with increased frequency on campuses across the country. Exploring consent within the context of yoga class allows the shift from conversation to embodied practice, as well as providing a place for consent to be taught in a space free of institutional politics and power dynamics. Spaces such as gyms, dance studios, conference rooms, student center spaces, and wellness centers are potentially good options. These spaces are more neutral in terms of power differentials often present in Greek houses, residence halls, and classrooms. If students are identifying as trauma-survivors by attending your class, then choose as discrete of a place as possible.

When offering classes on a college campus, location can significantly impact attendance. Because students often either lack access to vehicles or face parking restrictions, access via walking or public transit should be a key consideration when selecting a location. In particular, when offering classes during the daytime, try to hold classes in a location within close proximity of academic buildings. However, if classes

are being held early in the morning or later in the evening, consider choosing a location near student housing. If there are options, prior to scheduling a class, consider polling students on which location would be most convenient for them to attend classes.

> **Best Practice**
> Tailor the schedule of classes to accommodate the academic calendar and course schedules.

Typically, the daily schedule of college students vary. If possible, at the beginning of each semester after students have received their class schedules, send out a poll asking students what times would work best for them. If you have a collaborator at the college (such as the student wellness center) then request their assistance with distributing the survey to students on your behalf. Asking students directly can provide you with useful insight on why specific times might work or not work for students. For example, Mondays at 6:00 to 7:00 P.M. might be a popular class time for working adults because they could attend the class after leaving work and before going home for the evening. However, on a college campus, Mondays at 6:00 to 7:00 P.M. might conflict with the practice times for athletic teams or the weekly meetings of Greek organizations.

Sabeth Jackson, a campus yoga teacher, recalls, "I had a lot of classes with only a few students. I had better attendance when I moved to central campus: the social lodge. A common theme in all of the programs I've done, not just yoga, is problems with attendance. I tried a lot of different things, but the thing that helped most was feedback from students about the best days and times." It is also helpful to send students weekly reminders of the times and locations for classes that week, which can be done by listing the instructor's email on advertisements along with language such as "email [insert instructor's email] to sign up for weekly reminders."

> **Best Practice**
> To ensure maximum inclusivity, avoid using potentially alienating language.

Be mindful of the impact of using the word *om*, Sanskrit, Namaste, and hands in prayer, as all of these practices can be alienating for some students. If you do choose to use that language, then explain the intention and meaning, and use dual translation. Also, provide alternative options to hands in prayer – such as one hand over heart, one hand on abdominal muscles, placing hands on knees or thighs, or right hand holding left resting in lap. Be careful not to violate university policies around religion. Ask university personnel what policies exist and how to ensure your class does not violate them.

Utilizing Classes to Empower Survivors and Demonstrate a Culture of Consent

> **Best Practice**
> Decide as a class what it means to be safe and set expectations for group behavior.

Briefly discuss triggers and boundaries as a group. "Trigger" is a term used when a traumatic memory is activated by a known or unknown stimulus. The body creates the feeling of the traumatic experience in such a way as to be difficult or frightening to the survivor. When this happens in a trauma-informed yoga class, these occurrences can be discussed, normalized, and seen as opportunities to discern what is present moment reality, and what is a body memory.

Encourage students to practice self-care when they encounter triggers. Acknowledge the options students have during the class to help them ride the experience through. Offer some options such as making the choice to take any physical position that feels safe for them, such as child's form, laying on their stomach, or curling up into a ball (blankets are good for this). Furthermore, consider discussing replacing triggers with opportunities. In moments when triggers come up, encourage students to notice what is happening and remind themselves of the choices they can make in order to ride the trigger through.

In the discussion of boundaries, let people know if touch will be part of the class and describe what such touch will include. Touch is complicated and should be used judiciously if at all. See Chapter 4 for further discussion. If touch is utilized, consider providing chips as an option so that individuals may signal that they do not want to be touched. Encourage students to use their voices and to let you know what they need. Help students understand how movement and breath can be used as a way to practice and learn about their personal boundaries. Encourage them to observe those boundaries, notice how they may shift and change, and learn to recognize the boundaries with which they are comfortable. By normalizing the discussion of boundaries with students – encouraging them to allow their voice to be heard and respected – you are helping them not only reexamine the power relations on campus, but also specifically shift them back toward individual agency and bodily autonomy.

> **Best Practice**
> Be aware of the themes that characterize the college experience and utilize this awareness when structuring your sequence and/or curriculum.

Before designing a curriculum to be used with the college population, review the common characteristics of the college experience and the specific needs those characteristics produce, which are discussed earlier in this chapter. Consider the themes you plan to incorporate into your curriculum and ask yourself if they will create the type of experience or provide the messages college students need to hear. Remind yourself that the students are in the process of integrating new beliefs about self and others; reexamining what is "normal;" and consistently facing a judgmental, hierarchical, hyper-competitive, and comparison-prone environment in their regular campus life.

To help counteract the hierarchical environment, use invitational language to minimize the power differential and to empower your students. For example, you might say, "You are welcome to …" or "See if it feels more comfortable for you to …" To counteract the hyper-competitive and comparative-prone environment, offer cues to notice sensations in their body and bring their attention inward to keep their attention on themselves rather than others. For example, you might say, "Notice your breathing" or "Notice if you're feeling energized or feeling tired." Encourage the practice of observing without feeling the need to make any changes, accepting your own rhythm, and what is unique to you.

Create forms with options that will keep people interested, engaged, and challenged without compromising safety and support. Balance what will peak interest with what will make people feel safe. To accommodate the range of abilities you might have within a class, you could possibly divide classes by level of advancement, or offer multiple options for each form within a given class. Be sure to not value one level of difficulty over another.

> **Best Practice**
> Create a community that cultivates agency, connection, awareness, empowerment, and embodiment.

To effectively eliminate a culture of sexual trauma on college campuses, we must build and normalize a culture of consent. To do so, we need a radical new approach to programming – one that is not grounded in separation, but, rather, one that is rooted in connection. We need an approach that is radical precisely because of the degree to which it practices the principles of consent that acts of sexual violence completely disregard. Our programs, as well as the individuals running them and attending them, must embody these principles, and through communal practice, demonstrate the ability to generate a new culture.

This culture should be felt within each class through care and respect shown to one another. Care for one another may take the form of simply respecting a person's wishes expressed within a class, or it could be referring a student to student counseling services to ensure they have access to adequate support. If we are the sum of our experiences, then we must create experiences for people that will propel them to act in ways that contribute to a culture of consent.

The students attending our classes are at a time in their lives in which they are actively developing their identities, belief systems, and behavioral routines. They are deciding what they should stand up for, what compels them to action, and what they want to represent. The principles of consent practiced within the classes show students where the institution's culture could go.

It is not enough to speak out about the acts of sexual violence that we all should be fighting against. We must go further than speaking about the acts that we are standing up against, or even discussing consent as a concept that we should all employ. We need to explore consent through an embodiment of the practice that extends beyond the concept of sex. Embodied practice of consent within the safe container of a trauma-informed yoga class can help students recognize how it can be embedded within the foundation of their community and in every facet of life.

Conclusion

In our efforts to raise awareness of the pervasive acts of sexual violence taking place on college campuses, we cannot lose sight of the greater goal: to eliminate the culture that gives rise to these acts in the first place. We aim to do more than raise awareness of the culture of sexual violence at postsecondary institutions, or to effectively train bystanders on how to intervene in the moments before acts of sexual violence occur. We have perhaps lost sight of the greater truth, which is that we do not merely exist at these institutions. We *participate* in them, and our participation, in part, shapes their cultures.

In working in college settings, it is important to educate ourselves to the potential unique needs of this population. It is also important to recognize that there is no single profile of a college student; we should not limit our understanding of who students will be to any specific conceptualization. For example, while a college student is often pictured to be a young adult from the ages of eighteen to twenty-two, people attend college at all ages. We cannot and should not make assumptions as to what the needs of our students will be; we should instead engage stakeholders in shaping our practice. A process of active, intentional, and embodied engagement moves beyond merely *telling* students that they are safe, that they can set boundaries, and that they can choose how to engage with their own bodies; this process allows students to explore and control these experiences themselves. In the context of a college campus – which requires students to constantly renegotiate their sense of worth, sense of self, and personal priorities – showing oneself these things is a radical endeavor.

When a person experiences this process as part of a group – as one would in the context of a yoga class – they are given the opportunity to recognize a similarity between themselves and the others in the class: a common humanity. This common humanity bonds them together. Bonding through recognition of common humanity is a particularly phenomenal feat within the context of a college campus because almost all other "bonding" experiences rely on either the lubricant of alcohol, the evidence of intellect, or the competition of skill.

To experience bonding simply by virtue of shared humanity teaches individuals that they can find connection, commonality, and community without having to prove themselves worthy of it. It teaches them that they do not need to tolerate exploitation, change their ethical standards, assert a position of power, or renegotiate their identity to be worthy of connection. It shows them that though we are all always becoming – growing into ourselves, gaining more insight about our experiences and how they have affected who we are today, and intentionally shaping ourselves into the people we are meant to become – whoever that person may be today, in that very moment, is enough to be worthy of connection and belonging.

13

Author *Pamela Stokes Eggleston*

Contributors *Colleen DeVirgiliis, Beth Jones, Daniel Hickman, Emanuel Salazar*

"Serving requires us to know that our humanity is more powerful than our expertise."

– Rachel Remen

Introduction

The purpose of this Chapter is to address military sexual trauma – what it is, who suffers from it, and how to cultivate safe, brave spaces for veterans, military service members, and their families using awareness and humility, through yoga. In 2016, surveys revealed that approximately 14,900 service members had experienced some form of sexual assault. Individuals who reported assault feared retaliation and ostracism for speaking out about these crimes (DOD 2016). To be sure, military sexual trauma (MST) is an ongoing issue, as so often it is the institution of the armed forces that tends to re-trigger and re-traumatize the sufferer throughout the rigid military culture and traditional structure that maintains it. Thus, we surmise that yoga, through the application of best practices, is quite beneficial for the military and veteran populations.

Sexual harassment and sexual assault in the military is considered MST and is an increasing public health issue (Barth, et al. 2016: 77). This study focused on service men and women of Operation Iraqi Freedom (OIF) and Operation Enduring Freedom (OEF). It showed that about 41 percent of women veterans and 4 percent of men veterans reported experiencing MST (Barth, et al. 2016: 77). This and other studies (Castro, et al. 2015; Teeters, et al. 2017) shine a light on why MST is so pervasive within the armed forces.

The military culture's "code of silence" and chain of command are why victims often get triggered through the aftermath of the MST incident. This can be even further complicated when a perpetrator is party of one's chain of command. The many challenges that can arise after an assault compound the experience of trauma. In the wake of an epidemic that is often silenced, we face an ever-increasing public health issue. In addition, assault among female veterans in VA hospitals and facilities is notable. Recently, Andrea Goldstein, a navy intelligence officer veteran (and member of the Women Veterans Task Force of the House of Representatives) was assaulted at the Washington, DC VA Medical Center. "The department has scrambled to adjust to the rising population of female veterans by hiring more women's health care providers, expanding the health care service it offers women and trying to improve the culture. But Mr. Takano's letter did not mark the first time sexual harassment and assault at V.A. facilities have attracted the attention of Congress" (Steinhauer 2019). The task force that Goldstein is a member of was created in the spring of 2019 due in part to the issue of harassment and assault at VA facilities.

It is important to note that although the mindset among higher ranking officers and enlisted service members is shifting, for MST survivors, the change has not come quickly enough. Because of the complexity of military sexual trauma, it is imperative that yoga teachers, who work with veteran and military populations seek specialized training in trauma-informed practices for

Case study

About 4 years ago, I realized that I was not the same person. I couldn't sleep. I had more chronic pain than ever. I was dealing with medical issues from military service but they got worse and I was exhausted all the time. I had bad nightmares. My anger was uncontrollable and I couldn't maintain a steady relationship. I was frustrated because of the trauma that I did not know how to properly address: I used sex, hot baths, and VA prescribed medications to cope.

I trusted doctors to tell me what was going on instead of taking control of my own health. I tried CBT [cognitive behavioral therapy] and DBT [dialectical behavior therapy] training for my MST and PTSD [post-traumatic stress disorder] symptoms. My lymphedema and other health issues caused me difficulties in walking. I was experiencing anger outbursts and lack of sleep. I was getting sicker. Sometimes I couldn't even get out of bed. I used to pray to God that I just wanted to live for my daughter. But then, I had an epiphany and remembered that I used to meditate when I was younger! I used to dance and my dance teacher in high school introduced me to meditation. I was desperate because if I didn't take control of my health, I would have died.

I came across a video of an older lady that couldn't walk and she said yoga helped her dance again. I thought to myself that this is something like my story. My first yoga experience was hard: it was so difficult for me to do certain positions that I cried for two days. The yoga teacher told me not to give up and that there was more to yoga than just movement. Afterwards, I attended a free Yoga for Women Veterans session. After that first session I slept so well. I had never experienced anything like it. I saw yoga in a different light. I was able to finally sleep well after 6 years! I didn't have to use sleeping pills anymore. It calmed my anger. My relationship with my daughter improved and my mobility increased. No words can express my gratitude for yoga: it has changed my entire outlook on life.

survivors of sexual assault, and have specific awareness of or training in military culture.

Often it is the MST abuser who wields power, thereby leaving the MST survivor to fight for their rights without a sense of reprieve or agency. Yoga student Mojisola Adedayo Edu graciously shared this glimpse into her experience as a disabled army veteran:

Military Sexual Trauma (MST)

Military sexual trauma (MST) is the term that the Department of Veterans Affairs uses to refer to sexual assault or repeated threatening sexual harassment that occurred while the veteran was in the military. It includes any sexual activity in which one is involved against one's will.

Examples of military sexual trauma include:

- threats of negative consequences for refusing to be sexually cooperative or with implied faster promotions or better treatment in exchange for sex;

- inability to consent to sexual activities (for example, when intoxicated) or physical force into sexual activities;

- unwanted sexual touching or grabbing;

> - threatening, offensive remarks about a person's body or sexual activities; and/or
>
> - threatening or unwelcome sexual advances.
>
>   (DOD 2019)

Hazing

Hazing and bullying can be an unwanted component of military culture and is used to inflict humiliation, domination, retaliation, subjugation, and the removal of agency. Defined in the revised Army Regulation 600-20, *Army Command Policy*, hazing is "any conduct whereby one or more military members, family members and civilian members, regardless of service, rank, grade, or position, intentionally or recklessly and unlawfully endanger the mental or physical health or safety of another member or employee, regardless of service, rank, grade, or position, by any action taken, or situation created, that is cruel, abusive, humiliating, oppressive, demeaning or harmful" (Army Regulation 600-20 2014).

Hazing includes but is not limited to any form of initiation, "rite of passage," or congratulatory act, or excessive corrective measures that involve: physically striking another in order to, or resulting in, the infliction of pain or injury, piercing another's skin in any manner, forcing or requiring the consumption of excessive amounts of substances, or encouraging illegal, harmful, demeaning, or dangerous acts. Hazing can be verbal or psychological in nature.

Other considerations for hazing include the following:

- each service branch/unity has specific practices

- rooted in initiation practices

- specific to branches/units

- toxic masculinity

- threats and implications

- sexual humor/slang/sexualized language and innuendo

- cyber-bullying and harassment and stalking/social media/images/video/access/texts

- self-Identifying as LGBTQIA+, or being outed as such

- end of privacy and agency

- normalizing and desensitizing

- unwanted sexual contact

- forced nudity

- sodomy

- sexual perversion

- predatory behavior

- impact of combat

- frequent retraumatization due to contractual obligations of military service.

Best Practices

Survivors, in addition to grappling with the myriad challenges of living with MST, can also be living with PTSD, traumatic brain injury (TBI), and other service-related conditions. How this is applicable and translatable within the military and veterans' populations is: (1) constant awareness of possible triggers and trauma; (2) education and knowledge of military and veterans' culture prior to working with this population; (3) flexibility and adaptability; and (4) authenticity.

> **Best Practice**
> Yoga teachers should strive to create and maintain a classroom environment that maximizes a shared sense of safety, predictability, and agency.

Teaching yoga in a manner that maximizes a shared sense of safety, predictability, and agency is a cornerstone of trauma-informed yoga in general. It is particularly important for teachers working with veterans and the military to be aware that students with MST may be present. For students and clients with MST, a sense of agency and predictability helps to unpack the impact of traumatic experience, which is generally unsafe, unpredictable, and strip's one of a sense of agency.

> **Best Practice**
> Encourage teachers to be aware that pranayama can provoke or insight anxiety or panic; teach students to work with the breath in a way that helps regulate and balance the nervous system, so that they can take this skill into everyday life.

Individuals in the military have been trained for self-regulation and safety. However, we encourage teachers to be aware that certain breath practices may provoke anxiety and panic and hyperventilation. According to the Best Yoga Best Practices for Veterans (Horton 2016):

> Working systematically with the breath to positively impact physiological and psycho-emotional health is an integral part of a mindful yoga practice.

> Teachers should start with simple breath instruction to balance the nervous system. Providing simple, scientifically grounded explanations of why this works physiologically can be helpful.
>
> (Horton 2017: 42)

Pranayama that is simple and not complex should be used to balance heart rate and cultivate relaxation – diaphragmatic breath, guided breath, breath awareness, ujjayi, hara, spontaneous breath, and the natural breath – all of which can offer a felt sense/interoception for the yoga practitioner. Consider asana and other tactile movement like palming, somatics, and dancing, whether static or dynamic (Horton 2016: 42–3) to encourage interoception with intention setting and gratitude as the focal point. For further discussion, see Horton (2016).

> **Best Practice**
> Cultivate community through a check-in or sangha to support healthy relationships.

Cultivate community through a check-in or sangha using closed-ended questions, like have you noticed any changes in your practice? Leave time for feedback with finite language. Through this, teachers can create and foster healthy relationships with other members. Ask, "What do you hope to gain from this practice?" There is a level of trust or rapport to build and reckoning and meaning to cultivate post-traumatic growth.

> **Best Practice**
> Be aware of invitational language as often military and veterans are used to being told what to do.

Teachers should be aware of invitational language as often the military and veterans are used to being directed. Make sure that the language is not offensive or unappealing. Do not offer too many options that are confusing, ambiguous, and open ended. Be predictable in leading and teaching the class.

Best Practice
Dress modestly and appropriately when teaching and leading a class.

Teachers should dress appropriately and modestly: this can include neutral and layered clothing to accommodate varying temperatures in the room, no perfumes, no logos on clothes, following the guidelines of the facility that you are teaching in.

When choosing what to wear, consider what colors, styles, and fabrics are comfortable, practical, and uplifting for you and your students. Dress with the remembrance that you are a role model for your students. Avoid wearing camo-style clothing. "Yoga teachers would be wise to be dressed in a way that looks professional: clean, neat, and modest," advises Desiree Rumbaugh, a senior certified Anusara yoga teacher (Stover 2017). Modesty and appropriateness can have many different looks and faces. When you step into this, you embrace infinite possibility and the courage to radically accept and present yourself as you are, which is always a divinely unique being. Thus, appearance equals respect. For a further discussion of dress, see Chapter 4.

Best Practice
Take a course or training in military culture to be able to match teaching credentials to students' needs.

Yoga teachers should know the basics of military culture before embarking on teaching and leading veteran and military yoga classes. In addition, outreach to the specific MST and trauma survivor communities may require additional cultural training. Cultural considerations could also include decisions related to outreach, including how veterans are contacted or guidelines for any outreach to family members. Best Practice: Teach guided meditations that avoid long silences.

Meditations should be guided to avoid long periods of silence and include language that is body centric and grounding as opposed to visualization. This is so the student can remain focused, thereby not lamenting on negative thoughts, emotions, or beliefs. Meditation Studio App (by Muse) has an entire section of diverse meditations specifically for veterans dealing with trauma, current military service members, wounded warriors, and their caregivers (https://meditationstudioapp.com/collections/C6).

Best Practice
Offer options and modifications during the meditation session.

There are many different styles of meditation: to this end, techniques will vary so the teacher can choose what works best for the setting and space. For instance, the teacher should allow students the option to keep their eyes open or half-open, and focused on a particular point, or fully closed. Some students may feel more comfortable with their eyes either open or half-open, while others will prefer to close them completely.

Limiting your movement during the yoga practice is best while teaching. Consider staying on your mat more or, if you have to get up, let your students know that you are moving and then stay put for a time. This will help the student remain calm and in the present moment, so that they can focus on the yoga session.

Becoming familiar with the environment is important. Visit the space ahead of the time of the session, visiting areas around the space (for example, it may be near a police station or firehouse where sirens are often heard, which could be a trigger for some), and assessing what type of energy or vibe the space has. For instance, is this a studio that is constantly bustling and busy? Being fully prepared in a proactive manner will help to create safe predictability.

In order to respond to possible triggers that come up in class, it is recommended that yoga teachers have a solid plan in place. Know where the nearest medical or mental health professionals are, become familiar with the environment that you will be working in, as well as daily schedules and routines prior to teaching, and have your own safety plan. For many students, the world is full of triggers: the yoga studio or space is a part of that world – perhaps more so because we are working with the body. Simply being aware of the impact of triggers, along with helping survivors cope and manage them through yogic practices in the moment and an after-class discussion, can be extremely useful.

> [W]e have come to realize that our clients are being triggered all the time during yoga classes. While this is a reality, we have also come to trust the yoga practice as a way for many trauma survivors to manage these triggers successfully.
>
> (Emerson & Hopper 2011: 134)

The benefits of trauma-informed yoga can and commonly do extend well beyond the boundaries of teaching students suffering from clinical trauma. For yoga teachers working with veterans, it is useful to consider how the insights into the mind–body relationship that inform trauma-informed yoga can be applied to the experience of coping with MST.

Service members who have been sexually assaulted during training or in combat experienced lack of agency, and some remain traumatized as veterans. The pervasive military culture of acceptance, stemming from a "rigid chain of command and a perceived 'code of silence' can create an environment in which victims do not report or seek help because they believe nothing will be done or they fear retaliation or negative repercussions" (Castro, et al. 2015: 3).

> Interoception is "the [visceral] perception of the state of the body ... an umbrella term for the phenomenological experience of the body state, an experience which is ultimately a product of the central nervous system (CNS), regardless of what information the brain uses and does not use to construct this experience"
>
> (Ceunen, et al. 2016).

For many veterans, the relationship between the mind and body has been fractured after years of disciplining the body and overriding or compartmentalizing thoughts and feelings as necessary to put the mission first. An appropriately designed yoga class provides an opportunity to reconnect body and mind by developing new skills of proprioception (internal awareness of the physical body), interoception (internal awareness of feelings and sensations), self-regulation, and present-moment awareness. Over time, these resources support successful reintegration into civilian life.

Crisis Hotlines

Military and Veterans Crisis Line – Military Crisis Line at 1-800-273-8255 and Press 1, text to 838255, Hearing Impaired 1-800-799-4899

Rape, Abuse & Incest National Network (RAINN) – National Sexual Assault Telephone Hotline – 800.656.HOPE (4673)

Additional Resources

Healthystate.org (2012) Uniform betrayal: Rape in the military [video] [Online] Available: https://vimeo.com/46007403 15 August 2019].

Military Times (2018) The Marine Corps had the highest increase in sexual assault reports among the services [Online] Available: https://www.militarytimes.com/news/your-military/2018/04/30/dod-marines-had-highest-increase-in-reports-of-sexual-assaults/ [25 October 2018].

PBS (2019) Military sexual assault [Online] Available: https://www.pbs.org/newshour/tag/military-sexual-assault, 31 July [1 August 2019].

The Lion's Roar (2017) Helping, fixing, or serving? [Online] Available: https://www.lionsroar.com/helping-fixing-or-serving/ [15 November 2018].

The Washington Post (2017a) How the military handles sexual assault cases behind closed doors [Online] Available: https://www.washingtonpost.com/investigations/how-the-military-handles-sexual-assault-cases-behind-closed-doors/2017/09/30/a9df0682-672a-11e7-a1d7-9a32c91c6f40_story.html?noredirect=on [1 August 2019].

The Washington Post (2017b) In the military, trusted officers became alleged assailants in sex crimes [Online] Available: https://www.washingtonpost.com/investigations/in-the-military-trusted-officers-became-alleged-assailants-in-sex-crimes/2017/10/19/ec2cf780-ae9a-11e7-be94-fabb0f1e9ffb_story.html> [1 April 2019].

The Washington Post (2018) Sexual assault reports in the military spiked but the Pentagon thinks assaults are down [Online] Available: https://www.washingtonpost.com/news/checkpoint/

wp/2018/04/30/sexual-assault-reports-in-the-military-spiked-but-the-pentagon-thinks-assaults-are-down/ [10 October 2018].

Conclusion

MST stems from the abuse of rank, power, and status. Yoga providers who choose the admirable task of working with the military and veterans' populations must be considerate, compassionate, and cognizant of this critical reality, along with awareness of boundaries and countertransference at all times. Yoga teachers should contemplate conscious relationship with ourselves first, and then with our students and within the structures and cultures of the military and veterans' communities. Throughout this work, it is imperative that we remain steadfast, understanding that yoga is not a cure-all for MST or its survivors; rather, it is an inspirational modality that empowers and engenders transformation. In conclusion, we revisit the MST survivor's sentiment introduced at the beginning of this chapter:

> *"No words can express my gratitude for yoga: it has changed my entire outlook on life."*

Intimate Partner Violence

Author *Amanda J.G. Napior*

Contributors *Lisa Boldin, Anneke Lucas, Rosa Vissers, Kimberleigh Weiss-Lewit, Ann Wilkinson*

Introduction

During her first year teaching trauma-informed yoga, one of the contributors to this chapter taught at a yoga studio that partnered with a survivor advocacy center. She remembers what became a frequent experience: As dusk fell at the end of class, she would tidy up the room, her back turned. She anticipated checking in with students as they left. *Do you have any questions for me? Was this a useful practice for you?* But some people would slip out, unnoticed. She would turn around and know their absence, not their exit.

One of the volunteers from the advocacy center reminded this contributor that for some students, survival was a thing of the present, not the past. For them, getting home quickly was essential. Their partner may be expecting them gone for exactly seventy-five minutes, with travel. A late return could mean consequences. For the instructor, the awareness of why some students disappeared became a powerful one that conveyed more than the gravity of their circumstances. It showed how questions she had been holding, however lightly (Would her students come again next week? Had this class offered them sustenance? Were they safe?), were not hers to know, for now, or maybe ever. Their relationship with her would be one in which students could do what they needed to do. She would not become another person to whom anything was owed.

This chapter offers best practices for working with survivors of Intimate Partner Violence (IPV), whether such experience comprises the present or past. That abuse could be ongoing is, however, a unique feature of this context that service providers and teachers may encounter. Further, while the story above took place in connection with a survivor advocacy group, IPV is unfortunately common enough that practitioners can expect to be working with survivors wherever yoga is found. The forms IPV can take are diverse; the central feature is the context of intimate relationship in which it occurs.

A definition and some statistics about the prevalence of IPV will lend greater context to our discussion. The National Center for Injury Prevention and Control (NCIPC) defines intimate partner violence (IPV) as follows:

> IPV includes physical violence, sexual violence, stalking, and psychological aggression (including coercive tactics) by a current or former intimate partner. The violence may occur among cohabiting or non-cohabiting romantic or sexual partners and among opposite or same-sex couples.
> (Black, et al. 2011)

A report on the instance of IPV among (presumably cisgender) women and men, issued by

NCIPC, showed that about one in ten women in the United States has been raped by an intimate partner in her lifetime, "including completed forced penetration, attempted forced penetration, or alcohol/drug related completed forced penetration." One in forty-five men "has been made to penetrate an intimate partner in his lifetime" (Black, et al. 2011: 13). An estimated 16.9 percent of women and 8 percent of men "have experienced sexual violence other than rape ... by a sexual partner in their lifetime" (Black, et al. 2011: 2). The NCIPC's report indicates that while both women and men's experience of IPV may have involved or resulted in fear, women experienced certain elements with far greater frequency and intensity: concern for their safety, injury, post-traumatic stress disorder (PTSD) symptoms, and missing work or school (Black, et al. 2011: 39).

The National Coalition of Anti-Violence (NCAV) programs released a report in 2016, illuminating how LGBTQ and HIV-affected communities are disproportionately impacted by IPV. This report partially addresses the gap of studies focusing on (or assuming only the presence of) cisgender persons. A total of 60 percent of the IPV homicides as of 2016, for example, were perpetrated against LGBTQ and HIV-affected people of color. People of these identities also comprised 59 percent of 2016's survivors who reported to NCAV (Waters 2017: 10).

Taken together, these statistics reveal that women, people of color, LGBTQ-identifying people, HIV-affected persons, and people who inhabit a number of these identities, bear the traumatic impacts of IPV to a more frequent and often deleterious degree, however painful IPV is for anyone.

Survivors with whom you or your organization work may seek out yoga specifically, as a way to address their trauma from IPV. Other people who have experienced IPV may not recognize themselves as survivors of it, or their current relationships as abusive ones. Be mindful of this fact as you serve people who regard their experiences in various ways. Labeling experiences should remain the prerogative of the person who has them.

Also know that while you are likely to have survivors of IPV in your yoga studio or fitness center classes, you can serve them in settings designated for the support of people who are or have experienced it, like domestic violence hotlines and shelters, behavioral health institutions, and programs in schools, colleges, community centers, and hospitals. You will also encounter survivors incarcerated in jails and prisons, reentry programs, and community correctional programs, as well as living in halfway houses and rehabilitation centers. Be mindful that domestic violence shelters are often in undisclosed locations, but that an agency that yoga instructors are working with may connect them with advocates. Safe houses may also make arrangements for their clients to attend class in a behavioral health facility whose service providers are aware of the imperative of greater safety and caution.

We now turn to best practices for yoga with people who have experienced intimate partner violence.

Best Practices

Best Practice

Use language that describes the intended outcome, rather than the population being served.

Even if you are working in a setting where many yoga students are survivors of sexual trauma (such as a domestic violence shelter), keep in mind that some students may not think of themselves as survivors, or consider their situations to be abusive ones. For example, course titles like "Yoga for Peaceful Embodiment" (see Rhodes 2015) are preferable to "Yoga for Survivors of Violence." When discussing the benefits of or reasons for yoga in this setting, you might use language that points to the positive healing possibilities and benefits of yoga without using presumptuous language about the nature of students' experience, or why you think they would benefit.

> **Best Practice**
> Know the physical layout of the building and surrounding area.

Scope out the safety and security of the location where you are working, especially in the case of teaching night classes. Depending on the setting, it may not be safe to offer classes in the evening, or once most personnel – security or otherwise – have left. Establish a plan to lock the door once class has started, and notify people of protocol for entry after the space has been secured. Plan on having classes at a time when many other people are around. Consider leaving together or ensuring that no one exits the building alone.

> **Best Practice**
> Establish protocols and safe spaces.

There are several hypothetical situations for which establishing a protocol in advance will serve both students and the teachers who support them. Consider asking (and answering) the following questions, and brainstorming for more: If an intimate partner shows up to the location, who will be there for additional support? Is there a safe space where your class might wait, if not the practice space? How will you know whether it is appropriate to call the police? Learn about the existing protocols, policies, and helping hands in your setting and establish, ahead of time, how you and others can respond to these hypothetical situations, and others.

> **Best Practice**
> Anticipate that a client or student may one day disclose abuse to you.

Have a clear idea about what actions you must take or consider in the event that someone discloses abuse to you. This action plan is not one to decide in the moment. Your response includes a supportive reaction and legal obligations. First, be mindful of your own reaction to the disclosure. Focus on listening and being present so that the person feels heard and supported. Second, you may have an obligation to report the abuse. Ideally the person disclosing their situation to you knows what kind of confidentiality you can offer them. If you are a legally mandated reporter, you are required by law to inform your students or clients of this status and are then required to disclose the abuse to another person or agency, dependent upon the laws in your area. If you are not a mandated reporter, consider informing your clients or students, "Although I am not legally a mandated reporter, I function as one." You want to be able to support them in their time of need, and you want them to know what confiding in you entails. You might consider asking a client whether they want to share this information with you; give them a moment to pause for reflection and then accept their decision.

Best Practice

Recognize that creating safety and recovery from IPV are not linear. Be careful not to impose your own vision of "success" on someone undergoing IPV, as you support them.

What does "success," after or during IPV, look like? It may look like someone leaving their abuser and finding a safe home with loving friends or family. It may look like a friend or teacher intervening in a situation in which they can interrupt the abuse. Your role is not to get someone to realize your vision of liberation. It may or may not be appropriate or safe for you to directly intervene in someone's abusive situation. Leaving an abusive relationship can entail dangers of which you may not be aware. The process of finding safety and ending an abusive relationship is not linear. For example, perhaps your client or student starts to recognize their relationship as abusive. This may seem small. They go back into their relationship, but they go back knowing. This knowing may have to happen in their own timing. You can celebrate this

growing awareness as a little "success." Your role may not be to get someone out of their abusive relationship. Instead, your support says: "You have a voice; you have a choice; I'm here with you." Consider placing print material from local support organizations for domestic violence and sexual abuse in a common area, bathroom, or near the door, so that people can privately take a resource when they are ready.

Best Practice

Beware of the "savior complex"; know what goal you can affect.

Remember that the work and labor of showing up and being present for your client or student is yours, but the fruit of that labor belongs to them. Notice when a desire to hurry someone along to what you think is a *better* outcome arises, and instead practice being in the moment. In your work with survivors of IPV, you are not going to "give them agency." (In fact, you cannot *give anyone* agency.) Instead, you must allow people to make choices, which may

Case study

One of us is a social worker who supports girls and young women who are presently undergoing IPV and/or sex trafficking. She recalls accompanying one of her clients to the police station. The young woman client had been in a years-long relationship with an abuser against whom she had only recently become ready to file a restraining order. The process of supporting her client had already been an emotionally grueling one: the social worker had so much hope for the young woman's safety, and this trip to the precinct was characterized, at first,

by great relief. At the last minute, however, the young client changed her mind; she would not file a restraining order against her abuser, after all. The social worker felt deep disappointment and rage but recognized that expressing her emotions in that moment would not be beneficial for the young woman's journey. She recalls: "Instead of flying off the handle, I took a deep breath." She had to keep reminding herself that her job was to show up and support her client, but her client's decisions would be her own.

include choices you do not like. Share information, practices, and alternatives. Be firm in your support and abide in a practice of non-attachment and compassion. In *Trauma and Recovery*, Judith Herman sagely writes: "No intervention that takes power away from the survivor can possibly foster her recovery, no matter how much it appears to be in her immediate best interest" (Herman 1997: 133).

Best Practice
Be mindful that you may be working with persons who are still in relationships with their abusers.

Plan on the following, to ensure safety for you and the person you are supporting:

Begin sessions promptly and end on time

Having reliable timing of yoga sessions is important for many reasons. If someone is still in a relationship with their abuser, however, leaving later than they promised this partner can result in danger to their safety. Ending your class late is therefore a risk to your student or client.

Practice non-judgment of persons who may be going back into their abusive relationships

Know that leaving an abusive relationship is complicated. Leaving can come with new dangers and risks that you may not be aware of.

Titrate practices that involve moving into emotion and vulnerability

Somatic therapist Peter Levine recommends titration or "dipping" into a vulnerable or expansive feeling, which a breath or movement technique accesses (Levine 1997). This is a good practice for limiting the early intensity of practice, in student–teacher relationships. Recall that trust is the cornerstone of this relationship. Titration involves trying a practice for one or two minutes, checking in, and then going for longer, if deemed appropriate. (Allow trust to develop over time, before intentionally moving into deeply sensitive areas, energetically and emotionally.) This practice is also important, however, when someone may be going back home to an abusive situation. Going too quickly can overwhelm the practitioner, making it hard or impossible for someone to "hold it together." Having such "survival layers" at one's disposal is integral if one is not going to a safe home, irrespective of how safe the relationship between student and teacher is.

Help people close the practice in a way that reinstates their boundaries

Yoga practitioners may know the feeling of completing a yoga practice that leaves them feeling as if they were floating: the heart is open, the mind expansive, the boundedness of the self, soft. Consider that someone returning home to an abuser may need additional support in grounding this expansive feeling and redefining the boundaries around their own self and body, in order to be able to protect themselves. Ask them how they are feeling to discern what is appropriate. Consider a grounding closing practice to support this person who may be going back home to an unsafe environment. While you ultimately want them to be in a *safe* environment, you must be able to support them in the environment they are in in the present.

Case study

One of us was supporting a mother, daughter, and the mother's boyfriend as a Family Advocate at a community center. The mother had been working tirelessly to protect her daughter from the father, who had been abusive. One day, the mother showed up with bruises: the boyfriend had become violent with her. Legally, the Family Advocate could no longer offer this man support, by the terms of the grant which funded her community center; the grant had a stipulation that it would not support service of domestic abuse perpetrators.

Sadly, this man saw the Family Advocate's community center as his support system, as well, but she could no longer help him. "I was compassionate but clear he could not come to sessions. I had to hold a lot of anger (and some fear) ... I believe the director of the clinic gave him additional resources for addiction, but also backed up my program that he could not return. This situation tested my own boundaries, while breaking my heart. After the assault, the mother showed a resiliency I will never forget."

Be aware that the terms of your service may change if new abuse happens

If you are a therapist or yoga instructor working with an entire family, know that the terms of your engagement may change if abuse occurs.

Conclusion

Learning the above best practices in trauma-informed yoga will help you better serve not only survivors of IPV, but those of other contexts of abuse, as well. As ever, consider these practices to be touchstones as you continue to pursue your own training and collaboration with others. We now turn to best practices for yoga with survivors of sex trafficking.

Sex Trafficking

Author *Amanda J.G. Napior*

Contributors *Lisa Boldin, Anneke Lucas, Rosa Vissers, Kimberleigh Weiss-Lewit, Ann Wilkinson*

Introduction

The International Labor Organization (ILO) estimates that 4.5 million people are in situations of forced sexual exploitation, worldwide (ILO 2012). The National Human Trafficking Hotline, operated by the anti-human trafficking organization, Polaris Project, has received reports of 22,191 cases of sex trafficking in the United States, alone, between 2007 and the time of this writing (Polaris Project 2017). In a 2015 report by the Urban Institute, researchers estimated the 2007 underground sex economies of eight large US cities to range in worth from $39.9 to $290 million (Dank, et al. 2014).

This section offers best practices for yoga with people who have experienced the violence of sex trafficking. While our best practices mostly pertain to sex trafficking as an umbrella category, we also pay special attention to victims of two subcategories: the Commercial Sexual Exploitation of Children (CSEC), and ritual abuse. This introductory section aims to offer context for all three of these terms (sex trafficking, CSEC, and ritual abuse), while acknowledging that sex trafficking takes many forms whose range simply cannot be described in a couple of pages. Note that this section is not about sex work, which may be chosen for diverse and complicated reasons. Not everyone exchanging sex for money is being trafficked, although many are. While sex trafficking and sex work are not equivalent, the nature of consent may be especially complicated

for those who are economically disempowered. Remember that the voices and choices of those we serve must be our utmost priority, in order to foster dignity through self-determination. Here, the emphasis of our project is to provide teachers and service providers with best practices for those who are being or have been victimized by sex traffickers.

Sex trafficking is perpetrated against children and adults of all gender identities and orientations. The Polaris Project's definition of sex trafficking indicates:

> Sex traffickers use violence, threats, lies, debt bondage, and other forms of coercion to [force] adults and children to engage in commercial sex acts against their will ... The situations that sex trafficking victims face vary dramatically. Many victims become romantically involved with someone who then forces or manipulates them into prostitution. Others are lured in with false promises of a job, such as modeling or dancing. Some are forced to sell sex by their parents or other family members. They may be involved in a trafficking situation for a few days or weeks, or may remain in the same trafficking situation for years.

Traffickers most frequently target vulnerable populations, "including runaway and homeless youth, as well as victims of domestic violence, sexual assault, war, or social discrimination" (www.polarisproject.org). In a 2017 petition to

New York legislators, Anneke Lucas notes that many trafficked youth "don't realize they're being trafficked, because they think the abuse is part of a normal relationship" (Lucas 2017). Polaris's definition of trafficking, paired with Lucas's insight suggest that, as with IPV, service providers and yoga instructors working with youth or adult survivors of trafficking may expect that some may not consider their circumstances to be abusive or unusual.

Sex trafficking of children in particular is called the Commercial Sexual Exploitation of Children (CSEC). Meredith L. Dank describes commercially sexually exploited children as "juveniles (18 and under) who perform sexual acts in exchange for money, drugs, food, or shelter" (Dank 2011: 1). Discerning the number of children who are commercially sexually exploited is notoriously difficult, due to the stigmatized nature of this form of exploitation and the hiddenness of the population. The US Department of Justice estimates the number of commercially sexually exploited youth in the United States could be anywhere from 100,000 to three million children (Dank 2011). The authors of a 2001 report on CSEC, from the University of Pennsylvania, also cite the difficulty of learning actual numbers of currently exploited youth (Estes & Weiner 2002). However, their report found that 30 percent of youth living in shelters and 70 percent of youth living on the street engaged in prostitution in order to meet daily needs (Estes & Weiner 2001: 27). Sex trafficking in general and CSEC in particular most heavily impact persons who are already the most vulnerable in our society.

Finally, ritual abuse is another example of sex trafficking. The term *ritual abuse* invokes a controversial history. Therefore, in addition to defining this form of abuse, we must contextualize its history and problematic implications of its usage.

One of the reasons the term *ritual abuse* has been controversial is that when accusations become prevalent in the 1980s and 1990s, no forensic evidence was found by law enforcement agencies (Putnam 1991; Lacter and Lehman 2008). While there have been witness and survivor accounts, the absence of forensic evidence has caused accusations of such magnitude to appear dubious (Putnam 1991; Frankfurter 2003). Theories about therapists unwittingly planting these accounts in their child-clients by suggestion emerged, and much of the therapeutic community has resultantly come to look askance at rumors of such occurrences (Lacter & Lehman 2008; Frankfurter 2003). Invoking this term risks disbelief. However, not listening to survivors puts victims on trial for their own abuse, which is why we insist on the importance of naming it, here. Second, the ways in which *ritual abuse* has been described by advocates of survivors often involve language that promotes misunderstandings about (and thus discrimination against) minority religious communities. Much advocacy literature describes the sex-trafficking rings perpetuating these crimes as *cults*, a designation to indicate tacit violence (Lacter & Lehman 2008; Noblitt & Noblitt 2017). The word *cult* has been used in hateful rhetoric against minority communities, to indicate their tacit violence as well as to craft legislation against them. Three American examples include discrimination and often violence against Eastern European Catholic immigrants in the late nineteenth century, against the emerging new religious movement of Mormonism in the early nineteenth century (Frankfurter 2003), and against practitioners of the Afro-Cuban religion, Santería, in the late twentieth century (Eck 2001).

The West and the United States in particular also has a long history of *anti-ritualism*, which marks a popular prejudice against the centrality of religious rituals in some communities, as somehow outmoded or backwards (Douglas 2003; Seligman & Weller 2012). Last, Westerners coming into contact with shamanistic traditions of non-Western cultures, over the last many centuries, have called indigenous practices "satanic." These cultural misreadings have played a role in legacy of Western colonization of indigenous peoples. This history of reaction and naming between EuroAmerians and those deemed "other" is a part of the context out of which this form of abuse and survivor-advocate classifications of it have emerged. The failure of advocates of survivors to distinguish ritual abuse from non-abuse ritual contexts, or to contextualize the term in the storm of discriminatory anti-ritual accusations that have come before it, makes their work problematic.

An article by psychologist Ellen Lacter and psychiatrist Karl Lehman notes that *ritual abuse* is:

> often used broadly to include any organized abusive practice that furthers the abuser group's ideology. However, the term is usually restricted to organized physical or sexual assault, often including homicide and severe psychological abuse, within the context of a spiritual practice or belief. Some definitions encompass any spiritual belief, but most definitions use the term to refer to practices that involve physical and sexual abuse of children and adults, and human sacrifice, to propitiate and empower malevolent deities, such as Satan.
>
> (Lacter & Lehman 2008: 160)

For the purposes of providing best practices to survivors of sexual trauma in this context, we focus on ritual abuse as one form of sex trafficking, in which children are sold into sex rings whose practices include physical and sexual abuse, in a context designed to be spiritually terrorizing through evocation of ceremony and invocation of malevolent deities. This is a context of abuse characterized by incredible psychological manipulation and terror for the survivor. Lacter and Lehman note that survivors of ritual abuse are often misdiagnosed as schizophrenic or with Dissociative Identity Disorder (DID) without recognition of the trauma the person has suffered. In a 1995 survey of British psychotherapists working with survivors of sexual violence, 15 percent reported having worked with clients who reported ritual abuse. Eighty percent of the psychotherapists reported believing the allegations (Andrews, et al. 1995 cited in Noblitt & Noblitt 2017: 6).

Despite problematic aspects of the term *ritual abuse* detailed in the above footnote, we affirm that for survivors, the term continues to have power to meaningfully name the violence perpetrated against them. Service providers working with those who have survived ritual abuse must take a survivor-centered approach that at once accepts the terms by which people understand and describe their trauma, while keeping close at hand an understanding of how some language, this term included, can perpetuate injustices against misrepresented communities.

This section now turns to providing best practices for working with survivors of sex trafficking. We encourage our readers to remember that the commercial sexual exploitation of children (CSEC) and ritual abuse, described above, are but two specific manifestations of sex trafficking, and that working with survivors invites further education and training for the practitioner. As with serving people who have experienced IPV, practitioners may encounter survivors of sex trafficking in yoga classes and programs of diverse settings, from studios and fitness centers to shelters, behavioral health institutions, schools, colleges, community centers, hospitals, jails and prisons, reentry programs, community correctional programs, halfway houses, and rehabilitation centers. Be mindful that there are shelters specifically for people rescued from sex trafficking, whose locations, like those of domestic violence shelters, are undisclosed. Yoga instructors working for agencies serving survivors of sex trafficking will find these otherwise undisclosed settings through their host organization.

Best Practices

> **Best Practice**
> Be mindful of expectations that reflect harmful standards of success.

This best practice echoes others in this volume. For youth and adult survivors of this context, be mindful to recognize and celebrate small successes, and not to impose your own standards of success. As with IPV, remember that someone leaving an abusive or exploitative situation may come with dangers of which you may be unaware. This is why someone *recognizing* their situation as exploitation, through understanding what is going on, is a first, necessary step and a success worth celebrating. In most cases, intervening beyond sharing information and fostering understanding may not be appropriate. Someone directly asking you for help is an indication that you may need to intervene to a greater degree, by utilizing other official channels of support. Your and the student's safety requires that you seek help in doing so; do not go this alone.

> **Best Practice**
> Seek training appropriate to working with survivors of sex trafficking.

Please pursue extra training before working with survivors of sex trafficking. Remember that you *can* do harm by not having training specific to your setting, and that having good intentions is not enough. Get training through your facility. For example, you will receive Commercial Sexual Exploitation of Children (CSEC) training, working at a state agency that provides services to trafficked youth. If the organization you work with has their own training, you will be required to complete this before working with the population.

> **Best Practice**
> Hire wisely and assign teachers with care.

Facilities should create standards for hiring and training yoga instructors. Instructors need to be trauma-informed and keenly attuned to power dynamics. Do not offer mixed-gender classes for survivors of sex trafficking, and generally assign teachers to students of the same gender identity. Fear, love, sex, and power are likely commingled for people who have experienced this form of abuse, due to how they have learned to relate to someone in power. Therefore, while the right female yoga instructor may allow girls or women to take a break from these power dynamics, having even the most compassionate male teacher almost guarantees the reenactment of harmful dynamics.

Best Practice

Be aware of triggering language for survivors of human trafficking.

Certain language can be retraumatizing. Consider the following:

Be aware that posture names, including the word "pose," itself, can trigger recollections of exploitation

Consider not naming forms when possible and instead choose words that invite students into an exploration of sensation in movement and breath. For example, consider something like, "I am going to offer you a shape. I invite you to try this to stretch your shoulders. Or, you might try something like this…" Notice how such statements are invitations, rather than commands. Also notice how these invitational phrases can encourage self-inquiry through the cue's very format: students' engagement with this or that shape is framed as provisional, to begin with. They are only "trying" it; they are not locked in or committed, but, rather, in a process of discovery and exploration.

Keep in mind that being told how or when to breathe can be triggering

We recommend phrases that reduce the likelihood that breathing cues will feel coercive. The breath is our most powerful tool for self-regulation. Finding invitational and noncoercive language for breath will serve students in trauma recovery as well as help to build relational trust. First, help students simply come into relationship with their breath through observation.

"You might notice yourself breathing in your own manner – through your mouth, or through your nose." Instead of encouraging any particular modifications to breath, use words that normalize the way in which a person is already breathing. Second, avoid the language, "Breathe in and breathe out" – both for its command form, and for its ability to bring someone into an experience of their inner body (a potentially violated space) too quickly. Instead, consider language that invites self-observation. For example, consider the phrase, "You might notice that you're breathing." Second, bringing students' attention to external points of the body can be another way to draw attention to breath without forcing a specific pattern. "You might place your consciousness at your navel. What happens there when you breathe?" Finally, you might build to an invitational instruction and inquiry such as, "You may notice when you're breathing in. You may notice when you're breathing out. Is the breath supporting you?" See Chapter 4 for a foundational discussion of trauma-informed breath work.

Best Practice

Be mindful of certain movement and sensory stimuli that may be triggering.

A darkened room, the use of candles, and/or olfactory stimuli like incense, and even invocations may be triggering for a number of survivors of sexual violence, including survivors of ritual abuse. Instructors should maintain the same level of lighting throughout a class (for example, refrain from dimming the lights when people's bodies are at their most vulnerable resting forms, at the end). This will allow students for whom the lighting is not appropriate to know this at the beginning of class. (Likewise, you can honor requests to brighten a room if needed.)

Chapter 15

> **Best Practice**
> Create grounding practices to encourage present awareness and embodiment.

Consider practices that encourage *embodiment* and *present moment awareness* as a counterbalance for the dissociation that may become an unhelpful energetic pattern for survivors of sex trafficking. Practices that bring movement into the body (particularly the feet, legs, and hips), breath into the low belly, and consciousness of one's connection to the earth, can be especially grounding. Be careful, however, to draw awareness to these areas in ways that are unlikely to feel coercive or invasive. Instead, see what happens when you invite people to notice sensation in their feet, ankles, and knees, as they move in a particular way, as well as how their breath feels if they place their awareness on the *outside* of the belly or hips. Teachers might introduce guided visualizations that emphasize students' connection to earth, how the ground presses up as the feet press down, or how it can support our movement as we walk, run, or stand in yoga shapes. Be aware that some survivors of sex trafficking (as in other contexts) may not find their own bodies sufficiently interesting to pay attention to, as a result of low self-esteem, poor body-image, and dissociation. You may need to wait until students have had some experience with other embodiment practices before you can invite them into a body scan.

> **Best Practice**
> Teach how to notice pain and to back out of painful sensation.

Those who have experienced sex trafficking may have cultivated ways of presenting themselves as strong in order to eschew victimization. Be aware that these students may feel inclined to push through pain in a yoga practice. Take care with this understanding: Do not diagnose someone's situation or pain or assume you know what is going on for them. Instead, invite people to notice sensation, and suggest that if that sensation is painful, they can back out of a form and choose something else. You might inquire, "How does that feel for you?" to encourage dialogue about sensation. Teachers can model the practice of noticing and backing up by giving language to their own felt sensations and remarking upon stopping at their own limits.

> **Best Practice**
> Know that survivors of sex trafficking may act younger than their chronological age and have a distorted understanding of their body and its experience of pain.

Someone trafficked in their youth has likely had their emotional development arrested by trauma. Be mindful of this disruption in emotional development, as a survivor's maturity may not match the chronological age of the person in front of you. Use this understanding as a basis for cultivating compassion toward them, and possibly patience, if you find you need more. Also be mindful that someone who has experienced sex trafficking may have learned how to be comfortable in their pain. One of us, reflecting on her own experience, shared: "You expect it; you walk with it. Exploitation teaches you how to be strong in your brokenness." Yoga may enable a person to get more in touch with their physical pain; this growing awareness will also therefore come with newfound discomfort. Paradoxically, this person's yoga practice may help them develop tools and a capacity for meeting that pain in ways they could not before.

Best Practice
Reconsider rigorous practices; put them in new perspective.

Consider that a yoga practice utilized toward recovery and healing from sexual trauma may not also be a workout. A rigorous yoga practice, such as Ashtanga or other lineages influenced by it, can make for a fun practice and a spiritual one, too. However, be mindful that a highly rigorous and acrobatic practice can be a way to reenact the physicality and postures of sexual abuse. Therefore, these approaches may not represent models for offering trauma-informed yoga to survivors of sex trafficking. One of us who has experienced childhood sex trafficking recalls that when she first started practicing yoga, "I had no awareness of my body below the neck. I had to go so deep into the practice to feel anything. But I was doing postures that were replicating the … abuse." Incidentally, she *does* still practice Ashtanga sequences. However, she considers this soft, caring, listening work of trauma-informed yoga to be her true yoga practice. Indeed, this softer work can be the most challenging. We recommend that one's trauma-informed yoga practice prioritizes establishing a sense of safety and integrity in the body's systems, over getting cardiovascular exercise.

Best Practice
Ground meditation choices in the needs of the student.

Be sure your choice of meditation is guided by both theory and student feedback. Most trauma-informed literature will emphasize body-based meditations as key. Here, we echo their efficacy and also note the power and potential of visualizations. Body-based meditations (which use bodily sensation and breath as their object of attention) are known to increase a student's capacity for interoception, or one's felt awareness of the inner body. Increasing this capacity will help practitioners come "into their bodies," which we note can counteract a harmful dissociative pattern. This process of embodiment enables a person to feel at home in their body, as the body increasingly feels like a safer place for the person's consciousness to reside. Some survivors of sex trafficking, however, may find guided visualizations to be safer routes into meditation. Guided meditations can include having students conjure images of nature in order for students to create a sanctuary or safe place, alongside a body of water, or in a forest. Rather than going to the place, students might alternately practice bringing this landscape to their own location, which could help to create a sense of wholeness. This place can become a location in consciousness that students access in order to begin meeting their trauma. It can also become an outlet for creativity and a healthy use of imagination, to which many victims of abuse will have lost access. Note, however, that because this process of visualization *is* inherently dissociative; it can be used as a way to bypass trauma, if not firmly grounded in the needs of that student. As you explore how to best meet the needs of your students, consider titration your ally: For example, if body-based meditations do not seem to be offering your student access to themselves, you might walk slowly into a three- to five-minute visualization, and then check in. If it lands well, try extending the time.

Best Practice
Teach (and practice) how to shift attention.

Some survivors of sexual violence (and particularly in the contexts of sex trafficking and IPV) may have experienced a profound psychological manipulation that has engendered another layer of vulnerability. They may feel that their abuser has access to their thoughts, is in their head, or can control their actions. Teach mindfulness techniques for shifting attention away from this sense of another inhabiting one's mind, and to rebuild the integrity and inviolability of their consciousness. Students can learn not to give this external agent attention or energy – and that agent will lose access to them. As students learn more mindfulness exercises from practicing yoga movement and meditation, they will become more adept at depriving this external controller any attention. For example, such a shift in attention might be body-based. A student can use hands and fingertips for self-massage. This can be a way to connect with the body without contact from someone else, and can help ground the student's consciousness in their body. They can also pay attention to their fingertips or feet on the ground. When they notice the sense of an intruder, they might affirm to themselves: "I can feel my feet on the ground. I am whole, I am safe, I am independent; you have no power over me."

> **Best Practice**
> Adopt the job of "noticer"; be prepared to speak up.

Keep your eyes open

Part of your job is to observe. Perhaps a youth comes to your session with visible burns, cuts, bruises, or recent scars. Do you think it is a mistake that their shirt sleeve is rolled up just enough for you to see? Find a way to communicate to this person that you see them (and what they are revealing to you). Perhaps you take them aside at the end of class in a way that others will not find unusual. ("Do you have a minute? I'd like to go over something on your application …"). Learn not to gasp when you notice these wounds. Your natural reaction may be to pull back, from shock. Witness this inclination and then make a choice to stay present in that moment, instead. Now is the time to be present and ready to respond.

Collaborate with your team

Know the protocol where you are working. If you are a yoga instructor working in collaboration with clinicians, do not assume that the clinician is the more appropriate person to approach the client about whom you are concerned. Know that *you* noticed something. The clinician may not be the person the client wants to talk to. Whoever addresses the abuse, be sure to communicate with your team so that everyone who needs to be in the loop, is.

Know that you have the power to disrupt this situation, but you cannot do it alone

Sometimes we may be tempted not to call the police for fear that the officer who responds will abuse their power, putting your client in further danger. This is a possibility. However, keep in mind that you cannot interrupt the situation by doing nothing, so this is a time to put trust in official channels of support and to remain a witness in the process. The police are required to report the instance of trafficking to the district attorney, and to put the person who is being victimized in touch with the trafficking response team in your state. These are coordinated through Safe Harbor enactments as well as the federal Trafficking Victims Protection Act.

Safe Harbor enactments require that intercepted trafficked youth not be criminally charged but considered victims, and immediately given services. If you have reason to think this action is not being taken, you might stay involved as long as possible so that others know you are still there. Alternately, you can call the National Human Trafficking Resource Center Hotline (1-888-373-888); these helpers will also contact a local law enforcement agency. Consider yourself mandated to keep your eyes open outside your work as well. For example, if an older man comes into a yoga studio with three young girls, find a creative way to communicate with the girls, in order to ask if they need help.

Conclusion

One of our best practices in Chapter Five defines "holding space" as a practice of acceptance, non-attachment to outcome, non-judgment, and selective action. Working with people who may be currently experiencing sex trafficking calls for precisely this complex balance of awareness and activity: allowing and acting, letting be, and intervening. Knowing what this balance entails in any given moment is dependent upon context. By asking questions, checking in, listening to those you serve and following their lead, you can hold space not only for a particular yoga session, but also for the person's experience. Especially remember you do not need to hold these spaces alone.

Case study

In February of 2017, Alaska Airlines flight attendant, Shelia Frederick, rescued a teenage girl from sex trafficking. Frederick instinctively became suspicious when she saw the odd combination of a girl who looked "all disheveled and out of sorts," and by her side, the well-dressed, older man, with whom she was travelling. Frederick told the girl, in a whisper, to go to the restroom. There, she had left a note with her phone number, and the instruction to write whether the girl needed help. The girl did write "I need help," and Frederick was able to call law enforcement before the plane landed. The man was arrested at the gate, and the girl rushed to safety. Many of us may have a fear of pushing someone into a more dangerous situation, if we intervene in the wrong way. Sheila Frederick is testament to the importance of interrupting the situation. ("Flight Attendant Rescues Girl" 2017; Rosenblatt 2017)

Author *Amanda J.G. Napior*

Contributors *Lisa Boldin, Anneke Lucas, Rosa Vissers, Kimberleigh Weiss-Lewit, Ann Wilkinson*

Introduction

This chapter sheds light on best practices for working with survivors living in carceral settings. It recognizes that sexual trauma can arise during incarceration – in the form of abuse the law recognizes as sexual violence, as well as from carceral practices the law considers acceptable. It also recognizes that incarcerated people with whom practitioners work may have experienced sexual trauma in any of the other contexts of abuse this book treats. Like anyone else, people in prison have no more uniform experiences of sexual trauma than survivors elsewhere. At the same time, the greater prevalence of trauma among the incarcerated ought to inform our work in this setting.

Sexual Trauma and Incarceration

Sexual trauma is more prevalent among people in prison than among persons who are not incarcerated. In one year, 80,600 people reported being sexually assaulted or raped while incarcerated (rainn.org/statistics/scope-problem). One 2016 study investigating cumulative trauma and PTSD prevalence among people incarcerated in a Vancouver, Canada prison found that 48 percent of the prison sample exhibited symptoms of PTSD, compared with only 4 percent of the general US American population. While complex trauma was common for many incarcerated people, 70 percent of the incarcerated women sampled had experienced sexual abuse

as children, compared with 50 percent of men (Briere, et al. 2016). A 2013 study of complex trauma prevalence among incarcerated women in New Mexico found that 100 percent had been exposed to trauma, and 83 percent to physical and/or sexual trauma (Willging, et al. 2013). Trauma in general and sexual trauma in particular are more prevalent among people in prison and impacts cisgender women more heavily than cisgender men. For those who are transgender or non-binary, the numbers are staggeringly higher. Data from US federal facilities in 2011–12 demonstrated that transgender people are almost ten times as likely to experience sexual assault than the general incarcerated population.

Some indignities are unique to contexts of incarceration. While reported instances of abuse reflect illegal assaults, they are unlikely to capture sanctioned security practices, like strip and cavity searches or the use of solitary confinement. First, recent court cases in the United States have shown that state and federal courts have not come to agreement on whether strip and cavity searches constitute a violation of incarcerated people's – and particularly women's – Fourth Amendment rights. (See, for example, the July 2019 *Washington Post* article, "Female inmates were forced to expose their genitals in a 'training exercise.' It was legal, court rules.") Legality aside, firsthand accounts make clear that such experiences are traumatic. Second, federal statistics in 2015 showed that 28 percent of LGB incarcerated people were placed in solitary confinement compared with 18 percent of heterosexual prisoners (Bureau of Justice Statistics 2015 cited in NCTE 2018). Further, LGBTQ persons are often placed in solitary confinement for their protection from other prisoners ("protective custody"), effectively punishing them for their extreme structural vulnerability (NCTE 2018). While the mechanics of solitary confinement may not involve discrete sexually violent acts against individuals, the greater exposure to trauma it causes for sexual and gender minorities asks us to recognize such sexualizing and gendering practices under the rubric of collective trauma.

Working in Prison

The Yoga Service Council's last book, *Best Practices for Yoga in the Criminal Justice System*, offers a comprehensive look at best practices for yoga with people in prison. We recommend that those working in prisons consult this publication. In this present section, we will echo some recommendations from the previous book, as well as highlight new ones, specific to sexual trauma. Our present introductory task also warrants offering additional information about working in a prison. Specifically, we invite our readers to consider the possibility of themselves and others being impacted by vicarious trauma as well as the temptation some service providers may have to enter prisons with an antagonistic attitude toward correctional officers (COs) and staff.

Vicarious trauma (also called secondary trauma) can occur through learning the details of another person's or group's trauma or by witnessing violence against them. Its impacts and symptoms on the body and psyche can be similar to experiencing trauma first-hand. The trauma-informed service provider or yoga instructor in *any setting* is susceptible to experiencing

vicarious trauma, while working with survivors of sexual violence. A prison setting is unique in this regard, however, insofar as its systems can often do more to *re*traumatize than to foster recovery. Be mindful that COs and human services staff are also susceptible to vicarious trauma, and they can be impacted by it daily and over time. A study of correctional officers in Washington State has shown that 19 percent of COs also met diagnostic criteria for PTSD, with female-identifying, black, day-shift, and long-term employees showing greater symptoms than others (James 2018). Therefore, it is not only people living in prisons but also those working there who can benefit from the loving kindness of a trauma-informed yoga practice. Irrespective of whether a yoga program offers yoga classes to prison employees, service providers may keep in mind that bringing a trauma-informed approach to *all* people one encounters in a prison has the potential to engender trauma recovery for more people than just those incarcerated.

Note also that even though a prison is a setting that can retraumatize, many incarcerated people also receive beneficial services, like psychotherapy or basic health coverage, for the first time. In this way, the incredible domination of the carceral setting coexists with the possibility of care (including the services you may offer). The paradoxical realities of this setting require that we also recognize the thoughtful and many times trauma-informed people – staff and COs – who *already* work in prisons. Know that you have allies "on the inside," and that going into a prison with adversarial assumptions about employees is not only unstrategic but also a misrepresentation of who many people are. Finally, note that there are many different settings of incarceration, from prisons and residential hospitals to residential juvenile facilities. We use "prison," "carceral context," and "incarceration setting," as shorthand for a range of settings, in the best practices that follow.

Best Practices

> ### Best Practice
> Follow the rules of the institution, no exceptions.

Your actions reflect not only on you but also on other people in prison service and yoga service. Following rules only selectively (out of transgressive, justice-seeking intentions, no doubt) can shut down an entire program and limit your and others' ability to serve people in prison. Although we may sometimes feel as if shirking certain rules will better dignify someone, in the moment, know that its long-term effects far outweigh any short-term benefit.

> ### Best Practice
> Be aware that violence could be ongoing.

If an incarcerated person is being sexually abused during their imprisonment, the abuser may be a fellow incarcerated person, correctional officer, or staff member. Such a situation requires certain considerations and actions of you: you must know the Prison Rape Elimination Act (PREA), report the abuse accordingly and with discretion, and offer yoga classes with an awareness that any vulnerability that is born of the practice will need to be adequately addressed, with closing practices geared toward allowing students to put their "survival layers" back on.

> ### Best Practice
> Know PREA.

The Prison Rape Elimination Act (PREA) is a congressional act passed unanimously in 2003, which aims both to protect incarcerated people from rape and to conduct research on the incidence and effects of prison rape, in federal, state, and local carceral facilities (PREA Resource Center 2014). Request thorough training in PREA in the facility where you are working, if it does not already offer one, and find out which people and offices constitute the best channels for reporting abuse. Knowing the Act will serve you, in the event that someone discloses abuse to you. Knowing PREA in advance of such communication will provide you with steps you must take in your institution. See the best practice, "Anticipate that a client or student may one day disclose abuse to you" in Chapter 13 for insight on how you can be both a supportive listener and a responsive advocate. Last, review the PREA Resource Center's "Fact Sheet for Corrections Officials" online, which can serve as a resource in addition to your training materials.

> ### Best Practice
> Design yoga sessions with titration and boundary reestablishment, in mind.

See the best practices in Chapter 13, entitled "Titrate practices that involve moving into emotion and vulnerability" and "Help people close the practice in a way that reinstates their boundaries." These best practices are applicable here, as well, for they recognize that if abuse is ongoing, it may not be appropriate or safe to guide a student into emotionally vulnerable terrain, in their practice. First, titration – easing into a practice – can be a helpful way of assessing the appropriateness of a practice in the moment. Second, closing the practice in a way that emphasizes closure and inviolable boundaries will offer a student support in a situation that is far from desirable.

> ### Best Practice
> Celebrate and honor stories that may not reflect mainstream depictions of accomplishment.

Pausing to take a breath before reacting with anger is a success. So is getting a job while incarcerated, becoming a peer mentor, or deciding to join a yoga group. Leaving jail, finding one's own room, and getting a job are likewise successes to celebrate. Not going back to jail is another. That this person may face all-but-impossible odds to maintain such gains is knowledge you bear. Witnessing these (seemingly) small ways in which another's freedom has increased is but one of the rewards of working with currently and formerly incarcerated people. Our society is ever ready to lift up persons who conform to mainstream images of success: a family comprised of a man, woman, and kids, with a house in the suburbs, and enough money for vacations and weekend barbecues with friends. These mainstream images often reflect a (white) American middle-class nostalgia in which smiling kids and straight teeth testify to someone having pulled themselves up by their bootstraps. When doing advocacy work, notice whom you choose as your poster children. How representative are their "successes"? Are there other stories that also need sharing? Be sure you have permission to tell someone's story. If you invite someone to tell their own story, arrange to compensate them for their time. Experience is a source of expertise and should be honored in a way that helps a person, be it in the form of money or maybe a meal and a bus pass.

> ### Best Practice
> Make an honest self-assessment about working with certain populations.

Recognize and begin to address your own trauma around gendered and racialized violence before working in a prison, and do not enter into this work without the support of an organization. Having the support of a team is integral to your doing this work well. Do not enter into service in a prison with a goal of your own healing (however profoundly offering service can affect this). Keep active your self-assessment of how fit you are to be serving people in prison. They need your full attention, which you cannot offer if you are yourself overwhelmed. While your own self-work is ongoing, be sure that you are in an emotionally stable place when you enter. Next, you do not need to know the convictions of the people with whom you are working. You might have a general sense of this, however, if you are teaching a yoga program whose members are grouped together because of similar convictions, such as relating to drugs or sexual violence. If you find yourself too triggered by the knowledge of working with any particular group, excuse yourself from the work, knowing that someone whose own trauma is not actively firing will serve them better. If you find yourself able and willing to work with this group, your ongoing non-judgment and firm boundaries are integral.

> Non-judgment does not mean that you will accept unwelcome words or actions. Your boundaries are rock-solid, and your non-judgmental, compassionate service, fierce.

Best Practice
Teachers should be aware of safety measures for themselves.

Be aware of the possibility of the sexual abuse or harassment of instructors. Follow basic institutional protocols for safety, such as being closest to the door or having a pager. Also, be mindful that many institutional protocols for your own safety can sow seeds of distrust in an already paranoia-inducing setting. Be mindful of this effect and then use mindfulness to balance institutional alertness with trust in the people you are here to serve.

Best Practice
Be aware of institutional rules about touch and then practice extra care.

Some carceral contexts will not allow instructors and students to make physical contact, which necessarily precludes touch in yoga sessions. Be mindful that if you are in an institution that *allows* touch, incarcerated people cannot legally give you consent. Our recommendation is not to touch. Even with permission, risks of harm outweigh the benefits.

Best Practice
Plan yoga classes according to its location and layout.

People will likely feel more exposed in their yoga practice in a prison setting than in private spaces, due to the context of surveillance.

Most rooms are equipped with security cameras, and a correctional officer (CO) may be stationed in the room in which you are teaching. Therefore, set up the space in ways that will reduce the feeling of exposure. First, try to foster a working relationship with the CO stationed in the space. Include them energetically in the class, even though they are not on a mat. This will help reduce the intensity of the power dynamic and increase your ability to hold space for genuine community to unfold. Second, arrange mats in a circle, allowing students to face one another and to enable peer facilitation.

Best Practice
Offer sequences and shapes that avoid triggers and that make yoga practice less of a performance.

Consider shapes you are not offering because of the setting. For example, teachers might abstain from teaching Adho Mukha Svanasana (Downward Dog) if any student would have their backside to a correctional officer or security camera, as well as because of how this shape could itself trigger sexual abuse. Omitting this form will also alter the progression of a sun salutation or other sequence. Teachers might likewise avoid inviting students to clasp hands behind their backs, as in Salambhasana (Locust Form), because of how it may simulate the posture of being arrested. Pressing against the wall to lengthen or stretch the arms mirrors a strip search and should likewise be carefully considered or avoided altogether (Horton, et al. 2017: 42). Also structure your class in a way to make it less of a performance. As noted above, arrange mats in a circle to encourage a sense of community and non-competition, and build in opportunities for peer facilitation.

> **Best Practice**
> Be aware that a prison is a charged environment that necessarily changes how you teach and dress.

> *Carefully consider the gender of the instructor*

Ideally, yoga teachers will mirror the members of a group such as in their gender and racial identity. Such representation is important for reasons of both equity and healing. Consider, for example, that prisons usually segregate men and women, according to binary state designations of biological sex, and often place transgender or nonconforming persons in solitary confinement. As mentioned above, the official reason for putting people of non-normative gender identities in segregation is for their safety, but the effects are punitive. Know, therefore, that assigning male teachers to classes for men and female teachers to classes for women may exclude genderqueer people. Recruit genderqueer instructors when possible, so that everyone eligible at the prison can have access to yoga. Also consider placement of teachers a matter of healing. Many prison yoga organizations simply have more female instructors, and prisons tend to have higher male than female populations. Therefore, female instructors will often be assigned to classes of men. The right female-identifying instructor working with men can create the possibility for a healthy cross-gender relationship (which may be new for many). At the same time, female teachers need to be mature and have no confusion in their motivations for working with men in prison.

When working with sex offenders, consider team-teaching.

> *Wear clothing that desexualizes your body*

We offer this best practice not due to the people in prison, but rather to its setting. The prison is a highly controlled and neuter environment in which contact with and sometimes even seeing members of the so-called opposite sex is forbidden. These measures paradoxically and inherently sexualize the setting and the bodies in it. Therefore, take care with how you dress. Consider wearing a double-layered T-shirt with a high collar, and loose-fitting pants.

> *Build relationships in human services and know whom to ask for additional help*

We have already emphasized the importance of teaching in a team, and building relationships within and without an organization. Here, we highlight two stories that demonstrate the need to know people in human services who can offer additional support to yoga students. One of us had an incarcerated yoga student who was depressed and experiencing suicidal thoughts. The instructor asked if her student could talk to her therapist, but learned the student's appointment would not be for a week. The instructor was able to contact crisis-support personnel. They were able to support the student and bring her to a more stable place. Another one of us had a meditation student whose childhood sexual abuse resurfaced during a sitting practice. He was not currently meeting with a mental health clinician. However, the instructor was already in conversation with an on-site clinician who was then able to begin meeting with the student daily.

Best Practice
Manage your expectations about timing.

Know that things may take more time in carceral settings, due to lengthy processes for admitting visitors. You may need to arrive an hour or more ahead of time, as well as follow an equally lengthy process for leaving. Unexpected circumstances that arise at the facility might also necessitate a planned class happening behind schedule. Keep this in mind any time you prepare to work in new settings.

Conclusion

Trauma-informed yoga can be a tool for finding and cultivating infinitesimal degrees of freedom. Any of us who has benefited from its practice may know something of that experience first-hand: a first full breath, a prolonged stillness, a tight muscle letting go. In the presence of appalling limits, to exercise freedom can mean simply to endure. In offering yoga to incarcerated survivors, service providers can remember that on the inside, yoga can be a practice that offers strategies for survival and healing. On the outside, we can work together toward structural changes that will make larger degrees of freedom possible, for us all.

Abuse in Religious, Spiritual, and Intentional Communities

Author *Amanda J.G. Napior*

Contributors *Lisa Boldin, Anneke Lucas, Rosa Vissers, Kimberleigh Weiss-Lewit, Ann Wilkinson*

Introduction

The best practices of this chapter offer ways of thinking about the implications of sexual abuse (and possibilities for recovery) in the context of communities of belonging. Abuse occurring in a religious, spiritual, or intentional community (communities gathering around belonging and some form of shared practice and, often, belief) is a deep violation of the safety and shared values presumably central to the community itself. In this way, abuse by an authority figure like a pastor, teacher, or community leader, a fellow congregant or practitioner, or by a congregant or student one serves is a violation not only of an individual but also of the community. When a community is the context of abuse, individual survivors of sexual violence may find themselves thrown into existential crisis. They risk losing their sense of belonging in the world, as well as potentially losing the profound relationships formed within that community, which may include family or even the divine. Like incest or intimate partner violence in which the very persons meant to represent safety instead become perpetrators, sexual violence in a religious, spiritual, or intentional community may be experienced as a profound betrayal by those whom one loves, and potentially as abjection by divinity itself.

Commonality, Difference, and Shifting Categories

"Religious, spiritual, and intentional communities" names a broad and diverse field. Our claim about what these groups share in common must therefore be modest: they are communities of belonging. Communities are not simply a collection of individual persons. Rather, communities are notable phenomena in their own right (Durkheim 1999, 2019; Seligman, et al. 2008). Understanding abuse within community therefore requires a consideration of group dynamics and the ways in which people *"locate themselves in the world with reference to both ordinary and extraordinary powers, meanings, and values"* (Albanese 2007: 9; emphasis in the original). Examining group dynamics prompts us to consider how belonging to a community informs the fabric of who someone is, and how one's own threads are interwoven with those of others. In one way, the best practices of this chapter could be read as an invitation to notice how you may share more in common with survivors of other communities than you think, as well as to respect the fact of your differences.

When working with those who have suffered abuse in communities, it is important to pay attention to the language they use to describe their community. Adopt an attitude of curiosity, asking the individual to provide whatever background is meaningful to them. Do accept whatever words individuals and communities use to describe themselves and to make meaningful distinctions between themselves and others. While people may describe their communities as "religious," "spiritual," "intentional," or something else, recognize that these terms do not necessarily describe historically unchanging phenomena.

Nor does the invocation of religion mean that a community, ritual, or practice needs to "look religious" to function as religion in someone's life.

"Religion," as a phenomenon and concept, is multiple and constructed. This statement could use some unpacking. The word "religion," for example, can encapsulate so many discrete kinds of phenomena, from persons and material objects to experiences and ideas. Further, the category itself has had different meanings across time and place. Divinities, spirits, or God are not a concern in all religions. Nor do all traditions emphasize shared belief, even though popular understandings of religion in North America and beyond tend to prioritize "belief" due to the dominant role Protestant Christianity has played in creating cultural, legal, and scholastic definitions of religion.

Scholars of religion have recently turned their attention to forms of religious belonging that eschew institutions and instead embrace belief, understood as something internal and personal, as the core of religious, or perhaps spiritual, identity. In the last three decades, many people have started referring to themselves as "spiritual but not religious," in part, out of an effort to distance themselves from the institutional character of religions that have caused harm, or which may limit individuality and an ability to pick-and-choose (Barnes and Sered 2004; Mercadante 2014). And yet, "spirituality" cannot be considered at face value as an ahistorical, universal phenomenon. It, too, has been shaped out of historical processes of social power. Our understanding of "spirituality" as a seemingly universal, "individualistic, sometimes secular, interior experience" has developed over time (Barnes & Sered 2004: 8).

Understanding the new and shifting terrain of spiritual and/but-not religious identity is important for social workers, agency directors, yogis, and other healers of self-and-other to consider because it illuminates how people find religious significance and intentional community in seemingly secular places. For example, secular humanists or activist organizations alike might consider themselves participating in intentional communities, and model their belonging on religious organizations, while rejecting either "religious" or "spiritual" as descriptors (Stedman 2012).

Abuse can and has happened in all of these kinds of communities. While the most widely publicized cases of this abuse have been those of child sexual abuse by priests in the Catholic Church, the Catholic Church is not the only community of belonging in which sexual violence has occurred, nor the only institutional structure vulnerable to (and complicit in) abuses of power. Indeed, yoga communities are included in this history and present as well (Jain 2015; Remski 2019). Abuse within ideologically secular organizations shows that even a practiced skepticism is not panacea against outright abuse or power imbalances, as some might like to think (Mamone 2019; Hutchinson 2018). Last, our chapters on sexual trauma in the military and on college campuses remind us of two more (but not the only) examples of institutions troubled by sexual exploitation.

The type of problem we are looking at here seems much more caught up in our humanity than in any one way of belonging. Fortunately for us, so too is our capacity to heal.

The Particular: Two Examples

Abuse within a community often takes a shape that is distinctly *of* that community, an observation that is perhaps both obvious but also necessary. "'There is no one,' among the victims of clerical sexual abuse...'who was not abused in a Catholic way.'" These words were spoken to religion scholar Robert Orsi by his interlocutor, "Monica." For example, central components of mass, such as the Eucharist, have been used in the course of abuse itself. As a result, the meaning and embodiment of central, sacred components of religious practice have become entangled in the experience of abuse. For many survivors, finding their way back to the Eucharist has meant disembedding its practice, as adults, from the abuse that befell them as children. Further, because Catholics understand Catholic priests to be vicars of Christ – that is, earthly, contemporary presences of Christ himself, "being abused by a priest was to be abused at one degree of separation from God." Abuse within the Catholic context creates interrelational trauma for victims that extends to their relationship with the divine. While being abused by a priest may share similarities with abuse by a school-teacher or sports coach, the unique theological, ritual, and embodied valence of Catholic practice and relationships means abuse in this context is distinct and incomparable, in key ways, from any other (Orsi 2016: 216).

Similarly, abuse within yoga communities has taken a particularly yogic shape. In Ashtanga yoga community, guru-founder Pattabhi Jois's "*mulabhanda* assists," was the euphemistic justification for digital rape that he visited upon many female students. Such justifications depended upon a kind of mystification that surrounded Jois's charismatic leadership and the tradition by which he claimed authority (Remski 2019). Hands-on assists in yoga culture have arguably become mainstream in parallel with the assaultive touch of charismatic male leaders who helped to popularize postural yoga in the second half of the twentieth century. The example of abuse within yoga culture offers an interesting parallel and contrast to that within Catholicism: if abuse by a Catholic priest has occasioned a survivor's

interrelational trauma with a Catholic's lived experience of God, abuse in the modern postural yoga scene has produced trauma within a certain construction of the self. The "bodily isolation … of some practice experiences" can reinforce a theme of hyper-attentiveness to individuality and to "yoga as a personal journey of discovery" (Remski 2019: 73). If one's practices have not resulted in greater personal empowerment, then they might internalize the message that "you weren't really practicing hard enough" (Remski 2019: 74).

Both of these examples treat abuse by authority figures within communities variously considered by members as religious and spiritual. In both cases, victims' trauma manifested in interrelational ways. And yet, there are dimensions of each case that cannot be generalized across them both.

Many communities of belonging are in the midst of much needed soul searching. Offering yoga to people who have experienced sexual violence in the context of communities of belonging requires a respect for their relationship to their traditions and a willingness to follow the lead of people involved in the work of reclamation and liberation from within their traditions – whether they belong to communities that are Catholic, Ashtanga, or something else. As with other sections of this book, we hope the best practices of this chapter will offer our readers some grounding for meaningful understanding, reflection, and action, while also offering an invitation for continuing education and curiosity. We will close with a few words on the possibilities of healing and recovery.

Best Practices

Best Practice
Do not present yoga as a benevolent replacement for what your student lost; honor their religious identity.

Expect your student to be in a period of religious and relational negotiation. You may be supporting someone who has either remained a part of their religious community, or has left. If they came out about their abuse and the community responded well (a leader was fired and prosecuted, enabling factors were investigated, and a community asked this person for forgiveness), your student may still be part of their tradition. Alternately, the community may have silenced and castigated your student, in which case your student may feel especially ostracized. Perhaps more likely, your student straddles an ambiguous combination of these positions. Survivors may turn to yoga as a new community or to complement an existing spiritual practice.

> **Best Practice**
> Provide continuity and reliability in your service.

Continuity and reliability are important irrespective of context. However, be aware that your student may have lost their community and could be in the midst of rebuilding or exploring new communities. You have the responsibility to offer them continuity. Do not take on a student you cannot commit to working with for the duration of the series you are offering. Studio courses may not be set up in such a format; however, be mindful of the need for continuity if you enter into a more formalized relationship.

> **Best Practice**
> Be aware of religious illiteracy, including your own.

Religious traditions are internally diverse and change over time. However, we tend to ask things like, "What do Christians believe?" as if all Christians everywhere, throughout history, have always shared the same doctrines and individual beliefs (when, in fact, they have not). Further, mainstream culture in the so-called West tends to pit "spiritual" against "religious" and personal "authenticity" against "tradition." While we cannot go into the long history of how such misconceptions and dichotomies have developed, here, consider how religious illiteracy influences misunderstandings (and biases against) certain people and communities. Survivors of abuse in a religious tradition may distance themselves from their tradition as they negotiate their changing relationship to it. In the process, they may themselves vilify their own tradition, in an effort to understand how it was that a person they trusted, in a tradition they loved, could have so egregiously betrayed and violated them. In other words, they might suddenly lump their faith tradition in with the other "bad" ones. Give this person space to make meaning. At the same time, do not participate in reinforcing stereotypes about their estranged tradition. Doing so only drives a deeper wedge into distinctions between *us* and *them*.

> **Best Practice**
> Take responsibility for creating yoga spaces free of sexual harassment or abuse.

Modern postural yoga has a history of sexual abuse by community leaders. Creating safe yoga spaces means facing the conditions that have allowed such behaviors to take root in yoga culture and then having zero tolerance for their maintenance. Prior Ashtanga yogini Karen Rain has urged that *believing* victims is not enough. "Response to victims … needs to turn into action" (Rain 2018). Make reparations. Be accountable by confirming reports of abuse to which you may have been witness. And apologize for your own complicity, which may have included silence, denial, or enabling (Rain & Cooke 2019). Ideally, conversations about sexual misconduct in yoga studios and organizations should happen at their inception. But it is never too late to begin the conversation. Yoga studios, schools, organizations, and programs should be places where people can *be* in their bodies, free of sexualization and exploitation. While the publicized cases of sexual abuse in yoga communities have been ones in which leaders took advantage of their students or devotees, recognize that abuse can happen between peers, as well as to teachers by students. Offer trainings for your teachers in sexual trauma and abuse, and in spiritual bypassing. Also have a comment box, with persons other than the main teachers as the readers. Finally, make a pledge that proclaims the commitment of your yoga organization to being proactively and adamantly intolerant of sexual abuse or harassment. You can craft your own pledge or join a preexisting one, like the one created by the Yoga Service Council https://yogaservicecouncil.org/thepledge) or from Darkness to Light (https://fromdarknesstolight.live).

> **Best Practice**
> Recognize how relational and communal bonds constitute our humanity.

From one perspective, that which constitutes a community are shared, lived ways of understanding and embodying the sacred or the special. Maybe you share a context with your student; maybe you do not. If you do not, be curious in learning what this is about for them. If you do not necessarily identify with your student, recognize that you, too, have a sense of moral authority pieced together in similar ways. This authority becomes embodied in stories, practices, and in relationships. Consider ways in which the various communities to which you belong inform the many dimensions of who

you are, and of your connections to others within and beyond those communities. This best practice is an invitation to notice *both* how very much we all share in common, as well as the distinct differences that make us unique.

> **Best Practice**
> Anticipate possible rejection of the word "healing" among Christian survivors.

Not every person seeking recovery from sexual trauma will embrace the word "healing." This awareness may serve service providers in any context, but has particular weight here. In some Christian communities, emphasis on "healing" has worked to elide trauma survivors' suffering. "Healing" can work as an "imperative to silence" – an insistence that someone put their anger aside (Orsi 2016: 245). Further, the ongoingness of trauma can receive short shrift in a theology that places emphasis on the joy and hope of Christ's resurrection after crucifixion (Rambo 2017). In all parts of your yoga service, be attentive to the language people use to describe their own journeys. If you are uncertain about how your words land for a student, just ask!

> While the wounds of crucifixion stand as one of the central symbols of Christian faith, the articulations of the meaning of those wounds have often perpetuated rather than alleviated suffering. Paired with claims of resurrection, they often enact a story of life overcoming death, of alleviating suffering ... But these explanations are not sufficient to speak to the ongoingness of suffering, to wounds resurfacing within life.
>
> (Rambo 2017: 145–6)

> **Best Practice**
> Be open to adopting new language.

Maybe you put some language aside, and maybe you build your vocabulary. Working with someone for whom a faith tradition is a central feature of their life offers you an opportunity to try on other people's world-framing tools, as well as to teach more fully from your own. You can learn more about the ways in which your student's tradition informs their world, in part by listening to the language they use. For example, does your student use language for the divine? If so, you might ask how they understand divinity to work in the world, and how they would understand divinity to work in their yoga practice. Language is a tool. In any context of teaching, we can listen to how people use language to make their worlds and then join them in that creation.

> **Best Practice**
> Consider that the community is not the cause but the context of abuse.

A myriad of forces coalesce to enable abuse and silence its whistle-blowers. They are usually at least partially structural, with leaders having or seeming to have more specialized knowledge than others, as well as positions of privilege. But that does not mean that all hierarchy turns abusive. Elements of abuse can also be deeply steeped in practices of the tradition, but that does not make the Catholic Eucharist or all hands-on assists in a yoga class inherently bad. Separating the context from the cause will help you avoid stereotyping people, reducing them to the abuse that has violated their own community's values.

The distinction between context and cause is important for many reasons. Among them is that this same context may be a necessary eventual component of someone's healing.

> "The abuse crisis in modern Catholicism was not caused by the intimacies of the environment, but it arose within them."
>
> Robert Orsi (2016: 217)
> in History and Presence

> **Best Practice**
> Honor the mystery, ask questions, call it like you see it.

An air of mystique around charismatic leaders in various communities can heighten the potential for sexual abuse by allowing bogus explanations for bad behavior to hold together, or ostensibly inappropriate behavior to appear, instead, as a matter of a disciple's misunderstanding. You can honor a tradition's status positions and their varied meanings while also keeping your sense of appropriate boundaries and critical thinking skills intact. If you have a student you suspect may be in an abusive situation within their community, ask questions, voice your observations, and offer appropriate support.

> **Best Practice**
> Counter networks of complicity with networks of empowerment.

Abuse is able to persist for as long as it does due to "networks of complicity" (Remski 2019: 241). A victim may speak out, but fellow community members might dismiss and explain the victim's experience away. Further, those who have not been abused might stay silent in order to protect their privilege, rather than using their privilege to help those who most need support. When people do speak out and you and others listen, however, you can respond by helping to build connections (with legal aid, advocacy networks, and survivor networks). These connections extend and expand into "networks of empowerment." Matthew Remski observes that "the values expressed in an empowerment network directly oppose those in the abuse-enabling network, because the goal of victims and their allies is to deconstruct and redistribute power, rather than to capture and hoard it" (Remski 2019: 242). If you are in the community in which someone has experienced abuse, thank them for speaking up, ask how you can help, and then take action.

Conclusion
Healing off the Mat or in the Parish

Healing does not look the same for every person. When sexual abuse happens within a community of belonging, that very context may offer the necessary inroads of a person's healing journey. Alternately, a survivor may travel roads away from the community, never to return. But a survivor's changing relationship to their tradition invariably changes the community itself, whether through their absence, an active negotiation with tradition, or both.

A Catholic priest named "Frank" was abused by priests as both an altar boy and an adult seminarian. He has stayed within the Catholic tradition despite having had his ability to function as a parish priest revoked, for his agitation against clerical abuse.

An ongoing negotiation with his tradition and with God, Frank's faith is a brilliant, angry, stubborn, and vulnerable one. His theological position about clerical abuse is that "God had nothing to do with this." This is less a statement of classic Christian theodicy (that God gives humans free will but "is not responsible for the evil they do with it"), than it is a relational claim, Robert Orsi suggests. While survivors of this context may work through various human dimensions of their abuse in therapeutic relationships, the fact of abuse in "sacred spaces by men who were 'like a God,'" means their recovery may be as much about a healing relationship with the divine as with other human beings (Orsi 2016: 230). And so finding a way to approach God again may require new ways of understanding divine agency. "To have seen God at God's worst," writes Orsi, might make it possible to "to be liberated from the old relationship with an omnipotent and omniscient God," and instead to enter into a relationship among partners (Orsi 2016: 237). Frank advocates "praying angry," citing the Psalms as both "some of the angriest prayers we have," as well as the "most beautiful and loving prayers" (Orsi 2016: 232).

Karen Rain is a prior Ashtanga yogi who left Ashtanga in 2001, after having experienced repeated violation by Jois. She has not returned to the practice of Asana. Instead, she has pursued various forms of movement therapy to heal chronic pain related to yoga practice. She has also become a prolific critic of rape culture and victim blaming. Her writings began with her November 2017 #MeToo post in which she, "inspired by the importance of sharing experiences and naming names," disclosed Jois's abuse. Although Rain is no longer a yoga asana practitioner herself, her writings suggest a changing relationship to the tradition that has included dialogue with other yogis. From the perspective of this chapter, these conversations have formed several streams in a "network of empowerment," that is helping to make possible a yoga culture that will not accept sexual violence in its midst.

Our small glimpse into Frank's and Rain's stories offer us insight into the kinds of negotiations and changes happening within and without the Catholic and Ashtanga communities of belonging. Frank stayed. Karen left. Their doing so has helped form both in- and out-roads, into and from their current and past communities of belonging. They demonstrate varied orientations survivors may have, in relation to one's healing, and in relation to oneself, others, and the divine. "The spiritual journey," says Frank, "is all about people who have problems with God" (cited in Orsi 2016: 232).

Through the help of voices like Rain's, those of us who belong to yoga communities can reshape and reclaim yoga not only as a personal journey of discovery, but as an always already *inter*personal journey in which we must seek out, care for, and be accountable to one another.

PART
6

Conclusion

A Call to Action for Yoga

Authors *Danielle Rousseau and Dani Harris*

The reality of this book suggests that it is necessary to change the way we teach yoga and explore how we relate within a yoga community. We recognize that, in many ways, the modern practice of yoga falls short of the fundamental tenets of yoga's truest potential. People seek yoga for a variety of reasons, including a desire for connection or as a tool for increased well-being. In the wake of sexual trauma, survivors may turn to yoga in search of tools for coping and improved mental and physical well-being. Yet connection and well-being are not always offered. To the contrary, what is often found can include instances of appropriation, lack of accessibility, or even contexts of trauma perpetration.

We must challenge teachers to shift the way they think about, practice, and lead yoga through a radical approach that returns to focus on what is essential. This change is revolutionary not only because it questions existing power dynamics, but also because it takes care of the most vulnerable in a traditional yoga setting. It confronts the foundations of contemporary yoga practices and calls us to action. These shifts, we recognize, are no small feat, and is a process worthy of immense celebration.

This work is timely and overdue. The many impacts of sexual trauma are not new, nor are responses to its perpetration. Activists and social justice responders have long contested rape and violence against women. Feminist activism, rape crisis centers, and initiatives such as Take Back the Night are but examples of the ongoing efforts to combat sexual violence. More recently, and rooted in the efforts of Tarana Burke, the #MeToo movement has brought renewed interest in addressing sexual trauma. As far back as the civil rights movement survivors have wanted to be seen, heard, and create change. This book furthers the work of activists, researchers, and practitioners who voice a call to action to address the issue of sexual violence, sexual trauma, and power differentials.

In this work, we must fundamentally recognize that not all yoga spaces have been "safe." Yoga spaces, too, have been spaces marred by sexual violence. These spaces have served to keep people from accessing their healing. We must continue the work of creating safer and more inclusive space for the practice of yoga. Yoga exists within the context of multiple and complex challenges. Within our society, systemic structures exist that can perpetuate and even reward abuse and abusers. Yoga itself is situated within a historical structure of hierarchy and control. There is the potential for abuses of power in all places where yoga is being practiced and shared.

In discussing the role of yoga within a sexual trauma context, and within the context of trauma more generally, we must recognize both yoga's capacity to empower and support resilience as well as its place in a culture of trauma. We must acknowledge the role of problematic power differentials in the yoga community as well as the potential for harm through inadvertent re-traumatization by insensitive teachers or outright abuse by yoga teachers with poor boundaries or even predatory intent. As such, we have the highest responsibility to be very intentional in how our yoga is offered and to remain informed about the context in which yoga is taught.

In all of this, we must acknowledge that yoga is a vast field of practice, history, lineage, precepts, disciplines, texts, teachings, and approaches. Those working within the yoga community need to recognize both yoga's history and its contemporary place in service to trauma survivors, and to act accordingly with the deepest respect and humility.

Yoga can be a tool for well-being and help to foster resilience for practitioners. In the context of sexual violence, yoga can be a support for survivors, both in the wake of trauma and in negotiating the long-term impacts of trauma. It can offer an opportunity for people to rebuild a relationship with their own bodies in nonjudgmental and nonsexual ways. We believe that as an embodied practice, yoga is a tool that promotes an increased capacity for resilience, well-being, and connection. Further, we firmly believe that teaching yoga within a transparent, highly inclusive trauma-responsive framework has the potential to foster significant change.

We offer a call to action. In supporting survivors, and in addressing abuses within the yoga community itself, we suggest the need for implementation of trauma-informed practices rooted in an expanded understanding of how we conceptualize the trauma-informed practice, moving from trauma-understanding to resilience building. We further acknowledge the need to invite increased inclusion into yoga spaces and practices. Here we offer the concept of universal inclusion, an idea that grew out of the work of this project and that we will detail below. Finally, we suggest that yoga itself constitutes a tool for the change we seek.

Trauma-informed Yoga
Understanding trauma-informed perspectives

Trauma-informed yoga is a discipline of nuanced seeing and heightened understanding of how each yoga participant is experiencing the practice at any given moment, in any circumstance. It considers the safest possible experience of yoga to be the surest path for each person to become a stronger, more alert, and discerning individual. By understanding how trauma can impact the mind and body – and especially how it dysregulates the whole person – coupled with recognition of the barriers trauma often creates for survivors trying to access yoga, trauma-informed yoga allows teachers to respond to each student (and each class moment) in ways that create practices and spaces that see each participant as already whole, as opposed to broken, while accounting for each participant's needs for empowered choice, safety, and dynamic predictability.

Trauma-informed yoga specifically and intentionally takes the impact of trauma into account and recognizes the ways that yoga itself has the potential to traumatize and even re-traumatize. Yoga that is trauma-informed forefronts the needs of participants, creating an environment that is as safe as possible. Trauma-informed yoga offers yoga practice in a way that is consistent and predictable, while offering instruction in an invitational and nondirective manner. The primary focus is not on the physicality and exactness of bodily movement but instead on the internal experience of the student. Trauma-informed yoga takes into account the most vulnerable person in every setting and is structured around practices of orienting, containment, and body and brain positivity. It also builds on the great strengths that each person – including survivors of every sort – brings to their practice.

Seeking a Strengths-based Conceptualization of Trauma-informed Practice

We are indebted to early iterations of traditional trauma-informed yoga. The work done by the people who came before us is revolutionary, and as time, attitudes, and practices shift, we have greater capacity to change with it. We would suggest that traditional trauma-informed yoga has the propensity to see survivors of violence and trauma as being significantly disadvantaged when compared to more neuro-typical, "higher-functioning," "trauma-free," people. Truly inclusive yoga is yoga that accounts for every person in the room, including sexual trauma survivors. Inclusive teaching within a trauma-informed context means understanding each person's unique ability to cultivate and foster their resilience with raw, grounded courage, founded on strength and capacity. Yoga has a direct means to embolden this resilience building. Resilience then comes from yoga moving from catering to a survivor's perceived deficits (as a way to eliminate them), to working with an individual's highly attuned survival strategy and strengths.

Moving from seeing people as victims of trauma to whole, and unbroken people who have inherent strengths with resiliency within them dramatically shifts the paradigm of many contemporary trauma-informed yoga curriculums. Giving voice to previously silenced or misunderstood strategies a survivor has, trauma-informed inclusive yoga removes the barrier created in seeing those who have experienced sexual trauma as damaged. We have an opportunity to change our view as trauma survivors as having psychological or behavioral "gaps" to a celebration of those highly fine-tuned and valuable skills in survival.

It is essential to see that survivors are not broken. Truthfully, none of us are. The easiest purview into this way of beholding is to see people's survival strategies as strengths, no matter how maladaptive they may seem clinically. Seeing everyone as brilliant and unbroken is strengths-based building on already existing successes. These successes create a foundation for increased resilience that yoga as an embodied practice supports with abundant celebration.

Fundamentally, we need to celebrate, and not enter with the intention to "fix" people's survival strategies using yoga. This view acknowledges that all of us present have curated a set of finely attuned skills we carry with us for survival from our experiences in the world. This understanding is paramount as it is the foundation for the experience of increasing one's capacity for resilience. Celebrating the survival of others expands significantly when one experiences a sense of grounding, self-trust, and ease that yoga teaches us. This resilience grows when it is seen, heard, and celebrated from the inside out. In this way, yoga gives voice and agency to a survivor's successes.

Safety

We believe that understanding safety is at the core of providing yoga that is accessible to survivors of sexual trauma. Yoga creates space for people to "let down" both on the inside and the outside. This type of relaxation, or letting one's guard down in the most positive of ways, can be alarming for survivors; it shows a version of themselves they may not have experienced in many years, even decades. With yoga, we have an evident ability to create spaciousness for those we teach to see their strengths and their existing resilience. We are then able to use these felt-experiences each person has in our classes to illuminate and ease the stress dynamic playing out within nervous systems. Yoga creates a spaciousness that through practice poignantly connects them to the inner resourcing crafted as a way to survive. None of this is available unless a modicum of safety is present.

Being as safe as possible applies to so much more than being physically sound with yoga forms and sequences. It involves setting the space so that it feels welcoming and inclusive, striving to ensure that each person who comes to share yoga is seen, and honoring the needs that yoga can help meet.

Safety involves each teacher recognizing the extent to which people can hold past experiences in their body. It also means acknowledging how yoga can bring some of those to the fore and, with that, striving to be both challenging and conservative, so that people can safely grow in their practice. Being "safe" means recognizing that safety cannot be guaranteed, that it is a continual practice of action and reflection, mindful speech, and clear boundaries.

Individually and collectively, safety is multifaceted. When teaching survivors of sexual trauma, it is not appropriate to label yoga classes as safe spaces; it is false to say this. Instead, by suggesting that we can create spaces that are "as safe as possible," we create trust in our acknowledgment that none of us can either define or control what safety means to any one person. To suggest otherwise is faulty and unsafe as safety is situational, coming from mass amounts of internal and external understandings, emotional reactions, and biological responses. Creating as safe a space as possible means establishing an environment that promotes the capacity for positive regulation of the stress response. This safety extends itself to designing classes that are predictable, offering containment, strong teacher commitment, flexibility within the structure of a class as well as establishing norms around orienting people to the present moment. Finally, safety should not be

seen as an add-on or impediment to progress but rather an opportunity to explore the practice of yoga more deeply than ever before.

Universally Inclusive Yoga

Our united vision for universally inclusive yoga includes sharing and teaching yoga in ways that:

- are as safe as possible for everyone
- are accessible and welcoming to each person
- support all participants in being heard and seen
- help co-create an environment that fosters our individual and collective life journeys
- supports us living with brilliance, strength, and resilience
- always warmly include and support people who have experienced trauma, including critical life situations and sexual and/or family violence.

Facilitating universally inclusive trauma-informed approaches allows yoga to be offered in a conscious relationship between yoga service provider and diverse populations, and in every conceivable locale.

Universally Inclusive Yoga is as Safe as Possible for Every Person

To understand being as safe as possible, we have found it helpful to understand the opposite of that: feelings of un-safety that lead too many people – people who could most likely gain great measure for themselves if they had a place to practice that felt safe – to avoid yoga.

Safety (in this context) means that the body and mind do not panic or freeze during yoga, that breathing does not race out of control, that wariness goes down not up. Yoga, especially for people who have or are experiencing trauma, can increase feelings of vulnerability and trigger a stress response in one's nervous system. This triggering occurs because many people live their daily lives inside layers of survival strategies, and those survival strategies rely on the utmost predictability in moment-by-moment living. Since yoga invites personal inquiry and movement of body and breath that are outside the realm of everyday experience for most people, body, breath, and mind are subject to new sensations and perceptions. This can be unsettling for people for whom predictability is the cornerstone of their navigation through the day.

Yoga that is designed and practiced to be as safe as possible requires:

- real-time predictability

- orienting

- containment

- flexibility

- ongoing commitment.

Safety is a more complex idea than we may initially consider. In the context of yoga, there are a few core elements to safety that should be considered and implemented to ensure that the practices are supportive of each person's individual experience. To understand the core constructs of safety, one must consider:

- Safety is situational and depends on a large array of information, experience, biology, and more.

- Safety cannot be guaranteed; to promise otherwise is a potentially unsafe proposition.

- Any work to increase the safety of any situation must include all stakeholders.

- Safety is more likely when it is empowering and inclusive; this includes using language that reflects the diverse students in our spaces at any given time.

- Safety is not a tangible thing but rather a continually shifting experience of the present moment that grows from personal experience.

- Safety largely offers containment and predictability; structure is one of the surest ways to bring safety into any yoga service situation.

- Safety is enhanced when it includes personal choice; we can move toward this tenet by not creating hierarchies in language around forms and sincerely not assuming every person is going to have the same experience in every form or breathing practice.

- True safety must take into account the most vulnerable person in the room at all times; this includes the teacher and their ability to know themselves and their own shadow areas.

- Last, safety is the responsibility of everyone, including teacher and practitioner.

To co-create yoga that is universally inclusive and as safe as possible for every participant requires additional responsibility from the person offering the practices: the yoga teacher. This teacher should offer the forms, practices, and precepts from a place of great personal grounding, and continually affirm the ongoing well-being of the participants. This skill set includes listening to students, inviting questions, pacing classes spaciously, reading the energy of the room, remaining humble, and, most of all, focusing on approaches that give each participant the chance to glean from the practices exactly what they need in any given moment. To teach inclusively and safely like this then becomes a practice of its own, a continual opportunity to be mindful in each moment while teaching.

Universally Inclusive Yoga is Accessible and Welcoming to Each Person

Universally inclusive yoga includes the co-creation of spaces where people feel safe and supported to explore their own lives through yoga. We acknowledge that there are many thousands of people who struggle to access yoga in studio settings because of fear, doubt, physical limitations, financial limitations, or past traumas. We believe great good will come from expanding access to yoga and that such expansion will foster our capacity as human beings to learn from, and deeply support one another. When universally inclusive, yoga classes in community centers, studios, schools, and any other space where yoga is offered are welcoming and inclusive to everyone who has the curiosity and drive to explore life through yoga; classes are not limited to only those who appear capable of joining such a class.

Universally Inclusive Yoga Supports all Participants in Being Heard and Seen

One of the principles of inclusivity in its highest form is that it values the voice and input of each person. This does not mean that every yoga class will turn into a sharing circle. It simply means that each person in attendance is viewed as a full and important part of the class.

To be seen is a hallmark of inclusive yoga and is initially a responsibility of the person or people who are offering the yoga practice, class, or session. It may require deepened skills in observation of others, spaciousness, humility, and curiosity, blended with a willingness to provide opportunities for people to share their own

experiences in relation to yoga. Opportunities for shared experience can also help build community. To be heard involves creating ways for people to be able to speak their truths, add their opinions, ask questions, share stories, and more.

Universally Inclusive Yoga Helps Co-create an Environment that Fosters our Individual and Collective Journeys of Living into our Brilliance, Strength, and Resilience

This tenet is an opportunity for yoga spaces to embrace the sacred task of helping build community, while at the same time supporting each person on their journey of discovery and empowerment. This grows from a ceaseless awe at the vastness of what yoga has to offer joined with a rooted appreciation that each person can (and will) find their own path and their own understanding. Yoga teachers can help with this by using words that demonstrate a supportive appreciation for this vastness, rather than teaching that there are fixed or rigid truths.

Universally Inclusive Yoga Always Warmly Includes and Supports People Who Have Experienced Trauma, including Critical Life Situations and Sexual and/or Family Violence

One of the frequent ongoing aftereffects of significant trauma is that many survivors feel not only dissociation in the body but a parallel disconnection from society and healthy relations with others. As such, many people experiencing post-traumatic disruptions find it very stressful to take public yoga classes, to share space with others, or simply to go out in the world. Trust feels scarce for many survivors and, because of that, accessing yoga becomes a daunting endeavor.

One way to gently and continually counter this is to create *with* them a space where they can access and practice yoga. One example would be simple orientation practices before every class, very clear guidelines around permission to leave the class at any time, and pointing out all of the exits. Additionally, skillful use of words can make people of all genders and personal histories feel more welcome. Having thoughtful approaches to childcare, scheduling, cost, and duration can create added opportunities for inclusivity.

Yoga as Activism

Yoga service is activism. Through in-depth self-study and the co-creation of transparent relationships, we are better able to take care of the most vulnerable in any yoga setting. In its pages, this book offers a voice to populations who have been nearly silenced (although not entirely) through the perpetration of sexual violence. As such, the best practices in this book will increase the amount of safety in the world. By hearing the voices of those affected by sexual violence, including through breath and movement, we build safety. We believe that every studio and every space that offers yoga can become trauma-informed and accessible, offering the best of yoga's benefits to all.

Embodied practices, like yoga, have long been used in clinical and holistic settings to address not only myriad effects of sexual trauma but to aid the radical self-care needed to engage in and sustain the activism this book suggests as a tool for robust social transformation. We know that we can accomplish this in intentional and informed ways.

Yoga itself has a contribution to make in the pursuit of activism and positive social change. Yoga can impact change at the individual, collective, and even systemic levels and the potential change offered in yoga is complex and rich because it moves beyond the theoretical to the embodied. Yoga can foster a greater sense of agency; through tools and practices learned survivors may develop an improved capacity to advocate for self. The tenets of yoga themselves, if lived fully, call us to action. Yoga can also support activism at the community and even systemic levels. In its best and most universally inclusive, many voices are represented.

Choosing universally inclusive yoga is an active stance against injustice. Intentionality, inclusiveness, accessibility, empowerment, and accountability are all key tenets that will shape how yoga can be a vehicle for systemic change. Systemic change takes a community; it can only occur through connection. Yoga offers the potential for connection and systemic healing. Yoga, mindfulness, and other embodied practices provide an opportunity to consistently and conscientiously practice radical self-care, both as individuals and in relationship with others.

Community and Relationship

One of the most powerful aspects of contemporary yoga practice is that it so often takes place collectively: deep individual self-exploration in concert with others. With care and attention, this joined personal experience leads to building of actual community. As such, the Yoga Service Council has always supported every person seeking to do yoga, as well as communities and organizations small and large where yoga is offered and shared. In our work over the years, we have identified two of the most important aspects of building strong and vibrant communities: the willingness to put in the time to create strong relationships and the understanding that each person deserves the chance to be seen and heard. In yoga service, the practice of yoga is inextricably tied to conscious relationship.

Resilience and Trauma

A universally inclusive approach to yoga can serve as a tool to support resilience in the wake of trauma for both individuals and communities. Universally inclusive yoga works to foster an environment and support practices rooted in trauma-informed resilience building. In seeking a yoga community that promotes well-being, it is important to provide teachers with trauma-informed training and ongoing education. Equally important is promoting active self-inquiry and reflection. To support resilience, all teachers must actively pursue current and emerging best practices, seeking further education where there are gaps in one's understanding. We should support teachers and community members in pursuing both empirical and experiential expertise.

In sharing practices that promote well-being and resilience, we should be mindful of our words. Language is powerful. In teaching and in supporting yoga and mindfulness communities, we should strive to use language that is compassionate, inclusive, and inviting. We must also acknowledge and actively work to do better when we fall short of this. We must recognize and work to rectify the impact of intersectional disparities. We support resilience when we offer yoga practices and classes that engender strength and personal empowerment.

Empowering Policies

While yoga and mindfulness practices can embody a powerful and empowering tool for supporting resilience and building well-being, we must also recognize that the space of yoga is not immune to sexual violence and other abuses. Because yoga has the potential to offer tools for healing and, furthermore, because it offers a mechanism to seek connection and community, abuse in a yoga community can represent a double wound. It can be disempowering for an individual to have to disavow a support system. We must do the work to not only recognize and acknowledge but to actively eradicate problematic power differentials and abusive behavior.

There are clear and distinct practices that yoga providers and spaces can offer to empower participants and create a universally inclusive space. Studios and yoga spaces should establish, honor, and uphold clear sexual misconduct policies. Studios and providers should offer lines of communication with staff and management that are simple, clear, and open at all times. Providers should hear and actively investigate all complaints of sexual harassment and sexual misconduct by teachers. Yoga providers should recognize misconduct as a serious violation of trust, security, and ethics. Misconduct breaches student–teacher relationships. Providers should additionally pay attention to instances that include violation of the law and seek legal action if this is something agreed to by the complainant. Yoga community members should not only believe survivors, but take action where appropriate. Open awareness, action, and advocacy in response to the harms that can occur in the yoga community is part of the practice of yoga. Seeking awareness and just action is part of the yogic journey. Trauma-informed and trauma-responsive practices must go beyond teaching style and inform the character of yoga communities. Empowered justice should be a core component of the environment in which we offer yoga practice and service.

United Action

Collectively, our power comes when we stand together for a world free from sexual violence in every form. Help us co-create how we embody this pledge: share with us your raw material, your successes, practices, challenges, and opportunities. Together we will continue to build a world of compassion, joy, and abundance, a world that finally includes the well-being of all beings.

Conclusion

As mentioned, this work is unique in its creation. Over the course of two years, experts at the intersection of yoga service and sexual trauma have actively engaged in an ongoing process of inquiry (both individual and collective) and co-creation. The many voices that made up this journey are all reflected in the offering we present to you in this text. While we honor and are proud of the work that has been done, we also acknowledge that the journey has, in many ways, just begun.

As a practice, yoga's role in moving people towards increasing well-being in the wake of sexual trauma is gaining empirical support. The diversity among us, whether age, race, economic status, religion, sexuality, and gender, changes the approach we take in addressing population-specific outcomes of sexual trauma. This book works to offer recommendations for practice with a variety of populations and in diverse contexts. We also recognize that the list of offerings is not exhaustive; it is but a recommended starting point. We believe that yoga can create realities whereby each person's brilliance is shown, post-traumatic responses lessened, and where the connection between breath and body and

between individual and community become the seeds to healing. We hope that this book inspires ongoing self-inquiry and shared learning in these ways.

We can provide yoga that positively benefits survivors. We can do this through resilience building and a universally inclusive approach. This includes acknowledging the voices of survivors and valuing their experiences and insights. This approach represents radical resilience. We have watched the bravery of people in the #MeToo movement, and we can embody the same spirit and action within our yoga classes.

If there is any time, it is now. As yoga practitioners, studio owners, industry leaders, *and* students, we must move forward to actually meet people as they are. This begins by using methods and pedagogies that are inclusive, take care of the most vulnerable in any setting, and are trauma-informed and universally inclusive. The attention we place creating spaces that are as safe as possible for each person, does not take away from the practice we call yoga. In fact, it is a direct reflection of yoga in its truest form. Using trauma-informed best practices, including those that are orienting, predictable, and those that provide containment and flexibility, we can foster greater capacity for resilience in all who seek yoga as a way to bring their healing. Practices that are empowering and affirming become embodied experiences that move off the mat into daily living. We deeply honor, with the sincerest gratitude, the voices of activism, courage, and resilience that have influenced this book.

REFERENCES

References

Chapter 1

1. Childress T and Cohen Harper J (2016) What is yoga service? A working definition [Online] Available: https://yogaservicecouncil. org/community-resource-papers [29 October 2019].

2. Childress TM, Harper JC, Flesher A, Gonzalez A, Hyde AM and Kinder W (2015) Best practices for yoga in schools, Atlanta, GA: Yoga Service Council.

3. Horton C (2016) Best practices for yoga with veterans, Rhinebeck, NY: YSC/Omega Publications.

4. Horton C (2017) Best practices for yoga in the criminal justice system, Rhinebeck, NY: YSC/Omega Publications.

Chapter 2

1. American Psychiatric Association (2013) Diagnostic and statistical manual of mental disorders: DSM-5, Arlington, VA: American Psychiatric Association.

2. American Psychological Association (2019) Trauma [Online] Available: www.apa.org/topics/trauma/ [28 October 2019].

3. Barrett LF and Simmons WK (2015) Interoceptive predictions in the brain. Nature Reviews Neuroscience 16 (5) 419–429.

4. Borsini A, Hepgul N, Mondelli V, Chalder T, and Pariante CM (2014) Childhood stressors in the development of fatigue syndromes: A review of the past 20 years of research. Psychological Medicine 44 (9) 1,809–1,823.

5. Burgess AW and Holmstrom LL (1974) Rape trauma syndrome. American Journal of Psychiatry 131 (9) 981–986.

6. Clark DB, Chung T, Pajtek S, Zhai Z, Long E, and Hasler B (2013) Neuroimaging methods for adolescent substance use disorder prevention science. Prevention Science 14 300–309.

7. De Bellis MD and Zisk A (2014) The biological effects of childhood trauma. Child and Adolescent Psychiatric Clinics of North America 23 (2) 185–222.

8. Fallot R and Harris M (2009) Creating cultures of trauma-informed care (CCTIC): A self-assessment and planning protocol, Washington, DC: Community Connections.

9. Felitti VJ, Anda RF, Nordenberg D, Williamson DF, Spitz AM, Edwards V, Koss MP, and Marks JS (1998) Relationship of childhood abuse and household dysfunction to many of the leading causes of death in adults: The adverse childhood experiences (ACE) study. American Journal of Preventive Medicine 14 (4) 245–258.

10. Fergusson D, Mcleod G, and Horwood L (2013) Childhood sexual abuse and adult developmental outcomes: Findings from a 30-year longitudinal study in New Zealand. Child Abuse & Neglect 37 (9) 664–674. https://doi.org/10.1016/j.chiabu.2013.03.013.

11. Gazzangia MS, Ivry RB, and Mangun GR (2018) Cognitive neuroscience: The biology of the mind, New York, NY: W. W. Norton & Company.

12. Hopper EK, Bassuk EL, and Olivet J (2010) Shelter from the storm: Trauma-informed care in homelessness services settings. The Open Health Services and Policy Journal 3 80–100.

13. Justice L, Brems C, and Ehlers K (2018) Bridging body and mind: Considerations for trauma-informed yoga. International Journal of Yoga Therapy 28 (1) 39–50.

14. Levine PA (2008) Healing trauma: A pioneering program for restoring the wisdom of your body, Boulder, CO: Sounds True Inc.

15. Mate G (2003) When the body says no: Exploring the stress–disease connection, Hoboken, NJ: Wiley.

16. McCann IL and Pearlman LA (1990) Vicarious traumatization: A framework for understanding the psychological effects of working with victims. Journal of Traumatic Stress 3 (1) 131–149.

17. Richardson JI (2001) Guidebook on vicarious trauma: Recommended solutions for anti-violence workers, Ottawa: National Clearinghouse on Family Violence.

18. Rousseau D, Lilly M, and Harris D (2018) Creating a culture of universally-inclusive yoga. Yoga Service Council [Online] Available: https://yogaservicecouncil.org/community-resource-papers [10 October 2019].

19. Rousseau D, Weiss-Lewit K, and Lilly M (2019) #MeToo and yoga: Guidance for clinicians referring to trauma-informed yoga. Journal of Clinical Sport Psychology 13 (2) 216–225.

20. Substance Abuse and Mental Health Services Administration (SAMHSA) (2019) Trauma and violence [Online] Available: https://www.samhsa.gov/trauma-violence [10 October 2019].

21. Siegel DJ (2010) Mindsight: The new science of personal transformation, New York, NY: Bantam.

22. Streeter CC, Whitfield TH, Owen L, Rein T, Karri SK, Yakhkind A, Perlmutter R, Taylor AG, Goehler LE, Galper DI, Innes KE, and Bourguignon C (2010) Top-down and bottom-up mechanisms in mind-body medicine: Development of an integrative framework for psychophysiological research. Explore (New York, N.Y.) 6 (1) 29–41. doi:10.1016/j.explore.2009.10.004.

REFERENCES *continued*

23. Telles S, Singh N, and Balkrishna A (2012) Managing mental health dis-orders resulting from trauma through yoga: A review. Depression Research Treatment. Article ID 401513, 9 pages, 1–9. http://dx.doi.org/10.1155/2012/401513.

24. Van der Kolk BA (2006) Clinical implications of neuroscience research in PTSD. Annals of the New York Academy of Sciences 1,071 (1) 277–293.

25. Van der Kolk BA (2014) The body keeps the score, New York, NY: Viking.

26. Van Dernoot Lipsky L (2009) Trauma stewardship: An everyday guide to caring for self while caring for others, San Francisco, CA: Berrett-Koehler Publishers, Inc.

Chapter 3

1. American Psychiatric Association (2013) Diagnostic and statistical manual of mental disorders: DSM-5, Arlington, VA: American Psychiatric Association.

2. American Psychological Association (2019) Resilience [Online] Available: www.apa.org [2 October 2019].

3. Coutu D (2017) How resilience works. In resilience, Boston, MA: Harvard Business Review Press.

4. Equal Employment Opportunity Commission (EEOC) (2019) EEOC [Online] Available: https://www.eeoc.gov/ [2 October 2019].

5. Federal Bureau of Investigation (FBI) (2019) FBI: UCR [Online] Available: https://ucr.fbi.gov/crime-in-the-u.s/2018 [2 October 2019].

6. Grych J, Hamby S, and Banyard V (2015) The resilience portfolio model: Understanding healthy adaptation in victims of violence. Psychology of Violence 5 (4) 343–354.

7. Hamby S, Grych J, and Banyard V (2018) Resilience portfolios and poly-strengths: Identifying protective factors associated with thriving after adversity. Psychology of Violence 8 (2) 172–183.

8. Mohatt NV, Thompson AB, Thai ND, and Tebes JK (2014) Historical trauma as public narrative: A conceptual review of how history impacts present-day health. Social Science & Medicine 106 128–136 [Online] Available: https://www.ncbi.nlm.nih.gov/pmc/articles/PMC4001826/ [5 August 2019].

9. RAINN (2019) RAINN [Online] Available: https://www.rainn.org/ [2 October 2019].

10. Take Back the Night (2019) Take Back the Night Foundation [Online] Available: Takebackthenight.org. [2 October 2019].

11. Tedeschi RG and Calhoun LG (1996) The posttraumatic growth inventory: Measuring the positive legacy of trauma. Journal of Traumatic Stress 9 (3) 455–471.

12. Tedeschi RG and Calhoun LG (2004) Posttraumatic growth: Conceptual foundations and empirical evidence. Psychological Inquiry 15 (1) 1–18.

13. Yoga 4 Change (2019) Chartrand study: Short report, Jacksonville, FL: Yoga 4 Change.

14. Wolfe P (2006) Settler colonialism and the elimination of the native. Journal of Genocide Research 8 (4) 387–409.

15. Worthen MGF (2016) Sexual deviance and society: A sociological examination, London: Routledge.

Chapter 4

1. Bordoni B, Purgol S, Bizzarri A, Modica M, and Morabito B (2018) The influence of breathing on the central nervous system. Cureus 10 (6), e2724. doi:10.7759/cureus.2724

2. De Michelis E (2005) A history of modern yoga: Patanjali and Western esotericism, United Kingdom: Bloomsbury Academic.

3. Emerson D (2015) Trauma-sensitive yoga in therapy: Bringing the body into treatment, New York, NY: W.W. Norton & Company.

4. Feuerstein G (2011) The encyclopedia of yoga and tantra / Georg Feuerstein, rev. edn, Boston, MA: Shambhala.

5. Herman J (1992) Trauma and recovery, New York, NY: Basic Books.

6. Hopper EK, Bassuk EL and Olivet J (2010) Shelter from the storm: Trauma-informed care in homelessness services settings. The Open Health Services and Policy Journal 3 80–100.

7. Jain AR (2015) Selling yoga: From counterculture to pop culture, Oxford: Oxford University Press.

8. Jones S (2017) Mindful touch: A guide to hands-on support in trauma-sensitive yoga. Yoga Service Council 5 1–9.

9. Khalsa SS, Rudrauf D, Damasio AR, Davidson RJ, Lutz A, and Tranel D (2008) Interoceptive awareness in experienced meditators. Psychophysiology 45 (4) 671–677.

10. Ogden P, Minton K, and Pain C (2006) Trauma and the body: A sensorimotor approach to psychotherapy, New York, NY: W.W. Norton & Company, Inc.

11. Pascoe, MC and Bauer IE (2015) A systematic review of randomized control trials on the effects of yoga on stress measures and mood. Journal of Psychiatric Research (68) 9 270–282.

12. Rhodes AM (2015) Claiming peaceful embodiment through yoga in the aftermath of trauma. Complementary Therapies in Clinical Practice 21 (4) 247–256.

13. Singleton M (2010) Yoga body: The origins of modern posture practice, Oxford: Oxford University Press.

14. Smith SG, Zhang X, Basile KC, Merrick MT, Wang J, Kresnow M, and Chen J (2018) The National Intimate Partner and Sexual Violence Survey (NISVS): 2015 data brief – updated release, Atlanta, GA: National Center for Injury Prevention and Control, Centers for Disease Control and Prevention.

15. Substance Abuse and Mental Health Services Administration (SAMHSA) (2014) SAMHSA's concept of trauma and guidance for a trauma-informed approach (Report N0.SMA 14-4884), Rockville, MD. SAMHSA.

16. Tedeschi RG and Calhoun LG (2004) Posttraumatic growth: Conceptual foundations and empirical evidence. Psychological Inquiry 15 (1) 1–18.

17. Van der Kolk BA (2006) Clinical implications of neuroscience research in PTSD. Annals of the New York Academy of Sciences 1,071 (1) 277–93.

18. Van Dernoot Lipsky L (2009) Trauma stewardship: An everyday guide to caring for self while caring for others, San Francisco, CA: Berrett-Koehler Publishers, Inc.

19. West JI (2011) Moving to heal: Women's experiences of therapeutic yoga after complex trauma. ProQuest Dissertations Publishing [Online] Available: http://search.proquest.com/docview/914377530/ [29 October 2019].

Chapter 5

1. Alexander M (2012) The new Jim Crow: Mass incarceration in the time of colorblindness, New York, NY: The New Press.

2. Baptist EE (2014) The half has never been told: Slavery and the making of American capitalism, New York, NY: Basic Books.

3. Crenshaw K (1991) Mapping the margins: Intersectionality, identity politics, and violence against women of color. Stanford Law Review 43 (6) 1,241–1,299.

4. DiAngelo R (2018) White fragility: Why it's so hard for White people to talk about racism, Boston, MA: Beacon Press.

5. Flaherty J (2016) No more heroes: Grassroots challenges to the savior mentality, Chico, CA: AK Press.

6. hooks b (2015) Feminist theory from margin to center, New York, NY: Routledge.

7. Horton Carol A, Banitt Susan Pease, Bechtel Lilly, Danylchuk Lisa, Lillis Patricia, Huggins Michael, Eggleston Pam S, Yoga Service Council, and Omega Institute for Holistic Studies (2016) Best practices for yoga with veterans, Atlanta, GA: Yoga Service Council.

8. Johnson M (2017) Skill in action: Radicalizing your yoga practice to create a just world, Portland, OR: Radical Transformation Media.

9. Magee R (2019) The inner work of racial justice: Healing ourselves and transforming our communities through mindfulness, New York, NY: TarcherPerigee.

10. Margolin M (1997) The Ohlone way: Indian life in the San Francisco – Monterey Bay area, Berkeley, CA: Heyday.

11. Moraga C and Anzaldua G (2015) This bridge called my back: Writings by radical women of color, 4th edn, Albany, NY: SUNY Press.

12. Oluo I (2018) So you want to talk about race? New York, NY: Basic Books.

13. Peacock J (2018) Practice showing up: A guidebook for white people working for racial justice, Louisville, KY: Jardana Peacock.

14. Thích Nhất Hạnh (2006) The energy of prayer: How to deepen your spiritual practice, Berkeley, CA: Parallax Press.

Chapter 6

1. Augsburger DW (1982) Caring enough to hear and be heard: How to hear and how to be heard in equal communication, Ada, MI: Baker Publishing Group.

2. Biss E (2009) Notes from no man's land: American essays, Minneapolis, MN: Graywolf Press.

3. Chödrön P (2007) The places that scare you: A guide to fearlessness in difficult times, Boulder, CO: Shambhala Publications.

4. Click E (2014) Workshop on relational wisdom, lecture notes, Meaning Making: Thinking Theologically about Ministry Experience, Harvard Divinity School, delivered spring 2014.

5. Fisher-Borne M, Cain JM, and Martin SL (2014) From mastery to accountability: Cultural humility as an alternative to cultural competence. Social Work Education: The International Journal 34 (2) 165–181.

6. Implicit.harvard.edu. (2019) Project Implicit [Online] Available: https://implicit.harvard.edu/implicit/ [19 August 2019].

7. James L (2018) Prison employee PTSD. Public Health Post [e-journal] [Online] Available: https://www.publichealthpost.org/research/prison-employee-ptsd/ [19 August 2019].

8. Katzman F (2018) Lessons of the medicine wheel. Canadian Bar Association [e-journal] [Online] Available: https://www.cba.org/Sections/Alternative-Dispute-Resolution/Articles/2018/Medicine-wheel [21 August 2019].

9. Lawrence SM and Tatum DB (1999) White racial identity and anti-/racist education: A catalyst for change [Online] Available: https://www.teachingforchange.org/wp-content/uploads/2012/08/ec_whiteracialidentity_english.pdf [19 August 2019].

10. Le V (2015) Are you or your org guilty of trickle-down community engagement? [Online] Available: http://nonprofitwithballs.com/2015/01/are-you-or-your-org-guilty-of-trickle-down-community-engagement/ [19 August 2019].

11. Lee E (2011) Clinical significance of cross-cultural competencies (CCC) in social work practice. Journal of Social Work Practice 25 (2) 185–203.

12. Lipsky LD and Burk C (2009) Trauma stewardship: An everyday guide to caring for self while caring for others, San Francisco, CA: Berrett-Koehler Publishers.

13. Masters RA (2015) When spirituality disconnects us from what really matters, Berkeley, CA: North Atlantic Books.

14. Myers V (2014) How to overcome our bias? Walk boldly toward them [pdf] [Online] Available: https://www.ted.com/talks/verna_myers_how_to_overcome_our_biases_walk_boldly_toward_them [19 August 2019].

15. Pearlman LA and McKay L (2008) Vicarious trauma (Excerpted from Understanding and addressing vicarious trauma) [Online] Available: http://headington-institute.org/files/vicarious-trauma-handout_85433.pdf [19 August 2019].

16. radical (2019) Merriam Webster Online [Online] Available: http://www.merriam-webster.com [19 August 2019].

17. Rockwood L (2013) I am my own guru campaign launches in response to sex scandals [Online] Available: http://yogadork.com/2013/08/13/i-am-my-own-guru-campaign-launches-in-response-to-sex-scandals/ [19 August 2019].

18. Scopelliti I, Morewedge CK, McCormick E, Min HL, Lebrecht S, and Kassam KS (2015) Bias blind spot: Structure, measurement, and consequences. Management Science 61 (10) 2,468–2,486.

19. Stephens S (2018) White people: This is how to check your privilege when asking people of color for their labor [Online] Available: https://everydayfeminism.com/2018/07/white-people-this-is-how-to-check-your-privilege-when-asking-people-of-color-for-their-labor/ [19 August 2019].

20. Welwood J (1984) Principles of inner work: Psychological and spiritual. The Journal of Transpersonal Psychology 16 (1) 63–73.

Chapter 7

1. Birthroot Online Childbirth Class Blog (2019) LGBTQIA inclusive pregnancy and birth care [Online] Available: https://classroom.sandralondino.com/lgbtqia-inclusive-pregnancy-birth-care/ [26 August 2019].

2. The Birth Trauma Association (2018) What is Birth Trauma [Online] Available: http://www.birthtraumaassociation.org.uk/index.php/help-support/what-is-birth-trauma [23 October 2017].

3. Diaz-Tello F (2016) Invisible wounds: Obstetric violence in the United States. Reproductive Health Matters 24 (47) 56–64.

4. Grekin R and O'Hara MW (2014) Prevalence and risk factors of postpartum posttraumatic stress disorder: A meta-analysis. Clinical Psychology Review 34 (5) 389–401.

5. Pérez-D'Gregorio R (2010) Obstetric violence: A new legal term introduced in Venezuela. International Journal of Gynecology & Obstetrics 111 (3) 201–202.

6. Rhea T (2017) 8 gender-neutral birth terms and how to use them [Online] Available: https://www.tynanrhea.com/single-post/2017/02/13/8-gender-neutral-birth-terms-and-how-to-use-them [26 August 2019].

7. Roth LM, Heidbreder N, Henley MM, Marek M, Naiman-Sessions M, Torres J, and Morton CH (2014) Maternity support survey: A report on the cross-national survey of doulas, childbirth educators and labor and delivery nurses in the United States and Canada [Online] Available: www.maternitysupport.wordpress.com [26 August 2019].

8. Sufrin C, Mosher B, Beal L, Clarke J, and Jones R (2017) Incidence of abortion among incarcerated women in the United States: Results from the pregnancy in prison statistics study. Contraception 96 (4) 264–265.

9. Weiss-Lewit K (2019) Reflections on the experience of pregnancy [email] (Personal communication, 24 July).

Chapter 8

1. American Psychological Association (2014) Child sexual abuse: What parents should know [pdf] [Online] Available: http://www.apa.org/pi/families/resources/child-sexual-abuse.aspx [10 December 2018].

2. Anderson-McNamee JK and Bailey SJ (2010) The importance of play in early childhood development, Montana: Montana State University.

3. Barrett LF and Simmons WK (2015) Interoceptive predictions in the brain. Nature Reviews Neuroscience 16 (5) 419–429.

4. Bennett N and O'Donohue W (2014) The construct of grooming in child sexual abuse: Conceptual and measurement issues. Journal of Child Sexual Abuse 23 957–976. 10.1080/10538712.2014.960632.

5. Birdee GS, Yeh GY, Wayne PM, Phillips RS, Davis RB and Gardiner P (2009) Clinical applications of yoga for the pediatric population: A systematic review. Academic Pediatrics 9 (4) July–August 212–220. 10.1016/j.acap.2009.04.002 [10 March 2018].

6. Black M, Basile K, Breiding M, Smith S, Walters M, Merrick M, Chen J, and Stevens M (2011) The National Intimate Partner and Sexual Violence Survey: 2010 Summary Report. Centers for Disease Control and Prevention (CDC).

7. Breiding M (2015) Prevalence and characteristics of sexual violence, stalking, and intimate partner violence victimization – national intimate partner and sexual violence survey, United States, 2011. American Journal of Public Health 105 (4) E11–E12. https://doi.org/10.2105/AJPH.2015.302634

8. Buistand A and Janson H (2001) Childhood sexual abuse, parenting and postpartum depression – a 3-year follow-up study. Child Abuse & Neglect 25 (7) 909–921.

9. Butzer B, Ebert M, Telles S and Khalsa SB (2015) School-based yoga programs in the United States: A survey. Advances in Mind Body Medicine 29 (4) Fall 18–26. PubMed PMID: 26535474; PubMed Central PMCID: PMC4831047 [1 March 2019].

10. Butzer B, van Over M, Noggle Taylor JJ and Khalsa SB (2015) Yoga may mitigate decreases in high school grades. Evidence-Based Complementary and Alternative Medicine 1–8. https://doi.org/10.1155/2015/259814 [1 March 2019].

11. Childress T and Harper JC (2015) Best practices for yoga in schools, Atlanta, GA: YSC/Omega Publications.

12. Copeland WE, Keeler G, Angold A, and Costello EJ (2007) Traumatic events and post traumatic stress in childhood. Archives of General Psychiatry 64 (5) 577–584.

13. Cruise K and Ford J (2011) Trauma exposure and PTSD in justice-involved youth. Child and Youth Care Forum 40 (50) 337–343.

14. Epstein R, Blake J, and González T (2017) Girlhood interrupted: The erasure of black girls' childhood. Washington, DC: Georgetown Law Center on Poverty and Inequality [Online] Available: http://www.law.georgetown.edu/academics/centers-institutes/poverty-inequality/upload/girlhood- interrupted.pdf [19 July 2019].

15. Finkelhor D, Shattuck A, Turner HA, and Hamby SL (2014) The lifetime prevalence of child sexual abuse and sexual assault assessed in late adolescence. Journal of Adolescent Health 55 (3) September 329–333. Published online 25 February 2014. doi: 10.1016/j.jadohealth.2013.12.026

16. Flynn L (2013) Yoga for children: 200+ yoga poses, breathing exercises, and meditations for healthier, happier, more resilient children, New York, NY: Adams Media.

17. Frank JL, Kohler K, Peal A, and Bose B (2017) Effectiveness of a school-based yoga program on adolescent mental health and school performance: Findings from a randomized controlled Trial. Mindfulness 8 (3) 544. https://doi.org/10.1007/s12671-016-0628-3

18. Fromberg DP and Bergen D (2006) Play from birth to twelve: Contexts, perspectives, and meanings, 2nd edn, New York, NY: Routledge.

19. Galantino ML, Galbavy R, and Quinn L (2008) Therapeutic effects of yoga for children: A systematic review of the literature. Pediatric Physical Therapy 20 (1) Spring 66–80.

20. Goldberg L (2004) Creative relaxation: A yoga-based program for regular and exceptional student education. International Journal for Yoga Therapy 14 68–78.

21. Hagen I and Nayar US (2014) Yoga for children and young people's mental health and well-being: Research review and reflections on the mental health potentials of yoga. Front Psychiatry 5 35. 10.3389/fpsyt.2014.00035.

22. Jensen FE and Nutt AE (2015) The teenage brain: A neuroscientist's survival guide to raising adolescents and young adults, New York, NY: Harper-Collins Publishers.

23. Kaley-Isley LC, Peterson J, Fischer C, and Peterson E (2010) Yoga as a complementary therapy for children and adolescents: A guide for clinicians. Psychiatry (Edgemont) [e-journal] 7 (8) 20–32.

24. Kauts A and Sharma N (2009) Effect of yoga on academic performance in relation to stress. International Journal of Yoga 2 (1) 39–43. 10.4103/0973-6131.53860.

25. Kraag G, Zeegers MP, Kok G, Hossman C, and Abu-Saad HH (2006) School programs targeting stress management in children and adolescents: A meta-analysis. Database of Abstracts of Reviews of Effects (DARE): Quality-assessed Reviews [Internet]. York (UK): Centre for Reviews and Dissemination (UK) [Online] Available: https://www.ncbi.nlm.nih.gov/books/NBK73326/ [1 March 2019].

26. McAlinden NM (2006) "Setting 'em up": Personal, familial and institutional grooming in the sexual abuse of children. Social & Legal Studies 15 (3) 339–362. 10.1177/0964663906066613

27. Meggitt C (2012) Understand child development, London: Hodder Education.

28. Nunez N, Warren A and Poole D (2008) The story of human development, New Jersey: Prentice Hall.

29. Putnam FW (2003) Ten-year research update review: Child sexual abuse. Journal of the American Academy of Child and Adolescent Psychiatry 42 269–278.

30. Rousseau D, Weiss-Lewit K, and Lilly M (2019) #MeToo and yoga: Guidance for clinicians referring to trauma-informed yoga. Journal of Clinical Sport Psychology 13 (2) 216–225.

31. Siegel DJ (2013) Brainstorm: The power and purpose of the teenage brain, New York, NY: Penguin Group.

32. Solter AJ (2013) Attachment play. How to solve children's behavior problems with play, laughter, and connection, Goleta, CA: Shining Star Press.

33. Spinazzola J, Rhodes AM, Emerson D, Earle E, and Monroe K (2011) Application of yoga in residential treatment of traumatized youth. Journal of American Psychiatric Nurses Association 17 (6) November–December 431–444. 10.1177/1078390311418359.

34. Stanley B and Brown GK (2011) Safety planning intervention: A brief intervention to mitigate suicide risk. Cognitive and Behavioral Practice 19 256–264.

35. STAR Institute for Sensory Processing Disorder (STAR) (2018) Your Eight Sensory Systems [Online] Available: www.spdstar.org/ /basic/ your-8-senses/ [15 November 2018].

36. Sternberg EC (2017) The effects of daily yoga practice on the academic engagement and achievement of middle school students in a special education classroom. Theses and Dissertations. 2411.http:// rdw.rowan.edu/etd/2411 [15 January 2019].

37. Thomas RM (2001) Recent theories of human development, California: Sage Publications.

38. Trickett P, Noll J, and Putnam F (2011) The impact of sexual abuse on female development: Lessons from a multigenerational, longitudinal research study. Development and Psychopathology 23 (2) 453–476. https://doi.org/10.1017/S0954579411000174.

39. Wolf MR, Linn BK, and Pruitt DK (2018) Grooming child victims into sexual abuse: A psychometric analysis of survivors' experiences. Journal of Sexual Aggression 24 (2) 1–10.

40. Wolf MR, Linn BK, and Pruitt DK (2018) Grooming child victims into sexual abuse: A psychometric analysis of survivors' experiences. Journal of Sexual Aggression 24 (2) 215–224.

41. Zinzow HM, Resnick HS, McCauley JL, Amstadter AB, Ruggiero KJ, and Kilpatrick DG (2012) Prevalence and risk of psychiatric disorders as a function of variant rape histories: Results from a national survey of women. Social Psychiatry and Psychiatric Epidemiology 47 (6) 893–902.

Chapter 9

1. Brown T and Herman J (2015) Williamsinstitute.law.ucla.edu [Online] Available: https://williamsinstitute.law.ucla.edu/wp-content/uploads/Intimate-Partner-Violence-and-Sexual-Abuse-among-LGBT-People.pdf [19 May 2019].

2. Kessler RC, Avenevoli S, Costello EJ, Georgiades K, Green JG, Gruber MJ, He JP, Koretz D, McLaughlin KA, Petukhova M, Sampson NA, Zaslavsky AM, and Merikangas KR (2012) Prevalence, persistence, and sociodemographic correlates of DSM-IV disorders in the National Comorbidity Survey Replication Adolescent Supplement. Archives of General Psychiatry 69 372–380.

3. King M, Semlyen J, Tai SS, Killaspy H, Osborn D, Popelyuk D, and Nazareth I (2008) A systematic review of mental disorder, suicide, and deliberate self harm in lesbian, gay and bisexual people. BMC Psychiatry 8 70.

Chapter 10

1. 1in6 (2019a) The 1 in 6 statistic [Online] Available: https://1in6.org/ get-information/the-1-in-6-statistic/ [15 August 2019].

2. 1in6 (2019b) For family and friends of men [Online] Available: https://1in6.org/get-information/for-family-and-friends-of-men/ [15 August 2019].

3. Association of Alberta Sexual Assault Services (AASAS) (2018) Men and sexual assault [Online] Available: https://aasas.ca/support-and-information/men-and-sexual-assault/ [15 February 2019].

4. Arizona State University (ASU) (2008) *Caring men are happier than traditional "macho" men, study suggests* [Online] Available: https://www.sciencedaily.com/releases/2008/04/080429084317.htm [5 October 2019].

5. Barth F (2019) Toxic masculinity is terrible shorthand for a real problem plaguing men [Online] Available: https://www.nbcnews.com/think/opinion/toxic-masculinity-terrible-shorthand-real-problem-plaguing-men-ncna957941 [23 September 2019].

6. Clay R (2012) Redefining masculinity – three psychologists strive to "building" a better man [Online] Available: https://www.apa.org/ monitor/2012/06/masculinity [5 October 2019].

7. Fitzsimons T (2019) American Psychological Association links "masculinity ideology" to homophobia, misogyny [Online] Available: https://www.nbcnews.com/feature/nbc-out/american-psychological-association-links-masculinity-ideology-homophobia-misogyny-n956416 [2 October 2019].

8. Fortin J (2019) Traditional masculinity can hurt boys, say new A.P.A. guidelines [Online] Available: https://www.nytimes.com/2019/01/10/science/apa-traditional-masculinity-harmful.html?module=inline [23 September 2019].

9. French B (2014) Coerced sex not uncommon for young men, teenage boys, study finds [Online] Available: https://www.apa.org/news/press/releases/2014/03/coerced-sex [15 February 2019].

10. Holloway K (2015) Toxic masculinity is killing men: The roots of male trauma [Online] Available: https://www.salon.com/2015/06/12/toxic_masculinity_is_killing_men_the_roots_of_male_trauma_partner/ [23 September 2019].

11. Kimmel M and Bridges T (2011) Masculinity [Online] Available: https://www.oxfordbibliographies.com/view/document/obo-9780199756384/obo-9780199756384-0033.xml, 27 July [6 October 2019].

12. Lambert C (2019) Man up! Our "male code" fails boys and men – Recent research shows how the male code impacts men's mental health [Online] Available: https://www.psychologytoday.com/us/blog/mind-games/201903/man-our-male-code-fails-boys-and-men [5 October 2019].

13. Niiler E (2013) Why yoga is still dominated by women despite the benefit to both sexes [Online] Available: https://www.washingtonpost.com/national/health-science/why-yoga-is-still-dominated-by-women-despite-the-medical-benefits-to-both-sexes/2013/10/21/a924bed2-34f5-11e3-80c6-7e6dd8d22d8f_story.html?noredirect=on [15 August 2019].

14. Ptsd.va.gov (2019) U. S. Department of Veterans Affairs – PTSD: National Center for PTSD – sexual assault: Males [Online] Available: https://www.ptsd.va.gov/understand/types/sexual_trauma_male.asp [5 October 2019].

15. Rape, Abuse & Incest National Network (RAINN) (University (ASU) (2008) Caring 2019) Sexual assault of men and boys [Online] Available: https://rainn.org/effects-sexual-violence [15 August 2019].

16. Stiefel S (2019) 6 reasons men should do yoga [Online] Available: https://www.bodybuilding.com/content/6-reasons-men-should-do-yoga.html [15 August 2019].

17. Student Assault Prevention and Awareness Center (SAPAC) (2019) Male survivors of sexual assault [Online] Available: https://sapac.umich.edu/article/53 [15 February 2019].

18. Turner E (2019) Mental health among boys and men: When is masculinity toxic? [Online] Available: https://www.psychologytoday.com/us/blog/the-race-good-health/201902/mental-health-among-boys-and-men-when-is-masculinity-toxic [5 October 2019].

19. Weiss R (2016) Treating male survivors of sexual abuse [Online] Available: https://www.psychologytoday.com/us/blog/love-and-sex-in-the-digital-age/201606/treating-male-survivors-sexual-abuse [15 February 2019].

20. Worthen MGF (2016) Sexual deviance and society: A sociological examination, London: Routledge.

21. YJ Editors (2017) New study finds more than 20 million yogis in the U.S. [Online] Available: https://www.yogajournal.com/blog/new-study-finds-20-million-yogis-u-s [15 August 2019].

Chapter 11

1. Malmedal W, Iversen MH, and Kilvik A (2015) Sexual abuse of older nursing home residents: A literature review. Nursing Research and Practice [Online] Available: https://www.ncbi.nlm.nih.gov/pmc/articles/PMC4302365/ [23 July 2019].

2. Shapiro J (2018) In their own words: People with intellectual disabilities talk about rape. Abused and betrayed special series. National Public Radio [Online] Available: https://www.npr.org/2018/01/20/577064075/ [5 September 2019].

3. World Health Organization (2018) Elder abuse fact sheet [Online] Available: https://www.who.int/news-room/fact-sheets/detail/elder-abuse [5 September 2019].

Chapter 12

1. The Association of American Universities (2015) Report on the AAU Campus Climate Survey on Sexual Assault and Misconduct [Online] Available: https://www.aau.edu/key-issues/aau-climate-survey-sexual-assault-and-sexual-misconduct-2015 [3 November 2019].

2. The Association of American Universities (2019) Report on the AAU Campus Climate Survey on Sexual Assault and Misconduct [Online] Available: https://www.aau.edu/sites/default/files/AAU-Files/Key-Issues/Campus-Safety/FULL_2019_Campus_Climate_Survey.pdf [3 November 2019].

REFERENCES *continued*

3. Baker K (2015) Colleges are hard put to help students in crisis. Chronicle of Higher Education [Online] Available: http://chronicle.com/article/Colleges-Are-Hard-Put-to Help/232719/.jobs__topjobs-slider [3 November 2019].

4. Beiter R, Nash R, McCrady M, Rhoades D, Linscomb M, Clarahan M, and Sammut S (2015) The prevalence and correlates of depression, anxiety, and stress in a sample of college students. Journal of Affective Disorders 173 90–96.

5. Bergen-Cico D, Possemato K, and Cheon S (2013) Examining the efficacy of a brief mindfulness-based stress reduction (Brief MBSR) program on psychological health. Journal of American College Health 61 (6) 348–360.

6. Brown, Brené (2012) Daring greatly: How the courage to be vulnerable transforms the way we live, love, parent, and lead, New York, NY: Gotham Books.

7. For more on the Campus Save Act, see the website at http://campussaveact.org.

8. Cantor D, Fisher B, Chibnall S, Bruce C, Townsend R, Thomas G, and Lee H (2015) Report on the AAU campus climate survey on sexual assault and sexual misconduct, Rockville, MD: Westat.

9. Center for Collegiate Mental Health (2015) Center for Collegiate Mental Health 2014 Annual Report, University Park, PA: Center for Collegiate Mental Health.

10. Center for Collegiate Mental Health (2019, January) 2018 Annual Report (Publication No. STA 19–180).

11. Cieslak KJ, Hardy LE, Kyles NS, Miller EL, Mullins BL, Root KM, and Smith CM (2016) An environmental scan of mindfulness-based interventions on university and college campuses: A research note. The Journal of Sociology & Social Welfare 43 (4) [Online] Available: https://scholarworks.wmich.edu/jssw/vol43/iss4/7 [3 November 2019].

12. Coulter R, Mair C, Miller E, Blosnich JR, Matthews DD, and McCauley HL (2017) Prevalence of past-year sexual assault victimization among undergraduate students: Exploring differences by and intersections of gender identity, sexual identity, and race/ethnicity. Prevention Science: The Official Journal of the Society for Prevention Research 18 (6) 726–736. 10.1007/s11121-017-0762-8.

13. Deckro GR, Ballinger KM, Hoyt M, Wilcher M, Dusek J, Myers P, and Benson H (2010) The evaluation of a mind/body intervention to reduce psychological distress and perceived stress in college students. Journal of American College Health 50 (6) 281–287.

14. Eastman-Muller H, Wilson T, Jung AK, Kimura A, and Tarrant J (2013) iRest Yoga-Nidra on the college campus: Changes in stress, depression, worry, and mindfulness. International Journal of Yoga Therapy 23 (2), 15–24.

15. Federal Student Aid (n.d.) Glossary [Online] Available: https://studentaid.ed.gov/sa/glossary#Independent_Student [15 December 2016].

16. Fedina L, Holmes JL, and Backes BL (2016) Campus sexual assault: A systematic review of prevalence research from 2000 to 2015. Trauma Violence Abuse 1–18. https://www.ncbi.nlm.nih.gov/pubmed/26906086

17. Fisher BS, Cullen FT, and Turner MG (2000) The sexual victimization of college women [Online] Available: https://www.ncjrs.gov/pdffiles1/nij/182369.pdf [3 November 2019].

18. Flack WF Jr (2008) "The red zone": Temporal risk for unwanted sex among college students. Journal of Interpersonal Violence 23 (9) 1,177–1,196. 10.1177/0886260508314308.

19. Freitas D (2018) Consent on campus: A manifesto, Oxford: Oxford University Press.

20. Galatzer-Levy IR, Burton CL, and Bonanno GA (2012) Coping flexibility, potentially traumatic life events, and resilience: A prospective study of college student adjustment. Journal of Social and Clinical Psychology 31 (6) 542–567.

21. Gokhan N, Meehan EF, and Peters K (2010) The value of mindfulness-based methods in teaching at a clinical field placement. Psychological Reports 106 (4) 55–466.

22. Griffin MJ and Read JP (2012) Prospective effects of method of coercion in sexual victimization across the first college year. Journal of Interpersonal Violence 27 (12) 2,503–2,524.

23. Hindman RK, Glass CR, Arnkoff DB, and Maron DD (2015) A comparison of formal and informal mindfulness programs for stress reduction in university students. Mindfulness 4 873–884.

24. Holland D (2004) Integrating mindfulness meditation and somatic awareness into a public educational setting. Journal of Humanistic Psychology 44 (4) 468–484.

25. IWPR (2016) Institute for Women's Policy Research (IWPR) analysis of data from the U.S. Department of Education, National Center for Education Statistics, 2011–12 National Postsecondary Student Aid Study (NPSAS:12).

26. Jain S, Shapiro SL, Swanick S, Roesch SC, Mills PJ, and Schwartz GE (2007) A randomized controlled trial of mindfulness meditation

versus relaxation training: Effects on distress, positive states of mind, rumination and distraction. Annals of Behavioral Medicine 33 (1) 11–21.

27. Kerrigan D, Chau V, King M, Holman E, Joffe A, and Sibinga E (2017) There is no performance, there is just this moment: The role of mindfulness instruction in promoting health and well-being among students at a highly-ranked university in the United States. Journal of Evidence-Based Complementary & Alternative Medicine 22 (4) 909–918.

28. Kilpatrick D, Resnick H, Ruggiero KJ, Conoscenti LM, and McCauley J (2007) Drug-facilitated, incapacitated, and forcible rape: A National Study [Internet]. Jul. Report No.: 219181 [Online] Available: http://www.antoniocasella.eu/archila/Kilpatrick_drug_forcible_rape_2007.pdf [3 November 2019].

29. Krebs C, Lindquist C, Berzofsky M, Shook-Sa B, and Peterson K (2016) Campus climate survey validation study final technical report [Internet]. Bureau of Justice Statistics Research and Development Series, Report No.: NCJ 249545 [Online] Available: https://www.bjs.gov/content/pub/pdf/ccsvsftr.pdf

30. Mellins CA, Walsh K, Sarvet AL, Wall M, Gilbert L, Santelli JS, and Hirsch JS (2017) Sexual assault incidents among college undergraduates: Prevalence and factors associated with risk. PloS One 12 (11), 10.1371/journal.pone.0186471.

31. Messman-Moore TL and McConnell AA (2018) Chapter 13 – Intervention for sexual revictimization among college women, in Orchowski LM and Gidycz CA (eds) Sexual Assault Risk Reduction and Resistance, London: Academic Press, pp. 309–330.

32. Office for Civil Rights, Revised Sexual Harassment Guidance (66 Fed. Reg. 5512, Jan. 19, 2001) [Online] Available: https://www2.ed.gov/about/offices/list/ocr/docs/shguide.pdf [3 November 2019]. See also 20 U.S.C. § 1092(f).

33. Oman D, Shapiro SL, Thoresen CE, Plante TG, and Flinders T (2008) Meditation lowers stress and supports forgiveness among college students: A randomized controlled trial. Journal of American College Health 56 569–578.

34. Ramler TR, Tennison LR, Lynch J, and Murphy P (2016) Mindfulness and the college transition: The efficacy of an adapted mindfulness-based stress reduction intervention in fostering adjustment among first-year students. Mindfulness 7 179–188.

35. Read JP, Ouimette P, White J, Colder C, and Farrow S (2011) Rates of DSM–IV–TR trauma exposure and posttraumatic stress disorder among newly matriculated college students. Psychological Trauma: Theory, Research, Practice and Policy 3 (2) 148–156.

36. Rizzolo D, Zipp GP, Stiskal D, and Simpkins S (2009) Stress management strategies for students: The immediate effects of yoga, humor, and reading on stress. Journal of College Teaching & Learning (TLC) 6 (8) 79–88.

37. Rockefeller S (2006) Meditation, social change, and undergraduate education. Teachers College Record 108 1,775–1,786.

38. Sandars J (2009) The use of reflection in medical education: AMEE Guide No. 44. Med Teach 31 (8) 685–695.

39. Sears SR, Kraus S, Carlough K, and Treat E (2011) Perceived benefits and doubts of participants in a weekly meditation study. Mindfulness 2 167–174.

40. Shapiro SL, Brown KW, and Astin J (2011) Toward the integration of meditation into higher education: A review of research evidence. Teachers College Record 113 493–528.

41. Shiralkar MT, Harris TB, Eddins-Folensbee FF, and Coverdale JH (2013) A systematic review of stress-management programs for medical students. Academic Psychiatry 37 158–164.

42. Shirey MR (2007) An evidence-based solution for minimizing stress and anger in nursing students. Journal of Nursing Education 46 (12) 568–571.

43. Smith C, Hancock H, Blake-Mortimer J, and Eckert K (2007) A randomized comparative trial of yoga and relaxation to reduce stress and anxiety. Complementary Therapeutic Medicine 15 (2) 77–83.

44. Smyth JM, Hockemeyer JR, Heron KE, Wonderlich SA, and Pennebaker JW (2008) Prevalence, type, disclosure, and severity of adverse life events in college students. Journal of American College Health 57 (1) 69–76.

45. The White House (2014) Not Alone, The First Report of the White House Task Force [Online] Available: https://www.justice.gov/ovw/page/file/905942/download [3 November 2019].

46. U.S. Department of Education, National Center for Education Statistics, Biennial Survey of Education in the United States; Opening Fall Enrollment in Higher Education, 1963 through 1965; Higher Education General Information Survey (HEGIS), "Fall Enrollment in Colleges and Universities" surveys, 1966 through 1985; Integrated Postsecondary Education Data System (IPEDS), "Fall Enrollment Survey" (IPEDS-EF:86-99); IPEDS Spring 2001 through Spring 2018, Fall Enrollment component; and Enrollment in Degree-Granting Institutions Projection Model, 2000 through 2028. Prepared March 2019.

47. U.S. Department of Education, Office of Civil Rights (2011) Archived: Dear Colleague Letter from Office of the Assistant Secretary for Civil Rights Russlynn Ali [Online] Available: https://www2.ed.gov/about/offices/list/ocr/letters/colleague-201104.html [3 November 2019].

48. U.S. Department of Education, Q&A on Campus Sexual Misconduct, September 2017, 7 [Online] Available: https://www2.ed.gov/about/offices/list/ocr/docs/qa-title-ix201709.pdf [3 November 2019].

49. White House Task Force to Protect Students from Sexual Assault (2017) Preventing and Addressing Campus Sexual Misconduct: A Guide for University and College Presidents, Chancellors, and Senior Administrators [Online] Available: https://www.whitehouse.gov/sites/whitehouse.gov/files/images/Documents/1.4.17.VAW%20Event.Guide%20for%20College%20Presidents.PDF [3 November 2019].

Chapter 13

1. Army Regulation 600-20 (2014) Army command policy [pdf] [Online] Available: https://armypubs.army.mil/epubs/DR_pubs/DR_a/pdf/web/r600_20.pdf [16 October 2019].

2. Barth SK, Kimerling RE, Pavao J, McCutcheon SJ, Batten SV, Dursa E, Peterson MR, and Schneiderman AI (2016) Military sexual trauma among recent veterans: Correlates of sexual assault and sexual harassment 50 (1) 77–86 [pdf] [Online] Available: https://doi.org/10.1016/j.amepre.2015.06.012 [26 August 2019].

3. Castro CA, Kintzle S, Schuyler AC, Lucas CL, and Warner CH (2015) Sexual assault in the military [pdf] [Online] Available: http://cir.usc.edu/wp-content/uploads/2015/06/Sexual-Assault-in-the-Military.pdf [27 August 2019].

4. Ceunen E, Vlaeyen JWS, and Van Diest I (2016) On the origin of interoception [Online] Available: https://www.ncbi.nlm.nih.gov/pmc/articles/PMC4876111/ [26 August 2019].

5. Department of Defense (DOD) (2016) Annual report on sexual assault in the military [pdf] [Online] Available: http://snagfilms-a.akamaihd.net/8b/ea/d934a75d49f6a35e311dcaa14d00/dod-annual-report-on-sex-assault-in-the-military-fy2016.pdf [1 August 2019].

6. Department of Veterans Affairs (2019) [Online] Available: http://mentalhealth.va.gov [1 August 2019].

7. Emerson D and Hopper E (2011) Overcoming trauma through yoga: Reclaiming your body, Berkeley, CA: North Atlantic Books.

8. Healthystate.org (2012) Uniform betrayal: Rape in the military [video] [Online] Available: https://vimeo.com/46007403 [15 August 2019].

9. Horton C (2016) Best practices for yoga with veterans, Rhinebeck, NY: YSC/Omega Publications.

10. Military Times (2018) The Marine Corps had the highest increase in sexual assault reports among the services [Online] Available: https://www.militarytimes.com/news/your-military/2018/04/30/dod-marines-had-highest-increase-in-reports-of-sexual-assaults/ [25 October 2018].

11. PBS (2019) Military sexual assault [Online] Available: https://www.pbs.org/newshour/tag/military-sexual-assault, 31 July [1 August 2019].

12. Rape, Abuse, and Incest National Network (RAINN) (2019) [Online] Available: https://www.rainn.org/articles/military-sexual-trauma [1 August 2019].

13. Steinhauer J (2019) Woman trying to end sexual assault at V.A. centers says she is attacked in one [Online] Available: https://www.nytimes.com/2019/09/26/us/politics/women-veterans-sexual-assault-harassment.html [26 September 2019].

14. Stover SA (2017) Dress for success [Online] Available: https://www.yogajournal.com/teach/dress-for-success [26 September 2019].

15. Teeters JB, Lancaster CL, Brown DG, and Back SE (2017) Substance use disorders in military veterans: Prevalence and treatment challenges [Online] Available: https://www.ncbi.nlm.nih.gov/pmc/articles/PMC5587184/ [26 August 2019].

16. The Lion's Roar (2017) Helping, fixing, or serving? [Online] Available: https://www.lionsroar.com/helping-fixing-or-serving/ [15 November 2018].

17. The Washington Post (2017a) How the military handles sexual assault cases behind closed doors [Online] Available: https://www.washingtonpost.com/investigations/how-the-military-handles-sexual-assault-cases-behind-closed-doors/2017/09/30/a9df0682-672a-11e7-a1d7-9a32c91c6f40_story.html?noredirect=on [1 August 2019].

18. The Washington Post (2017b) In the military, trusted officers became alleged assailants in sex crimes [Online] Available: https://www.washingtonpost.com/investigations/in-the-military-trusted-officers-became-alleged-assailants-in-sex-crimes/2017/10/19/ec2cf780-ae9a-11e7-be94-fabb0f1e9ffb_story.html> [1 April 2019].

19. The Washington Post (2018) Sexual assault reports in the military spiked but the Pentagon thinks assaults are down [Online] Available: https://www.washingtonpost.com/news/checkpoint/wp/2018/04/30/sexual-assault-reports-in-the-military-spiked-but-the-pentagon-thinks-assaults-are-down/ [10 October 2018].

Chapter 14

1. Black, MC, Basile KC, Breiding M, Smith SG, Walters ML, Marrick MT, Chen J, and Stevens MR (2011) The National Intimate Partner and Sexual Violence Survey: 2010 summary report, Atlanta, GA: National Center for Injury Prevention and Control Centers for Disease Control and Prevention [pdf] [Online] Available: https://www.cdc.gov/violenceprevention/pdf/nisvs_report2010-a.pdf [15 January 2018].

2. Herman JL (1997) Trauma and recovery, rev. edn, New York, NY: Basic Books.

3. Levine PA (1997) Waking the tiger: Healing trauma: The innate capacity to transform overwhelming experiences, Berkeley, CA: North Atlantic Books.

4. Rhodes AM (2015) Claiming peaceful embodiment through yoga in the aftermath of trauma. Complementary Therapies in Clinical Practice 21 (4) 247–256.

5. Waters E (2017) Intimate partner violence in 2016: Lesbian, Gay, Bisexual, Transgender, Queer, and HIV-affected intimate partner violence in 2016. National Coalition of Anti-Violence Programs [pdf] [Online] Available: http://avp.org/wp-content/uploads/2017/11/NCAVP-IPV-Report-2016.pdf [15 January 2018].

Chapter 15

1. Andrews B, Morton J, Bekerian DA, Brewin CR, Davies GM, and Mollon P (1995) The recovery of memories in clinical practice. The Psychologist 8 209–214.

2. Dank ML (2011) The commercial sexual exploitation of children, Criminal Justice: Recent Scholarship. El Paso, TX: LFB Scholarly Pub.

3. Dank ML, Khan B, Downey PM, Kotonias C, Mayer D, Owens C, Pacifici L, and Yu L (2014) Estimating the size and structure of the underground commercial sex economy in eight major US cities. Urban Institute [Online] Available: https://www.urban.org/research/publication/estimating-size-and-structure-underground-commercial-sex-economy-eight-major-us-cities/view/full_report [2 January 2018].

4. Douglas M (2003) Natural symbols: explorations in cosmology, New York, NY: Routledge.

5. Estes RJ and Weiner NA (2002) The commercial sexual exploitation of children in the U.S., Canada, and Mexico: Executive summary of the U.S. national study [pdf] [Online] Available: https://abolitionistmom.org/wp-content/uploads/2014/05/Complete_CSEC_0estes-weiner.pdf [28 August 2019].

6. Frankfurter D (2003) The satanic ritual abuse panic as religious-studies data. Numen 50 (1) 108–117.

7. International Labour Organization (2012) New ILO global estimate of forced labour: 20.9 million victims [pdf] [Online] Available: https://www.ilo.org/global/topics/forced-labour/news/WCMS_182109/lang--en/index.htm [27 August 2019].

8. Lacter EP and Lehman KD (2008) Guidelines to diagnoses of ritual abuse/Mind control traumatic stress. Attachment: New directions in psychotherapy and relational psychoanalysis journal 2 (2) 159–181.

9. Lucas A (2017) I was sex trafficked at age six. Help me stand up for trafficking victims in New York. Care 2 Petitions [Online] Available: https://www.thepetitionsite.com/559/755/353/i-was-sex-trafficked-at-age-6.-help-me-stand-up-for-trafficking-victims-in-new-york/ [20 October 2019].

10. Noblitt JR and Noblitt PP (2017) Empirical and forensic evidence of ritual abuse, with personal introduction by Ellen Lacter, PhD [Online] Available: http://endritualabuse.org/empirical-and-forensic-evidence-of-ritual-abuse/ [2 January 2018].

11. Polaris Project (2017) Sex trafficking [Online] Available: https://polarisproject.org/sex-trafficking [20 October 2017].

12. Putnam FW (1991) The satanic ritual abuse controversy. Child Abuse & Neglect 15 (3) 175–179.

13. Rosenblatt K (2017) Flight attendants train to spot human trafficking. NBC News [Online] Available: https://www.nbcnews.com/news/us-news/flight-attendants-train-spot-human-trafficking-n716181 [2 January 2019].

14. Seligman AB and Weller RP (2012) Rethinking pluralism: Ritual, experience, and ambiguity, New York, NY: Oxford University Press.

15. Williams R (2017) Safe harbor: State efforts to confront child trafficking, National Conference of State Legislatures [pdf] [Online] Available: http://www.ncsl.org/Portals/1/Documents/cj/SafeHarbor_v06.pdf [27 August 2019].

Chapter 16

1. Briere J, Agee E, and Dietrich A (2016) Cumulative trauma and current posttraumatic stress disorder status in general population and inmate samples. Psychological Trauma: Theory, research, practice, and policy 8 (4) 439–446.

2. Bureau of Justice Statistics (2015) Use of restrictive housing in U.S. prisons and jails, 2011–12. Washington, DC: Department of Justice Statistics [pdf] [Online] Available: https://www.bjs.gov/content/pub/pdf/urhuspj1112.pdf [5 December 2019].

3. Flynn M (2019) Female inmates were forced to expose their genitals in a "training exercise." It was legal, court rules. The Washington Post [Online] Available: https://www.washingtonpost.com/nation/2019/07/19/female-inmates-were-forced-expose-their-genitals-training-exercise-it-was-legal-court-rules/ [26 August 2019].

4. Horton C (ed.) (2017) Best practices for yoga in the criminal justice system, Rhinebeck, NY: YSC-Omega Publications.

5. James L (2018) Prison employee PTSD. Public Health Post [Online] Available: https://www.publichealthpost.org/research/prison-employee-ptsd/ [1 November 2018].

6. National Center for Transgender Equality (NCTE) (2018) LGBTQ people behind bars: A guide to understanding the issues facing transgender prisoners and their legal rights [pdf] [Online] Available: https://transequality.org/transpeoplebehindbars [26 August 2019].

7. PREA Resource Center (2014) Third-party reporting under the PREA standards: Fact sheet for corrections officials [pdf] [Online] Available: https://www.prearesourcecenter.org/sites/default/files/library/third-partyreportingfactsheet.pdf [27 August 2019].

8. Willging CE, Malcoe LH, St Cyr S, Zywiak WH, and Lapham SC (2013) Behavioral health and social correlates of reincarceration among Hispanic, Native American, and White rural women. Psychiatric Services 64 (6) 590–593.

Chapter 17

1. Albanese CL (2007) America, religions, and religion, 4th edn, Australia and Belmont, CA: Thomson/Wadsworth.

2. Barnes LL and Sered SS (2004) Religion and healing in America, Oxford: Oxford University Press.

3. Durkheim É (1999) Suicide: A study in sociology, trans. George Simpson, New York, NY: Free Press.

4. Durkheim É (2019) The elementary forms of the religious life, Middletown, DE: Pantianos Classics.

5. Hutchinson S (2018) Atheists miss another #MeToo moment. Rewire. [Online] Available: https://rewire.news/religion-dispatches/2018/09/11/movement-atheism-misses-another-metoo-moment/ [19 October 2019].

6. Jain A (2014) Branding yoga, in Selling yoga: From counterculture to pop culture. Oxford: Oxford University Press, p. 29.

7. Mamone T (2018) Why are secular skeptic communities failing to address sexual crime? The Establishment [Online] Available: https://theestablishment.co/why-are-secular-skeptic-communities-failing-to-address-sexual-crime-26cddb5ce63b/index.html [19 October 2019].

8. Mercadante LA (2014) Belief without borders: Inside the minds of the spiritual but not religious, New York, NY: Oxford University Press.

9. Orsi RA (2016) History and presence, Cambridge, MA: The Belknap Press of Harvard University Press.

10. Rain K (2017) "#MeToo." Facebook.

11. Rain K (2018) "I don't need 'I believe you.' I need 'I'll stand up for you.'" Human Parts [Online] Available: https://humanparts.medium.com/i-dont-need-i-believe-you-i-need-i-ll-stand-up-for-you-c6f9a2cc8d35> [31 October 2019].

12. Rain K and Cooke J (2019) How to respond to sexual abuse within a yoga or spiritual community with competency and accountability. Yoga International [Online] Available: https://yogainternational.com/article/view/how-to-respond-to-sexual-abuse-within-a-yoga-or-spiritual-community [31 October 2019].

13. Rambo S (2017) Resurrecting wounds: Living in the afterlife of trauma, Waco, TX: Baylor University Press.

14. Remski M (2017) Karen Rain responds to Mary Taylor's post about the sexual misconduct of Pattabhi Jois. Decolonizing Yoga [Online] Available: https://decolonizingyoga.com/karen-rain-responds-mary-taylors-post-sexual-misconduct-pattabhi-jois/ [19 October 2019].

15. Remski M (2019) Practice and all is coming: Abuse, cult dynamics, and healing in yoga and beyond, Rangiora, New Zealand: Embodied Wisdom Publishing.

16. Seligman AB, Weller RP, Puett M, and Bennett S (2008) Ritual and its consequences: An essay on the limits of sincerity, Oxford and New York, NY: Oxford University Press.

17. Stedman C (2012) Faitheist: How an atheist found common ground with the religious, Boston, MA: Beacon Press.

INDEX

INDEX *continued*